T0327743

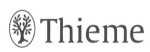

Complications in Minimally Invasive Facial Rejuvenation

Prevention and Management

Paul J. Carniol, MD, FACS
Clinical Professor
Department of Otolaryngology
Rutgers New Jersey Medical School;
Plastic Surgeon
Carniol Plastic Surgery
Summit, New Jersey, USA

Mathew M. Avram, MD, JD
Associate Professor
Department of Dermatology
Massachusetts General Hospital/Harvard Medical School
Wellman Center for Photomedicine
Boston, Massachusetts, USA

Jeremy A. Brauer, MD
Clinical Associate Professor
Ronald O. Perelman Department of Dermatology
New York University
New York, New York, USA

262 illustrations

Thieme
New York • Stuttgart • Delhi • Rio de Janeiro

Library of Congress Cataloging-in-Publication Data is available with the publisher.

Thieme Publishers New York
333 Seventh Avenue, New York, NY 10001 USA
+1 800 782 3488, customerservice@thieme.com

Georg Thieme Verlag KG
Rüdigerstrasse 14, 70469 Stuttgart, Germany
+49 [0]711 8931 421, customerservice@thieme.de

Thieme Publishers Delhi
A-12, Second Floor, Sector-2, Noida-201301
Uttar Pradesh, India
+91 120 45 566 00, customerservice@thieme.in

Thieme Publishers Rio de Janeiro,
Thieme Publicações Ltda.
Edifício Rodolpho de Paoli, 25º andar
Av. Nilo Peçanha, 50 – Sala 2508,
Rio de Janeiro 20020-906 Brasil
+55 21 3172-2297

Cover design: Thieme Publishing Group
Typesetting by TNQ Technologies, India

Printed in USA by King Printing Company, Inc.

ISBN 978-1-68420-013-9

Also available as an e-book:
eISBN 978-1-68420-014-6

Important note: Medicine is an ever-changing science undergoing continual development. Research and clinical experience are continually expanding our knowledge, in particular our knowledge of proper treatment and drug therapy. Insofar as this book mentions any dosage or application, readers may rest assured that the authors, editors, and publishers have made every effort to ensure that such references are in accordance with **the state of knowledge at the time of production of the book**.

Nevertheless, this does not involve, imply, or express any guarantee or responsibility on the part of the publishers in respect to any dosage instructions and forms of applications stated in the book. **Every user is requested to examine carefully** the manufacturers' leaflets accompanying each drug and to check, if necessary in consultation with a physician or specialist, whether the dosage schedules mentioned therein or the contraindications stated by the manufacturers differ from the statements made in the present book. Such examination is particularly important with drugs that are either rarely used or have been newly released on the market. Every dosage schedule or every form of application used is entirely at the user's own risk and responsibility. The authors and publishers request every user to report to the publishers any discrepancies or inaccuracies noticed. If errors in this work are found after publication, errata will be posted at www.thieme.com on the product description page.

Some of the product names, patents, and registered designs referred to in this book are in fact registered trademarks or proprietary names even though specific reference to this fact is not always made in the text. Therefore, the appearance of a name without designation as proprietary is not to be construed as a representation by the publisher that it is in the public domain.

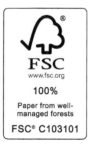

This book could not have been achieved without the encouragement and support of our entire family. Many thanks to my wife, Renie, and: Michael, Stephanie, Maddie, Alan, Andrea, Lucelia, Eric, Aliza, and David. Thanks to the co-editors, Dr. Mathew M. Avram and Dr. Jeremy A. Brauer for all of their thoughtful contributions. Finally, thanks to Thieme and their excellent staff, especially Stephan Konnry and Madhumita Dey who have provided their excellent editorial skill and dedicated numerous hours to production of this book.

-Paul J. Carniol

To my amazing parents, Morrell and Maria Avram, who have provided me with love, inspiration, and support for my entire life. You are the best example of everything I hope to become. To my wife, Alison, and my wonderful children, Rachel, Alexander, and Noah, thank you for the gifts of love, joy, fun, and happiness you give me daily. I finally want to thank my outstanding, tireless co-editors, Drs. Paul J. Carniol and Jeremy A. Brauer as well as our team at Thieme, Stephan Konnry and Madhumita Dey.

-Mathew M. Avram

To my wife, Anate–the love of my life, nothing in this world would be possible without you. Words cannot express how much I appreciate your support and all that you do for our family, so that I can pursue all of my personal and professional dreams. To our daughters, Maddie, Noa, and Sophie–you are the lights of our life, who keep us young, smiling, and exhausted! To my mother, Bobbi-your unconditional love, guidance, and unwavering support have made me the person I am today. Lastly, I'd like to thank Drs. Carniol and Avram–it has been an honor and pleasure to work with you.

-Jeremy A. Brauer

Contents

Section I: Complications Prevention Essentials

Section II: Injectables: Avoiding and Managing Complications

11   Vascular and Pigment Laser and Light Sources. 116
Elizabeth F. Rostan

12   Radiofrequency and Microneedle Radiofrequency. 127
Steven F. Weiner

13   Complications of Platelet-Rich Plasma and Microneedling 131
Amit Arunkumar, Anthony P. Sclafani, and Paul J. Carniol

Videos

Foreword

As specialists practicing facial plastic surgery and aesthetic medicine, we are continually challenged to maintain our clinical expertise on the cutting edge. With each innovative technique, pharmaceutical, or device comes the aspiration, often accompanied by lofty assurances, that Nirvana has arrived to meet a specific patient need.

At times, the ubiquitous presence of "new" advances can overwhelm our ability to choose what procedures and practices are truly best for us and our patients. Furthermore, it is axiomatic that each established treatment, let alone innovation, carries with it not only the potential for enhanced patient outcomes but also the risk of unfortunate complications.

So how do each of us acquire our integral knowledge and desired expertise that will enable us to effectively, and safely, become the best that we can be?

In their new textbook, *Complications in Minimally Invasive Facial Rejuvenation: Prevention and Management*, Drs. Avram, Brauer, and Carniol have assembled an acclaimed group of clinicians and academicians in our field who have created a tome to solve this conundrum for us. Together, as facial plastic surgeons, dermatologists, plastic surgeons, and oculoplastic surgeons, they have covered both the breadth and depth of this demanding and exciting field.

Most impressively, this has been accomplished in a textbook that is, at once, both holistic and subject specific. The young practitioner will absorb himself or herself by reading from cover to cover and, in doing so, will build a firm knowledge base to grow a successful practice in noninvasive facial aesthetics. The experienced practitioner will utilize the chapters for their specific details and nuances of demonstrated empirical wisdom. All readers will discover delightful pearls of knowledge and tips on clinical finesse to enhance their skill set and their patients' outcomes.

The text appropriately begins by recognizing that complications should best be avoided. After all, it is important to operate well; but it is even more important not to operate poorly. Chapters on selecting patients wisely, anesthesia, anatomy, and the significance of laser and cautery smoke lay a basic foundation and emphasize the importance of safe practice. They are practical and provide necessary information all practitioners should have. Injectables, including fillers, neuromodulators, fat transfer, and deoxycholic acid, each have their own chapter covering the most popular and effective modalities. Skin resurfacing in the form of laser and chemical peels, as well as chapters on vascular and pigment laser and light sources, followed by radio frequency and micro needling round out the detailed overview of minimally invasive subjects. Finally, surgical procedures such as liposuction, cryolipolysis, thread lifting, face lifting, blepharoplasty, and hair transplantation complete the book.

What is truly impressive is the content of the chapters. The authors organize basic information, state specific principles, emphasize procedural planning, and articulate how to technically achieve maximum results while minimizing potential complications. The writing is clear, concise, and crisp. The book is replete with superb, demonstrative patient photographs, along with detailed illustrations to enhance understanding of the subject matter. There are a plethora of tables, graphs, and algorithms which simplify, consolidate, and summarize the text. They are clear and colorful, and command the reader's attention. Each chapter is very well referenced for the scholar seeking even more insight into a particular subject.

Another pleasure in reading this book is the neat organization of each chapter, beginning with a summary and keywords, following with numbered subject headings, and closing with a conclusion. The Thieme Gulliver font is simple, contemporary, and soothing on the eyes.

Every practitioner committed to the science and art of minimally invasive facial rejuvenation will want to own this outstanding and beautiful book. This collaborative effort of esteemed surgeons and physicians brings to us an invaluable resource imbued with fundamental knowledge, clinical pearls, and acquired wisdom. It also emphasizes the potential perils of these sometimes simpler, but never trivial, procedures.

Complications in Minimally Invasive Facial Rejuvenation: Prevention and Management is an invaluable literary addition to our specialty. It will be a utilitarian library treasure for both the nascent and accomplished practitioner for many years to come.

Peter A. Adamson, OOnt, MD, FRCSC, FACS
Professor
Division of Facial Plastic and Reconstructive Surgery
Department of Otolaryngology-Head and Neck Surgery
University of Toronto;
President
International Board for Certification in Facial Plastic and Reconstructive Surgery;
President and Founder
Face the Future Foundation
Toronto, Ontario, Canada

Preface

Looking at this preface you may be wondering, "Why should I read this book?" The answer to this question is best answered by asking the question, "Why did the editors create this book?"

In brief, this book needed to be written. It needed to be written for our patients and for the physicians who treat them. A recent procedural 2019 survey by the American Academy of Facial Plastic and Reconstructive Surgery revealed that 80% of the cosmetic facial procedures performed by their surgeons were minimally invasive in 2019. Although we do not have similar survey results from the American Society for Dermatologic Surgery, or the American Society of Plastic Surgery, we suspect that their members might report similar statistics. Considering this, the issue of avoiding and managing complications of minimally invasive procedures becomes even more important. Important for both our patients and the physicians who care for them.

Thus, the editors have come together to create this book. If read carefully, it will help you, the reader, to minimize the risk or decrease the incidence of complications and, if they occur, give some of the best information available on how to manage them.

This book should not be considered a cookbook but rather a helpful reference and it must be left to each physician who uses this book to determine and decide on the optimal technology, procedure, product, and/or technique for the patient. If complications do occur, it is up to each physician to decide whether the management discussed in this book is appropriate for his or her patient. We are optimistic that both our patients and readers will benefit from this.

The book is in an easily accessible format, so that sections which are appropriate for your practice can be easily referenced. The majority of the chapters include videos which are also valuable. This is especially beneficial as the multiple videos in this book help to illustrate and emphasize many of the points found within the chapters.

Based on the unpredictable incidence of complications as well as the associated management issues, we suggest that in addition to having a hard copy of the text sitting on your shelf, it would be beneficial to have a copy on your mobile device so that you always have it available.

We have made all efforts to create an easily referenced comprehensive text which includes every minimally invasive procedure currently being performed. The text opens with perhaps the first important technique for minimizing complications, namely patient selection.

This chapter starts with patient consultation. The importance of the consultation cannot be overemphasized. This consultation is your opportunity to evaluate whether the patient is psychologically and medically a good candidate for a procedure. It also gives you the opportunity to meet a potential patient, evaluate his or her concerns and/or problems, and decide on the optimal treatment. During this initial visit, it is important to listen to your patient. Then, in addition to evaluating their anatomical areas of concern, you have the opportunity to determine if their goals and expectations are aligned with realistic outcomes.

After you have met with your patient, and reviewed the procedure, with the associated variable results, risks, alternatives, and complications, for many of these procedures it is time to move on to consideration of anesthesia if or as needed. This leads us naturally to a discussion on this topic in our second chapter. The second chapter is on anesthesia for these procedures, which is an important consideration. After all, significant systemic reactions, including toxicity, to anesthesia including topical anesthesia have been reported.

The third chapter gives an important review of the relevant anatomy, including extensive illustrations providing wonderful visual detail. For many procedures, in addition to setting realistic expectations and selecting appropriate patients, it is the knowledge of the relevant anatomy that will help to optimize outcomes and reduce the incidence of complications.

The remainder of this text is dedicated to the discussion of the minimally invasive procedures. The first procedure discussed is injection of fillers. Fillers are frequently utilized for aesthetic reasons by physicians from multiple training backgrounds, as well as for less commonly performed fat transfers. Significant complications are uncommon but can include some serious events. These serious events include, but are not limited to: cerebrovascular accidents, visual loss, skin loss, and infection. Considering how significant these are, it is important to know how to avoid and manage them.

The next chapter is about fat transfers. Although used less commonly than fillers, they too have significant related issues, and are discussed in the subsequent chapter.

Neuromodulators are perhaps the most commonly used injectable agent, and fortunately major complications are rare. However, although not typically life-threatening, diplopia, ptosis, deformities, and asymmetry can develop from these treatments. Therefore, understanding how to minimize the incidence of these problems is also important.

Considering the risks of burns, scarring, deformity, and pigmentary disorders, it is important to know how to avoid, minimize, and/or treat complications associated with lasers, light, and energy-based devices. This includes discussion on selection of the optimal technology for the particular issue and the associated challenges.

The same issues of risks and complications are important in order to avoid or minimize the incidence of complications from chemical peels, and it is important to have a full understanding of the various components and best techniques. This is discussed in the chapter on chemical peels.

There are multiple lasers which can be used to treat vascular or pigmented lesions. It is important to understand the use of these devices for the treatment of these lesions. Recently there has been a lot of interest in radiofrequency. Avoiding and managing complications of these procedures are also discussed in detail.

Other minimally invasive facial procedures include reduction of excess adiposity by utilizing an injectable. There are also chapters dedicated to deoxycholic acid, heat with lasers and energy, and cryolipolysis for treatment of excess adiposity.

Thread lift procedures, although initially introduced years ago, have made a strong comeback with better materials and techniques. Considering this increased use, it is important to have a chapter dedicated to these procedures. The chapter on thread lift procedures includes techniques to minimize complications of these procedures.

Beyond injectables and devices, the next three chapters discuss the avoidance and management of complications reported in more minimally invasive surgical procedures such as facelift, hair transplants, and blepharoplasty.

Plumes can be associated with the use of cautery, some radiofrequency, and lasers. The last chapter of this text specifically addresses these plumes as they can have associated risks. Considering this, the chapter discusses how to minimize these risks. There are also multiple videos with this book to illustrate and emphasize many of the points in the chapters. In summary, this book provides an invaluable and needed reference for healthcare providers who perform any of these procedures. Read on, and feel free to send the editors any comments.

Paul J. Carniol, MD, FACS
Mathew M. Avram, MD, JD
Jeremy A. Brauer, MD

Contributors

Seden Akdagli, MD
Resident
Department of Anesthesiology
State University of New York-Downstate
    Health Sciences University
Brooklyn, New York, USA

Murad Alam, MD, MSCI, MBA
Professor and Vice-Chair
Department of Dermatology;
Professor
Department of Otolaryngology-Head
    and Neck Surgery;
Professor
Department of Surgery;
Feinberg School of Medicine
Northwestern University
Chicago, Illinois, USA

Kaete A. Archer, MD
Assistant Clinical Professor
Department of Surgery
Columbia University
New York, New York, USA

Christian Arroyo, MD
Plastic Surgeon
West Houston Plastic Surgery
Houston, Texas, USA

Amit Arunkumar, MD
Resident
Department of Otolaryngology—Head and
    Neck Surgery
Weill Cornell and Columbia University
New York, New York, USA

Mathew M. Avram, MD, JD
Associate Professor
Department of Dermatology
Massachusetts General Hospital/Harvard
    Medical School
Wellman Center for Photomedicine
Boston, Massachusetts, USA

Alfonso Barrera, MD, FACS
Clinical Assistant Professor
Department of Plastic Surgery
Baylor College of Medicine
Houston, Texas, USA

Sydney C. Butts, MD, FACS
Associate Professor and Chief-Facial Plastic and
    Reconstructive Surgery
Department of Otolaryngology
State University of New York-Downstate Health
    Sciences University
Brooklyn, New York, USA

Eric T. Carniol, MD, MBA
Facial Plastic Surgeon and Hair Restoration Surgeon
Department of Facial Plastic Surgery and
    Otolaryngology Head and Neck Surgery
Carniol Plastic Surgery
Summit, New Jersey, USA

Paul J. Carniol, MD, FACS
Clinical Professor
Department of Otolaryngology
Rutgers New Jersey Medical School;
Plastic Surgeon
Carniol Plastic Surgery
Summit, New Jersey, USA

Jason E. Cohn, DO
Fellow and Instructor
Department of Otolaryngology-Head and
    Neck Surgery
Division of Facial Plastic Reconstructive Surgery
Louisiana State University Health
Shreveport, Louisiana, USA

Lisa Coppa-Breslauer, MD
Associate Attending-Dermatology
Department of Internal Medicine
Morristown Memorial Medical Center
Morristown, New Jersey, USA

Louis M. DeJoseph, MD
Adjunct Assistant Professor of Otolaryngology
Department of Otolaryngology and Head and
    Neck Surgery
Emory University School of Medicine
Atlanta, Georgia, USA

Dennis P. Dimaculangan, MD
Clinical Associate Professor
Department of Anesthesiology
State University of New York-Downstate
    Health Sciences University
Brooklyn, New York, USA

Fred G. Fedok, MD, FACS
Adjunct Professor
Department of Surgery
University of South Alabama
Mobile, Alabama;
Plastic Surgeon
Fedok Plastic Surgery
Foley, Alabama, USA

George Ferzli, MD
Attending
Department of Otolaryngology
Lenox Hill Hospital
New York, New York, USA

Timothy M. Greco, MD, FACS
Director
Department of Facial Plastic and
    Reconstructive Surgery
Center of Excellence in Facial Cosmetic Surgery
Bala Cynwyd, Pennsylvania;
Adjunct Assistant Professor
Department of Otorhinolaryngology and
    Head and Neck Surgery
Division of Facial Plastic Surgery
Perelman School of Medicine at the University
    of Pennsylvania
Philadelphia, Pennsylvania, USA

Kian Karimi, MD, FACS
Double-Board Certified Facial Plastic Surgeon
Head and Neck Surgeon
Medical Director and Founder
Rejuva Medical Aesthetics
Los Angeles, California, USA

Rachel L. Kyllo, MD
Dermatologist
Meramec Dermatology, LLC
Arnold, Missouri, USA

Phillip R. Langsdon, MD
Professor and Chief of Facial Plastic Surgery
Department of Otolaryngology—Head and
    Neck Surgery
University of Tennessee Health Science Center
Memphis, Tennessee, USA

Devinder S. Mangat, MD, FACS
Clinical Professor
Department of Orolaryngology and Head and
    Neck Surgery
University of Cincinnati
Cincinnati, Ohio, USA;
Facial Plastic Surgeon
Mangat Plastic Surgery
Vail, Colorado, USA

Aubriana M. McEvoy, MD, MS
Resident
Department of Dermatology
Washington University
St. Louis, Missouri, USA

Rebecca C. Metzinger, MD
Associate Professor
Department of Ophthalmology
Tulane University School of Medicine;
Chief
Section of Ophthalmology
Department of Surgery
Section of Ophthalmology
Southeast Louisiana Veterans Health Care Center
New Orleans, Louisiana, USA

Stephen E. Metzinger, MD, MSPH, FACS
Aesthetic Surgical Associates;
Clinical Associate Professor
Department of Surgery
Division of Plastic and Reconstructive Surgery
Tulane University School of Medicine
New Orleans, Louisiana, USA

Basia Michalski, MD
Resident Physician
Department of Medicine
Division of Dermatology
Washington University
Saint Louis, Missouri, USA

Helen M. Moses, MD, ABFPRS
Graduate Fellow
Facial Plastic and Reconstructive Surgery;
Private Practice
Palmetto Facial Plastics
Columbia, South Carolina, USA

Sunny S. Park, MD, MPH
Plastic Surgeon
Sunny Park Facial Plastic Surgery
Newport Beach, California, USA

Nikunj Rana, MD
Fellow
Department of Facial Plastic Surgery
Premier Image Cosmetic and Laser Surgery
Atlanta, Georgia, USA

E. Victor Ross, MD
Director of Laser and Cosmetic Dermatology
Division of Dermatology
Scripps Clinic
San Diego, California, USA

Elizabeth F. Rostan, MD
Charlotte Skin and Laser
Charlotte, North Carolina, USA

Ronald J. Schroeder II, MD
Fellow
Department of Otolaryngology—Head and
  Neck Surgery
University of Tennessee Health Science Center
Memphis, Tennessee, USA

Anthony P. Sclafani, MD, MBA
Professor
Department of Otolaryngology
Weill Cornell Medical College
New York, New York, USA

Sidney J. Starkman, MD
Facial Plastic Surgeon
Private Practice
Starkman Facial Plastic Surgery
Scottsdale, Arizona, USA

Aria Vazirnia, MD, MAS
Laser and Cosmetic Dermatology Fellow
Department of Dermatology
Massachusetts General Hospital/Harvard
  Medical School
Wellman Center for Photomedicine
Boston, Massachusetts, USA

Steven F. Weiner, MD
Facial Plastic Surgeon
The Aesthetic Clinique
Santa Rosa Beach, Florida, USA

Brandon Worley, MD, MSc, FRCPC, DABD
Fellow
Mohs Micrographic Surgery and Dermatologic
  Oncology;
Fellow
Cosmetic Dermatologic Surgery
Northwestern University
Chicago, Illinois, USA

Daniel A. Yanes, MD
PGY-3, Dermatology
Department of Dermatology
Massachusetts General Hospital
Boston, Massachusetts, USA

Section I

Complications Prevention Essentials

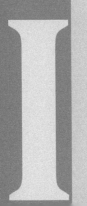

1 General Approach: The Consultation—Patient Evaluation

Eric T. Carniol

Summary

The preoperative stage of a surgeon-patient relationship is important in order to assess physical and psychological candidacy for a procedure and establish realistic expectations. Surgeons must be prepared to deny treatments to patients who are not candidates as well as build trust with patients with whom they would like to continue with treatment. The surgeon-operated patient relationship is permanent, and both parties must understand and willingly enter into this relationship.

Keywords: consultation, preoperative planning, preoperative assessment, psychological evaluation

1.1 Introduction

The goal of minimally invasive facial rejuvenation or aesthetic/cosmetic procedures is to enrich a patient's life by improving a perceived flaw in function or appearance. The initial consultation is important in avoiding and minimizing complications from procedures. This first meeting between the physician and new patient is an important opportunity to establish a strong enduring relationship. For the physician, it is imperative to identify the patient's goals and aspirations and to determine the appropriate potential procedure or procedures. For the patient, it is imperative to express those goals and establish realistic expectations. Patient selection is of paramount importance, and the issues related to patient selection can be challenging. There are four main components. First, how likely is the identified procedure(s) going to yield the change that the patient is seeking? The answer to this and other related issues will be discussed in the chapters that follow. The second component is patient selection. The third component is procedure execution, and the final component is any care, if appropriate, that is required after the procedure.

Patients today can do extensive research on both a desired procedure and their potential physician. It is important for the physician to recognize that the patient will probably present with a fair amount of information about the procedure being requested. This comes with additional challenges, as some of the information may not be accurate or may not be applicable to the patient or their concerns. The physician should be prepared to discuss the risks, benefits, and alternatives to the procedure in addition to respectfully addressing any misinformation that the patient may have acquired from their own research. It is important to demonstrate expertise when addressing any misinformation.

Many patients seek multiple opinions and consultations prior to deciding upon a physician and procedure; therefore, during this time, it is imperative for the physician to ensure that she/he engages the patient in a physician–patient relationship. As the aphorism goes, "The preoperative period is finite. The postoperative period is infinite."

Once goals and expectations are identified, discussed, and agreed upon, the physician should pursue a structured conversation regarding the remainder of the treatment experience. A well-described and adapted structured discussion is the R-DOS model, adapted from Daniel Sullivan, founder of "The Strategic Coach."[1]

The first question (The R-Factor) is "If we were to meet here in one year and look back over the year, what would have happened, both personally and professionally, for you to be satisfied with your progress in life?" While the answer usually has little to do with the requested procedure or displeasing bodily feature, the answer will reflect whether the physician and the patient will have an ongoing relationship that will last at least one year. The answer, as with all answers, is important to note as precisely as possible. This allows the physician to utilize the patient's own language, a process known as reflective listening.[2] If a potential patient has difficulty answering this question, it is worth asking if they anticipate that the procedure being discussed has the potential to change their future. This may be the situation for a patient with a significant deformity or problem. However, for a more frequent, relatively straightforward cosmetic procedure, it is unlikely that the procedure will change their future. Patients who anticipate that a relatively small cosmetic procedure will change their lives expect too much from the procedure and may become unhappy with the outcome when their life does not change. Therefore, these patients should be avoided.

The second question relates to the patient's perceived risks of the procedure. "When thinking about [the procedure/body part], what specific questions or concerns do you have?" Writing down these questions also imparts to the patient that you are listening and that you are attentive to their concerns. These questions also give the physician an insight into the emotionality that the procedure or the disliked feature plays on the psyche of the patient. The concerns or questionsare the only negative part of the interaction. The physician should go over every question with the patient for completeness. Once addressed, the discussion can be (permanently) shifted to the positive.

Opportunities: Once the concerns have been addressed, attention in the conversation can be moved to the future. "Pretend that it is one year in the future and that you have had the successful procedure, what will that do for you?" Although this question can seem similar to the R-Factor, it instead shifts the patient's focus to the future, once the procedure and the recovery are finished.

Strengths: Many times, patients have already addressed their personal strengths in the consultation. However, this is the time to address strengths specifically and continue to build on them. "What are your strengths and how will this procedure build on them?"

The R-DOS conversation allows the physician to gain key insight into the patient. By assessing these, the physician can decide whether a patient is a candidate for surgery. There are some patients who are unable to provide quality responses to these questions, or are so apprehensive about these questions that they will refuse.

If the patient is unable to imagine their future and their place in it, they may also be unable to imagine their postprocedure recovery and may have increased difficulty adjusting to their postoperative result. Some prospective patients may also describe secondary gains from surgery such as change in social stature, renewal of love or attention from a significant other, or maintenance/attainment of a job. These responses help the physician identify a potentially unhappy patient. The physician may also determine that the prospective patient is not someone with whom they would like to engage in a permanent physician-operated patient relationship.

This conversation can help a patient frame their surgery as not just an outcome or a good that is purchased, and instead as an experience that they will use to continue to improve their life. After going through the R-DOS conversation, patients have increased engagement and higher rates of conversion to and satisfaction from their procedure.

1.2 Assessment of Expectations

Management of expectations is also important in order to obtain a happy patient. If a patient's expectations are greater than what is usually attainable from a procedure or even what a given procedure can achieve, there is no way to please the patient.

For example, a patient in her fifties who comes in requesting facial rejuvenation and shows you a photo of a celebrity in her twenties probably will not be able to look like the celebrity. As well, a patient with a prominent nose and thick skin should not expect a petite ultra-defined nose after a rhinoplasty as their soft tissue envelope may not contract down after the procedure.

1.3 Assessment for Body Dysmorphic Disorder

Care must be taken with patients with body dysmorphic disorder. Although early studies demonstrated increased rate of this disorder in men, more recent research demonstrates that this purported increased risk may not be present.[3] Patients with body dysmorphic disorder often have other psychiatric comorbidities. In one study, more than 75% had a lifetime history of major depression, 30% history of obsessive compulsive disorder, 25 to 30% history of substance abuse, and 7 to 14% history of an eating disorder. More than half of these patients fulfilled criteria for at least one personality disorder.[4]

In patients with body dysmorphic disorder, it is important to recognize that cosmetic procedures do not usually improve symptoms, and can often worsen them.[5] For patients with concern for previous psychopathology, open-ended questions about body image and perceived appearance can often be helpful, as well as degree of dissatisfaction compared to the physician's measure. Assessment of appropriate motivations is also important as otherwise discussed in this chapter.

1.4 Accurate History Taking

It is important to ask patients about their medical history in different ways. Patients can be intentionally or unintentionally forgetful about medical comorbidities. Intake questions that are specific about particular organ systems are more effective in obtaining accurate histories. As well, separate questions on prescription and over-the-counter medications, vitamins and other supplements can also serve as a valuable resource to determine other disease processes that are ongoing. It can be frustrating for the physician to find out, just prior to a procedure, about a portion of the patient's medical history that was not previously disclosed. Particularly, history of infectious diseases, such as HIV and hepatitis C, should be asked specifically. In some states, patients are mandatory reporters of their viral status but this should not be solely relied upon, as many patients are unaware of their viral status.

Today, as the cultural and political landscape shifts about marijuana and related products, it is also important to question patients on this in addition to alcohol and other drug use. Recent research has demonstrated that certain marijuana-related products can alter patient's pain tolerance, with some patients requiring increased dosages of anesthesia during surgery and also increased postoperative narcotic requirements.[6]

Patient's support systems can be very important during the immediate preoperative, postoperative, and the long-term postoperative periods. Having emotional backing prior to undergoing a procedure can decrease preoperative stress and allow the patient to focus on instructions for example, easing the recovery period. After a procedure, patients who have less support are more likely to have challenges associated with their recovery. They are at greater risk of being noncompliant, and therefore may be more likely to encounter post-procedure problems, exacerbate postoperative symptoms, and possibly delay recovery resulting in suboptimal outcomes. Finally, encouragement from a patient's support system can aid the transition to their new, rejuvenated appearance.

1.5 Preoperative Counseling

The preprocedure period is an important time to counsel patients on the postprocedure course. If a physician discusses with a patient a potential complication that they could have before surgery, it is *counseling*. However, a discussion with a patient about an issue that they are having after a procedure is a *complication*.

For more major procedures, after the consultation an additional preprocedure appointment can be beneficial to confirm the treatment plan, expectations, and discuss postoperative recovery. The interval between the two visits is important for both the patient and the physician to decide that they wish to proceed with the procedure. During this interval, the physician can also elicit feedback from staff on their interaction with the patient. Often a patient can "put on a show" for the physician, but may be completely different toward staff, potentially cluing the physician to an underlying personality or other psychiatric disorder.[2]

At the preoperative visit, we review the indications, contraindications, procedure itself, risks, and recovery from surgery. One key area of risk to focus on during this period is the probability of revision. This inherent risk of surgery can be a difficult discussion with patients, as many physicians believe that this discussion pierces the veil of confidence. However, by addressing it with the patient (and documenting this discussion), physicians can more effectively manage the patient's expectations. Even for a surgery with a 5% revision rate, for 5% who fall in that subset of patients, 100% of them are having a revision. As well, there is some percentage of patients within the 95% who are not totally satisfied with the outcome, but not dissatisfied enough to undergo the revision surgery. Therefore, the physician must also anticipate that any given patient could be in the dissatisfied/ revision group. If a patient does experience such an issue, then the follow-up for the patient will be at a much higher frequency than that of a patient who does well. Therefore, the physician must be prepared for spending significant portions of time with the patient postoperatively.

For some patients who are not psychologically ready for a procedure, a psychiatrist, psychologist, or counselor can be very helpful. Such patients may over the course of therapy become ready for the procedure, or acknowledge that they are not ready. It is important for the physician to partner with the patient and the mental health team. Any patient who returns for surgery after counseling should allow the physician to discuss the patient directly with the counselor.

1.6 Conclusion

The preoperative evaluation (the consultation and the preoperative planning meeting) is an important area for physicians to carefully select patients for a procedure. Overall, most patients will do well and be happy with a given procedure. However, it is the physician's responsibility to do her/his best to wean out the patients who are significantly more at risk of poor outcomes. The physician should never be fearful of saying no to a patient, as the physician-operated patient relationship is permanent.

References

[1] Constantinides M. The rhinoplasty consultation and the business of rhinoplasty. Facial Plast Surg Clin North Am. 2009; 17 (1):1–5, v

[2] Sykes J, Javidnia H. A contemporary review of the management of the difficult patient. JAMA Facial Plast Surg. 2013; 15 (2):81–84

[3] Daines SM, Mobley SR. Considerations in male aging face consultation: psychologic aspects. Facial Plast Surg Clin North Am. 2008; 16(3):281–287, v

[4] Phillips KA, McElroy SL. Personality disorders and traits in patients with body dysmorphic disorder. Compr Psychiatry. 2000; 41(4):229–236

[5] Crerand CE, Phillips KA, Menard W, Fay C. Nonpsychiatric medical treatment of body dysmorphic disorder. Psychosomatics. 2005; 46(6):549–555

[6] Huson HB, Granados TM, Rasko Y. Surgical considerations of marijuana use in elective procedures. Heliyon. 2018; 4(9): e00779

2 Anesthesia for Minimally Invasive Facial Aesthetic Surgery

Seden Akdagli, Dennis P. Dimaculangan, George Ferzli, and Sydney C. Butts

Summary

A variety of anesthetic techniques are used for facial plastic procedures. Laser treatment of facial lesions is a subset of these procedures that require unique considerations and planning. Procedural anesthesia and laser treatment may both be performed by the same practitioner; anesthesia of the region to be treated may be accomplished in a short period of time or can take an extended period of time requiring dedicated preprocedural preparation; procedures that require deep levels of sedation will require nursing staff and anesthesia personnel; and finally, there are numerous safety considerations unique to laser therapy that may dictate the type of anesthesia provided. Patient factors to consider include type and extent of lesions to be treated, overall health status of the patient, and prior experiences with laser treatment or other procedures requiring anesthesia. The type of anesthesia approaches needed can range from noninvasive methods using topical agents to invasive techniques that require infiltration of anesthesia with or without the addition of sedation (monitored anesthesia care [MAC]) to the use of general anesthesia in certain situations.[1] In this chapter, we discuss the commonly used anesthesia methods that are employed in treating laser resurfacing patients and review potential complications associated with these anesthetic techniques.

Keywords: local anesthesia, nerve blocks, cryoanesthesia, monitored anesthesia care (MAC), local anesthetic systemic toxicity (LAST)

2.1 The Office-Based Surgery Setting

The number and complexity of elective surgical procedures performed outside the hospital setting in the United States has expanded rapidly in the last 30 years. Part of the reason for this growth is the development of newer surgical and anesthesia techniques that allow more invasive and complex procedures to be performed safely in ambulatory surgery centers and in surgeons' offices.[2] Following this trend, facial aesthetic surgery procedures are being routinely performed in the office-based settings.[3] In 2017, 17.5 million cosmetic procedures were performed in the United States. Out of these, 15.7 million or 70% were cosmetic minimally invasive procedures that were mostly done in the office.[4]

Office-based surgery (OBS) and anesthesia offer many advantages to both patients and their healthcare providers. Procedures can be more conveniently and economically done in the office setting compared to the hospital. Patients get more personal attention and privacy, while surgeons enjoy more flexibility in scheduling and greater productivity.[5]

For OBS facilities, regulations differ compared to hospital-based surgical facilities. Regulations vary from state to state and at the local government level.[5] The American College of Surgeons (ACS) issued guidelines listing ten core patient safety principles for OBS in a joint consensus statement with the American Medical Association (AMA) in 2003.[6] One principle requires that OBS facilities be accredited by one of a number of recognized regulatory organizations. The American Academy of Facial Plastic and Reconstructive Surgery, the American Society of Plastic Surgeons (ASPS), and the American Society of Aesthetic Plastic Surgery have mandated its members perform outpatient surgery only in accredited facilities for procedures needing intravenous and/or general anesthesia. Surgical cases that require local anesthesia and possibly some oral sedation are exempt.[7]

2.2 Preprocedure Preparation

The ideal patient for a procedure performed in an office-based facility or ambulatory surgery center should have few or no comorbidities to avoid anesthesia complications.[8] The American Society of Anesthesiologists (ASA) Physical Status Classification status of I or II are associated with the lowest 30-day morbidity and mortality rates.[8] Patients with higher physical status ratings, associated with significant systemic disease, are considered poor candidates for deep sedation and general anesthesia and include patients with morbid obesity, obstructive sleep apnea, congestive heart failure, recent myocardial infarction (within the last 6 mo), severe chronic obstructive pulmonary disease, seizure disorder or stroke within the last 3 months.[8]

Patients undergoing procedures involving the face may be more anxious and concerned than the general patient population. Discussions about pain management, expectations of pain levels, and patient's prior experiences with procedural pain are increasingly appreciated as important to overall patient satisfaction.[9] Recent studies have shown communication about postoperative analgesia to be associated with decreased opioid consumption after procedures.[9] Patients who received preoperative education (including materials about pain control and opioids) were less likely to fill narcotic prescriptions, using non-narcotic analgesia more often than a comparison group receiving no preprocedure pain counseling. Pain scores of the counseled group were also lower postoperatively compared to the alternate group.[9]

2.3 Local Anesthesia

Laser treatment of the skin of the face can be performed using local anesthesia with or without oral sedation that can be provided by the surgeon.[10] MAC with moderate-to-deep intravenous or general anesthesia administered by an anesthesiologist is employed for more extensive procedures.[11]

Local anesthetics (LAs) are used to block transmission of nerve impulses, thereby reducing or eliminating sensation.[8,12] LAs may be applied topically, injected via subcutaneous tissue infiltration, injected to perform specific peripheral nerve blocks of the face, and used for tumescent anesthesia of the areas to be treated.[10,13,14,15]

LAs are divided into esters and amides based on the chemical structure of the compounds. The majority of LAs in use are in the amide class (lidocaine, bupivacaine, ropivacaine, levobupivacaine, prilocaine) while cocaine and tetracaine are types of esters.[8,10] The metabolism of an LA differs between ester and amide classes.[10,12,13] The most

commonly used LAs are lidocaine and bupivacaine (► Table 2.1). Lidocaine has a duration of action of 2 to 3 hours compared to a longer duration of action of bupivacaine (3–8 h, prolonged duration with the addition of epinephrine). In the 1990s, two additional long-acting amides were introduced: levobupivicaine and ropivacaine which are the S-isomers of bupivacaine, a racemic mixture of S and R isomers.[12] These new agents—similar in potency, onset of action, and duration of effect to bupivacaine—have decreased central nervous system and cardiac toxicities.[16] The cardiac toxicity associated with bupivacaine plasma levels at toxic doses can be resistant to treatment with reported fatalities.[16]

Esters are hydrolyzed by plasma cholinesterase while amides are metabolized by the cytochrome P450 system in the liver.[8,12] Any condition that reduces hepatic enzymatic function or hepatic blood flow can delay the metabolism and prolong the duration of action of amides. The dose of LA must be reduced in these patients.[8,12] LAs differ in their potency, onset and duration of action, and potential for toxicity. Several injectables are combined with epinephrine which increases the dose that can be safely given[10] (► Table 2.1).

Allergic reactions to LAs are rare and many reactions described by patients as allergies most likely are idiosyncratic nonallergic reactions such as vasovagal and anxiety reactions. The reactions to additives such as epinephrine (flushing, palpitation) are often misconstrued or interpreted as allergies.[8,10] True allergies from LAs are from type I and IV hypersensitivity reactions. Anaphylaxis and immediate allergic reactions are examples of type I reactions, which typically begin within 1 hour after drug administration, but are very rare. Contact dermatitis and delayed-onset localized swelling are examples of type IV, delayed-type hypersensitivity reactions. Symptoms develop 1 to 3 days after drug

Table 2.1 Local anesthesia dosing, duration of action

Anesthetic agent	Maximal dose (mg/kg)	Onset of action	Duration of action (h)
Lidocaine 1% (10 mg/mL)	5	Rapid	1.5–2
Lidocaine 1% + epinephrine	7	Rapid	2–3
Bupivacaine .25% (2.5 mg/mL)	2	Slow	3–6
Bupivacaine, 25% + epinephrine	3	Slow	6–8
Bupivacaine .5% (5 mg/mL)	2	Slow	3–6
Ropivacaine .5% (5 mg/mL)	3	Moderate	3–8
Levobupivacaine .5% (5 mg/mL)	3	Moderate	3–8

Source: Used with permission from Armstrong.[18]

administration and can be evaluated with patch testing. Allergic reactions to amide LAs are extremely rare, with the ester class of LAs most often the cause of allergies in patients.[8,12] One special circumstance can be encountered in patients who report allergies to sunscreen and other cosmetics. These products contain methylparaben– a preservative that is contained in some amide LAs and is metabolized to *para*-amino-benzoic acid (PABA). PABA can bind to tissue protein that is antigenic and can cause allergic dermatitis. PABA is also a metabolite of ester LAs.[8,12] Because of this common pathway, cases of cross-sensitization between ester and amide LAs have erroneously been reported.[8,12,13] If a patient is allergic to an ester-type LA, the patient should be given preservative-free amide. Proper screening with appropriate tests for ester or amide preservatives is important to clarify the basis for allergic reactions to LAs.[8,12,13]

2.3.1 Topical Local Anesthesia

EMLA Cream

Eutectic mixture of local anesthetics (EMLA) is a topical anesthetic cream that contains a mixture of two amide LAs: 2.5% lidocaine and 2.5% prilocaine.[10,17] It is used to provide sensory anesthesia to intact normal skin. Its depth of penetration is 3 mm at its peak effect of 60 minutes and up to 5 mm after 1.5 to 2 hours. It is recommended that 2 g of EMLA cream be applied per 10 sq. cm of skin and covered with occlusive dressing for 60 minutes to attain adequate anesthesia for dermal procedures.[10]

Known sensitivity to lidocaine, prilocaine, or other amide LAs and any predisposition to methemoglobinemia such as glucose-6-phosphate dehydrogenase deficiency are contraindications to the use of EMLA.[17] Most reactions associated with EMLA are mild, transient skin irritations. However, adverse reactions including methemoglobinemia can occur if EMLA is applied to large areas of skin for prolonged periods of time.[8,12]

Liposomal Lidocaine

Liposomal lidocaine (LMX) is a topical cream preparation with a prolonged period of drug absorption and delay in its metabolism. LMX comes in two preparations: either 4% lidocaine (LMX 4) or 5% lidocaine (LMX 5).[1] The mechanism of action and effectiveness is similar to EMLA but it has a more rapid onset of analgesia than EMLA and its application does not require an occlusive dressing. Adequate anesthesia can be attained within 30 minutes after application. Contraindications for LMX include lidocaine hypersensitivity or allergy to any amide-type LA.

2.3.2 Subcutaneous or Tissue Infiltration

Lidocaine is the most commonly used anesthetic for local infiltration. It is usually given as a 1% solution (10 mg/mL). If large volumes are needed or a smaller dose is desired, the clinician may use a 0.5% solution. Large volume tissue infiltration should be executed in a way that does not distort tissue anatomy or obscure treatment landmarks. Needle gauge and injection technique are important factors in the pain associated with injections of local anesthesia.[10] Slow rates of injection decrease pain associated with infiltration.[10,11] Distraction techniques have been shown to decrease the anxiety and discomfort that patients experience during injection of local anesthesia. Tactile stimulation of the injection site by the injector or with a handheld vibratory device help distract the patient and decrease the stimulus perceived by the central nervous system.[8] Verbal distraction focusing and breathing techniques by the patients are other adjuncts that can be employed to deal with the anxiety of the injection.[10]

Buffering of lidocaine with sodium bicarbonate decreases the pain of injection, and can shorten the time to anesthetic effect.[14] The basis for these effects is the increased pH of the solution from the addition of bicarbonate.[18] A ratio of 9 mL of lidocaine (with or without epinephrine) to 1 mL of 8.4% sodium bicarbonate is recommended.[10,18,19] A systematic review of randomized trials comparing levels of pain between patients receiving plain lidocaine and buffered lidocaine showed significantly decreased discomfort when bicarbonate was added to the LA.[18] Adding bicarbonate to bupivacaine may result in precipitation of the medications.[10,18,19]

Local anesthetic systemic toxicity (LAST) stems from administration of large doses of LA. Increased plasma levels from local infiltration or inadvertent intravascular injection can result in adverse reactions. Initial signs of toxicity involve the central nervous system (CNS) including circumoral numbness, tinnitus, and agitation. Progression results in seizures and CNS depression with respiratory depression.[20] Cardiac toxicity initially manifests as tachycardia and hypertension, progressing to arrhythmias and cardiopulmonary collapse.[8,12,20] Treatment of systemic toxicity begins with support of the airway and blood pressure which may require the initiation of ACLS protocols. Benzodiazepines are a first-line therapy for seizures.[21] Cardiac arrhythmia secondary to local anesthesia toxicity, with bupivacaine toxicity being most refractory to treatment, can be treated with lipid rescue therapy.[12,20] Lipid emulsion therapy (administered intravenously) acts to bind and sequester plasma anesthetic. It should be administered at the first signs of LAST.[12,20]

2.3.3 Regional Nerve Blocks

LA injections are used for regional nerve blocks of branches of the trigeminal nerve: supraorbital, supratrochlear nerves = V1; infraorbital nerve = V2, mental nerve = V3[13,22,23] (▶ Fig. 2.1). One to 3 mL of 1% or 2% lidocaine with epinephrine 1:100,000 can be injected at the landmark for each nerve. When performing the desired regional block of the

trigeminal nerve, the clinician should aim the needle to the base of the nerve as it is exiting the bone. This direction will provide the most efficacious block and also will not alter the surrounding tissues appearance.[23] Blockade of the forehead and scalp can be accomplished by blocking the supratrochlear and supraorbital nerves as they exit their foramina at the supraorbital rim (▶ Fig. 2.2). Blockade of the infraorbital nerve (V2) will anesthetize the medial cheek, nasal sidewall, and ala and upper lip (▶ Fig. 2.1). It can be approached transcutaneously by piercing the skin at the inferior orbital rim along a line dropped from the medial limbus (or the junction of the medial and middle 1/3 of the infraorbital rim) and aiming the needle 10 mm below the infraorbital rim.[13,23] The nerve can also be approached from an intraoral route, inserting the needle through the mucosa of the gingivobuccal sulcus at the level of the first maxillary premolar[10,13,23] (▶ Fig. 2.3). Anesthesia of the chin and lower lip can be accomplished with a block of the mental nerve (V3) most easily approached intraorally by injecting the mucosa between the

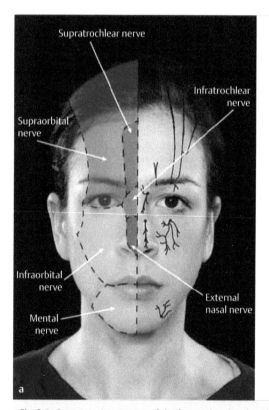
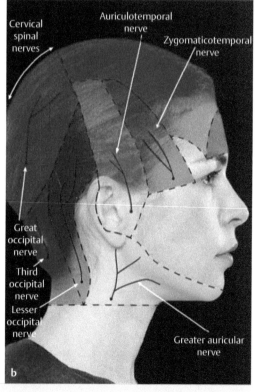

Fig. 2.1 Cutaneous innervation of the face and scalp. Identified are branches of the trigeminal nerve that innervate the face **(a)** as well as innervation of the lateral cheek and scalp **(b)**. (Source: Used with permission from Davies et al.[19])

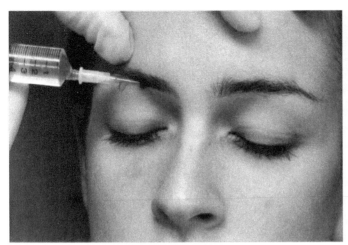

Fig. 2.2 Supraorbital and supratrochlear nerve blocks. Local anesthesia injected at the supraorbital rim—the nerve exits the bone about 2.5 cm from midline, and the supratrochlear nerve exits at the same level 1.5 cm from midline. (Source: Used with permission from Davies et al.[19])

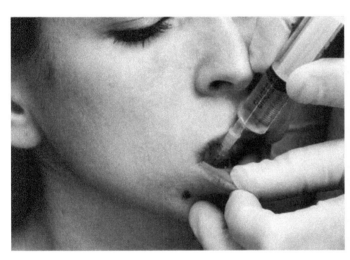

Fig. 2.3 Local anesthetic injection of the mental nerve (V3) which results in anesthesia of the lower lip and chin. Mucosa of the gingivobuccal sulcus adjacent to the mandibular second premolar is injected. (Source: Used with permission from Davies et al.[19])

mandibular first and second premolars.[13,22,23] Additional blockade of the lateral cheek, forehead, and lateral nose may be accomplished by injecting peripheral nerves at well-described landmarks as shown in ▶ Fig. 2.1. The advantage of regional blocks is achieving large areas of anesthesia without using large volumes of anesthetic which can distort tissues and lead to high doses that approach toxic levels. It is often necessary to infiltrate local anesthesia closer to the primary site of treatment to more fully anesthetize the area and in situations where the regional block does not cover the entire treatment area.[12,13]

2.3.4 Tumescent Anesthesia

Tumescent anesthesia is a technique that has been employed in liposuction surgery. It takes advantage of the slow rate of absorption of the injected local anesthesia from the adipose tissue. Large volumes of crystalloid with dilute concentrations of lidocaine (.05–.2%) and epinephrine (1:1,000,000) are injected into the target tissues, resulting in a unique appearance of the tissue due to turgor and stiffness from injection. Combinations of tumescent techniques, which results in significant levels of anesthesia, with regional nerve blocks have been reported for laser resurfacing.[1,12,14]

2.3.5 Cryoanesthesia

Skin cooling is another effective approach used to decrease pain during laser treatment.[15,17,24] The direct effect from cooling and the mental distraction provided by the coolant application are benefits of this technique. Coolants can also be applied to reduce the pain associated with injection of LAs. Cryoanesthesia techniques are broadly divided into contact cooling and noncontact cooling.[24,25] Contact cooling includes application of ice packs, cooled gels, or laser cooling tips: the sapphire cooling tip for the long-pulsed laser, metal cooling finger for the ruby laser, and the sapphire lens for the diode laser.[18,19,20] Noncontact cooling is often accomplished with forced cold air anesthesia(FCAA).[11,24,26] Cooling devices disperse cool air over the skin surface, and wide areas can be cooled rapidly by moving the handpiece over the area to be treated. An advantage of FCAA is the ability to pretreat the skin and continue to cool the skin during lasering and afterward for post-procedure analgesia.[11,24,25,26] The added benefit of cooling is the thermal protective effect to the surrounding skin which can result in decreased post-procedure pain, erythema, and scarring.[15,24,25,26] Contraindications to skin cooling are patients with hypersensitivity to cold, area of impaired sensation or circulation, or open wounds.[24,25,26]

2.3.6 Oral Sedation

Oral sedation is easy to administer and convenient for patients. It has been proven to be effective for conscious sedation during facial cosmetic procedures.[27]

Oral diazepam is a long-acting benzodiazepine that has anxiolytic and amnestic properties. Diazepam is the prototypical benzodiazepine with 100% oral bioavailability. It has an onset of action of 20 to 40 minutes. Flumazenil, a competitive benzodiazepine receptor antagonist, is an antidote that can be used in cases of inadvertent overdose.[12]

2.3.7 Monitored Anesthesia Care

Ablative laser procedures and nonablative procedures can be associated with moderate-to-severe levels of pain requiring sedation with oral or intravenous agents in the presence of an anesthetist.

Intravenous Sedatives

A variety of intravenous sedative hypnotics are available for use during MAC or to induce general anesthesia. Benzodiazepines, opioids, propofol, dexmedetomidine, and/or ketamine can be used as a sole agent or in combination with another.

Benzodiazepines[1,8,15]

Midazolam is a frequently used benzodiazepine for premedication before surgery in the ambulatory setting. It is an anxiolytic, amnestic, and can be titrated when used during MAC sedation. It is an intermediate-acting sedative with a half-life of 1.5 to 2 hours, peak effect of 5 to 10 minutes, and a duration of action range of 16 hours. Caution should be exercised when midazolam is used in the elderly because benzodiazepines have been associated with postoperative cognitive dysfunction in this patient population.

Opioids[1]

Intravenous fentanyl and morphine are commonly used opioid analgesics. These can also be used as agents during sedation under MAC. Fentanyl is ten times more potent than morphine. It is intermediate acting with a half-life of 2 to 4 hours, and duration of action of 11 to 22 hours. Both can be reversed with naloxone in case of overdosing. Disadvantages of opioids include adverse side effects like postoperative nausea and vomiting (PONV), pruritus, constipation, and respiratory depression. PONV is the most common side effect that can delay recovery and discharge in the office and ambulatory setting.

Propofol[1,8,15]

Propofol is a lipid-based sedative hypnotic that has a quick onset and offset of action. It is used as an induction agent for general anesthesia and as a sedative hypnotic for MAC. Because of its short duration of action, it allows for fast recovery and thus is ideal for use as a sedative in the ambulatory setting. It can be delivered in titrated boluses or as a continuous infusion between 25 and 150 µg/kg/min. The disadvantages of propofol include pain on injection, hypotension, and respiratory depression. This can be problematic in a facial or head-and-neck procedure setting where the airway is away and not readily accessible to the anesthesia provider to manage in case of sudden respiratory depression. The most common complication in the office setting is respiratory depression under MAC.

2.4 Laser-Anesthesia Complications

2.4.1 Fire

Fire and facial burn are a particular risk in facial procedures that require laser or routine cautery, due to the presence of supplemental oxygen in combination with combustible materials such as paper drapes and alcohol prep. When laser or cautery is used for surgery in a setup where oxygen is insufflated via nasal cannula under the drapes, it constitutes as a prime setup for fires to occur. Preventive measures include avoidance of the use of nitrous oxide[28] or avoidance of the use of supplemental oxygen[29] if possible, allowing sufficient time for alcohol prep to dry or use of nonalcohol-based prep all together and proper time-out verification procedures assessing the presence and mitigation of identified risks to fires if present.

2.5 Recovery and Discharge

Anesthesia goals in the ambulatory and office-based setting include the use of quick onset and quick offset sedatives that would allow quick recovery and have minimal risk of side effects like PONV for faster discharge.

Provisions for adequate analgesia using multimodal techniques with minimal or no opioids and the use of oral sedatives and topical and local anesthesia allow for a quick recovery and discharge.

Minimizing the use of general anesthesia (GA) is recommended to reduce the risk for PONV from exposure to N_2O and volatile agents which are known to be emetogenic agents.[28,29] The use of opioids for pain control can also increase the risk for PONV but can be minimized by using a multimodal approach to postoperative pain management using other agents such as NSAIDS, acetaminophen, and longer acting LAs for nerve blocks or local infiltration.[30]

2.6 Conclusion

Providing adequate anesthesia during laser treatment begins with familiarity with patient's history with procedures, experience with anesthesia, and counseling about postprocedure analgesia regimens. The extent of laser therapy (focused lesion on the face vs. full-face laser resurfacing) will dictate the level of anesthesia required. Topical options include topical EMLA, LMX cream, and skin cooling. Injection of LAs, via local infiltration or regional nerve blocks, offers wide areas of anesthesia which can last for several hours after the procedure, contributing to analgesia in the immediate postprocedural period. Several of these methods can be used in combination to enhance comfort for the patient and may achieve enough pain control so that additional sedation is not required. The laser surgeon must be able to recognize complications of LAs and treatment, especially allergic reactions and systemic toxicity.

The addition of sedation (MAC) or the need for general anesthesia may provide the best options in extensive procedures. Numerous additional clinical considerations include anesthesia monitoring, patient co-comorbidities, and adverse effects of agents that patients will need to be counseled about.

References

[1] Gaitan S, Markus R. Anesthesia methods in laser resurfacing. Semin Plast Surg. 2012; 26(3):117–124

[2] Shapiro FE, Punwani N, Rosenberg NM, Valedon A, Twersky R, Urman RD. Office-based anesthesia: safety and outcomes. Anesth Analg. 2014; 119(2):276–285

[3] Chuang J, Barnes C, Wong BJF. Overview of facial plastic surgery and current developments. Surg J (N Y). 2016; 2(1): e17–e28

[4] Shapiro FE, Osman BM. Office based anesthesia. www.uptodate.com. Accessed February, 2018

[5] Lapetina EM. The migration of care to non-hospital settings: have regulatory structures kept pace with changes in care delivery? American Hospital Association; July 2006. http://www.aha.org/research/reports/tw/twjuly2006migration.pdf

[6] Lapetina EM, Armstrong EM. Preventing errors in the outpatient setting: a tale of three states. Health Aff (Millwood). 2002; 21(4):26–39

[7] Vila H, Jr, Soto R, Cantor AB, Mackey D. Comparative outcomes analysis of procedures performed in physician offices and ambulatory surgery centers. Arch Surg. 2003; 138(9): 991–995

[8] Eichorn JH, Goulson DT. Anesthesia complications in facial plastic surgery. In: Capone RB, Sykes JM, eds. Complications in Facial Plastic Surgery. 1st ed. New York: Thieme; 2012:17–38

[9] Sugai DY, Deptula PL, Parsa AA, Don Parsa F. The importance of communication in the management of postoperative pain. Hawaii J Med Public Health. 2013; 72(6):180–184

[10] Kouba DJ, LoPiccolo MC, Alam M, et al. Guidelines for the use of local anesthesia in office-based dermatologic surgery. J Am Acad Dermatol. 2016; 74(6):1201–1219

[11] Raulin C, Grema H. Single pass CO2 laser skin resurfacing combined with cold air cooling. Arch Dermatol. 2004; 140: 1333–1336

[12] Armstrong K. A primer on local anesthetics for plastic surgery. Clin Plast Surg. 2013; 40(4):515–528

[13] Davies T, Karanovic S, Shergill B. Essential regional nerve blocks for the dermatologist: part 1. Clin Exp Dermatol. 2014; 39(7): 777–784

[14] Hanke CW. The tumescent facial block: tumescent local anesthesia and nerve block anesthesia for full-face laser resurfacing. Dermatol Surg. 2001; 27(12):1003–1005

[15] Pabby N, Pabby A, Goldman M. Anesthesia for cutaneous laser surgery. In: Goldman M, ed. Cutaneous and Cosmetic Laser Surgery. 1st ed. Philadelphia: Elsevier;2006:311–324

[16] Casati A, Putzu M. Bupivacaine, levobupivacaine and ropivacaine: are they clinically different? Best Pract Res Clin Anaesthesiol. 2005; 19(2):247–268

[17] Sari E, Bakar B. Which is more effective for pain relief during fractionated carbon dioxide laser treatment: EMLA cream or forced cold air anesthesia? J Cosmet Laser Ther. 2018; 20(1): 34–40

[18] Strazar AR, Leynes PG, Lalonde DH. Minimizing the pain of local anesthesia injection. *Plast Reconstr Surg.* 2013;132(3):675–684

[19] Guo J, Yin K, Roges R, Enciso R. Efficacy of sodium bicarbonate buffered versus non-buffered lidocaine with epinephrine in inferior alveolar nerve block: a meta-analysis. J Dent Anesth Pain Med. 2018; 18(3):129–142

[20] Lönnqvist PA. Toxicity of local anesthetic drugs: a pediatric perspective. Paediatr Anaesth. 2012; 22(1):39–43

[21] Sekimoto K, Tobe M, Saito S. Local anesthetic toxicity: acute and chronic management. Acute Med Surg. 2017; 4(2):152–160

[22] Suresh S, Voronov P. Head and neck blocks in infants, children, and adolescents. Paediatr Anaesth. 2012; 22(1): 81–87

[23] Zide BM, Swift R. How to block and tackle the face. Plast Reconstr Surg. 1998; 101(3):840–851

[24] Tierney EP, Hanke CW. The effect of cold-air anesthesia during fractionated carbon-dioxide laser treatment: prospective study and review of the literature. J Am Acad Dermatol. 2012; 67(3):436–445

[25] Das A, Sarda A, De A. Cooling devices in laser therapy. J Cutan Aesthet Surg. 2016; 9(4):215–219

[26] Kelly KM, Nelson JS, Lask GP, Geronemus RG, Bernstein LJ. Cryogen spray cooling in combination with nonablative laser treatment of facial rhytides. Arch Dermatol. 1999; 135(6):691–694

[27] Butz DR, Gill KK, Randle J, Kampf N, Few JW. Facial aesthetic surgery: the safe use of oral sedation in an office-based facility. Aesthet Surg J. 2016; 36(2):127–131

[28] Haith LR Jr, Santavasi W, Shapiro TK, et al. Burn center management of operating room fire injuries. J Burn Care Res. 2012; 33(5):649–653

[29] Phillips BT, Wang ED, Rodman AJ, et al. Anesthesia duration as a marker for surgical complications in office-based plastic surgery. Ann Plast Surg. 2012; 69(4):408–411

[30] Rosero EB, Joshi GP. Preemptive, preventive, multimodal analgesia: what do they really mean? Plast Reconstr Surg. 2014; 134(4) Suppl 2:85S–93S

3 Anatomy

Kaete A. Archer

Summary

Facial anatomy is highly complex and intricate. A strong knowledge of facial anatomy is the foundation for performing facial plastic surgery. This in-depth knowledge and understanding of facial anatomy is necessary to safely perform facial plastic and reconstructive surgery. Therefore, this chapter thoroughly reviews facial anatomy.

Keywords: epidermis, frontalis, facial nerve, levator aponeurosis, SOOF, zygomatic ligament, upper lateral cartilage, lower lateral cartilage, lateral nasal artery, submusculoaponeurotic system

3.1 Introduction

As facial plastic and reconstructive surgeons, our goal is to provide the highest level of care and safety to our patients. An in-depth knowledge and understanding of facial anatomy is necessary to avoid complications when performing facial plastic surgery procedures. The objective of this chapter is to examine the face by region and discuss the anatomy relevant for safely performing facial plastic surgery procedures.

3.2 Skin Anatomy

3.2.1 Epidermis

Layers

The epidermis is divided into five layers. From superficial to deep, the outermost layer is the stratum corneum which represents the terminal differentiation of keratinocytes into anucleate, flattened keratinocytes.[1] The stratum lucida is an eosinophilic acellular layer beneath the stratum corneum in acral skin (palms and soles).[1] The stratum granulosum contains deeply basophilic keratohyalin granules important for the cornification of the stratum corneum.[1] The stratum spinosum layer contains polygonal cells with abundant eosinophilic cytoplasm named for small, spiny intercellular desmosomal attachments seen under light microscopy.[1] The deepest layer is the stratum basale. This is a single mitotically active layer of cuboidal to columnar-shaped basophilic keratinocytes that attach to the basement membrane by hemidesmosomes and give rise to the more superficial epidermal layers.[1]

Composition

The epidermis contains keratinocytes, melanocytes, Langerhans cells, and Merkel cells.[1] Keratinocytes make up 80% of the epidermal cells and originate in the basal layer.[1] Melanocytes are neural crest derived, pigment-producing, dendritic cells found in the basal layer.[1] They produce melanin to protect the mitotically active basal keratinocytes from UV radiation.[1] Langerhans cells are bone marrow–derived antigen-processing and antigen-presenting cells found mainly in the stratum spinosum layer.[1,2] These cells are characterized by intracytoplasmic tennis racket–shaped structures called Birbeck granules.[1] Merkel cells are mechanoreceptors of neural crest origin involved with touch sensation.[1,2] They are found in the basal layer of palms, soles, oral and genital mucosa, nailbeds, and the follicular infundibulum.[1]

3.2.2 Dermis

Layers

The dermis is composed of two layers: the papillary dermis (superficial) and the reticular dermis (deep). The papillary dermis is thinner than the reticular dermis. The dermis is organized into upward projecting papilla that intercalate with the downward projecting rete ridges of the epidermis.[1]

Composition

Collagen is the primary structural component of the dermis.[1] Collagen is synthesized by dermal fibroblasts and provides tensile strength and elasticity.[1] The majority of dermal collagen is type I (80–90%).[1] Dermal elastic tissue is composed of multiple substances including elastin protein, microfibrillar matrix with fibrillin, and a glycoprotein.[2] Ground substance of the dermis includes proteoglycans, glycosaminoglycans, and filamentous glycoproteins.[1] The cellular components of the dermis include fibroblasts, phagocytic cells (monocytes, macrophages, and dendrocytes), and mast cells.[2]

Vasculature

The skin has two vascular plexuses connected by communicating vessels. The superficial vascular plexus is in the superficial reticular dermis and receives its vascular supply from the deep vascular plexus.[2] It gives rise to the capillary loop system in the papillary dermis.[2] It abuts the epidermis and provides nutrients by diffusion.[2] The deep vascular plexus is at the junction of the dermis and subcutaneous fat and receives its vascular supply from the musculocutaneous arteries perforating from the subcutaneous fat.[2] Arterioles from the deep vascular plexus supply the epidermal appendages and the superficial vascular plexus.[2]

3.3 Forehead Anatomy

3.3.1 Central Forehead and Glabella

Topography

Presenting as early as the 20s, the central forehead can develop dynamic horizontal lines due to underlying frontalis muscle contraction and creasing of the forehead skin (▶ Fig. 3.1). Likewise, the glabella develops vertical lines (corrugator creases) related to repeated creasing of the skin from underlying corrugator contraction (▶ Fig. 3.2) and horizontal lines from underlying procerus contraction. The corrugator crease is a landmark for the vertical course of the supratrochlear artery, which supplies the soft tissue of the central forehead (▶ Fig. 3.3).

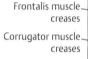
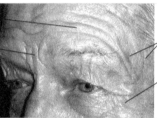

Frontalis muscle creases
Corrugator muscle creases
Oblique temporoparietalis muscle creases
Orbicularis oculi muscle creases

Fig. 3.1 Dynamic horizontal forehead creases. (Source: Chapter 6 The Temporal Fossa. In: Pessa J, Rohrich R, ed. Facial Topography: Clinical Anatomy of the Face. 1st Edition. Thieme; 2012.)

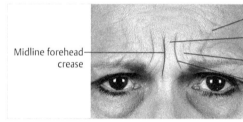

Midline forehead crease
Supraorbital crease
Medial corrugator compartment
Lateral corrugator compartment
Corrugator crease

Fig. 3.2 Dynamic glabella creases. (Source: Chapter 2 The Central Forehead. In: Pessa J, Rohrich R, ed. Facial Topography: Clinical Anatomy of the Face. 1st Edition. Thieme; 2012.)

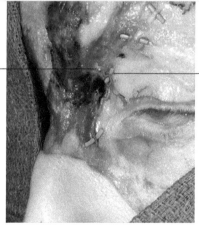

Corrugator crease
Supratrochlear artery

Fig. 3.3 Corrugator crease as landmark for vertical supratrochlear artery. (Source: Chapter 2 The Central Forehead. In: Pessa J, Rohrich R, ed. Facial Topography: Clinical Anatomy of the Face. 1st Edition. Thieme; 2012.)

Soft Tissue

The scalp is composed of five soft tissue layers: skin, subcutaneous tissue, galea, loose areolar tissue, and periosteum.[3] The skin of the forehead is the thickest of the face. The galea aponeurotica of the scalp divides into a superficial and deep layer to envelope the frontalis muscle.[3,4] The deep layer of the galea attaches to the supraorbital margin.[5] Between the deep galea plane and periosteum is a plane of loose areolar tissue.[4] The periosteum and galea fuse approximately 1 cm above the supraorbital rim.[3]

Muscles

Frontalis

The frontalis muscle is the primary brow elevator with a central attenuation.[4] The frontalis originates from the galea aponeurotica of the scalp, penetrates through the overlapping orbicularis muscle, and inserts into the subcutaneous tissue deep to the eyebrows.[6] Medially, it becomes confluent with the vertical procerus muscle.[3] The lateral frontalis margin stops or markedly attenuates over the temporal line. The frontalis muscle is firmly fixed to the overlying dermis by transverse-oriented fibrous septae.[6] These are thought to play a role in the transverse forehead furrows that occur across the forehead.[6]

Corrugator Supercilii

In the medial canthal area, the bulky corrugator supercilii is located deep to the frontalis.[7] It originates from the nasal process of the frontal bone and extends obliquely over the supraorbital rim where it interdigitates with fibers from the frontalis and orbicularis muscle and inserts into the dermis of the forehead skin behind and just superior to the middle one-third of the eyebrow.[4] Medially the corrugator is congruent with the procerus.[7] Its action is to pull the eyebrow in an inferomedial direction.

In cadaver dissections by Pessa, the corrugator muscle was identified with two muscular bellies, a transverse and an oblique (▶ Fig. 3.4).[8] The thickest portion of the muscle is at the medial canthus. Substantial bulk was still present at the midpupillary line, but no distinct corrugator fibers were detectable at the lateral canthus.[7]

Depressor Supercilii

The small, vertically oriented depressor supercilii muscle originates on the medial orbital rim, near the lacrimal sac, and inserts on the medial aspect of the bony orbit, inferior to the corrugators (▶ Fig. 3.5). It acts as an accessory depressor of the medial eyebrow.[6] Of note, not all reports have identified this muscle.

Procerus

The procerus is a small, thin pyramidal muscle arising from the fascia of the inferior portion of the nasal bone and the upper lateral nasal cartilage.[6] It inserts into the glabellar skin, between the paired

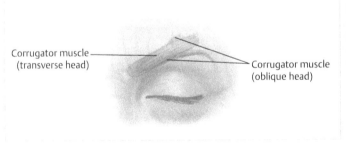

Corrugator muscle (transverse head)

Corrugator muscle (oblique head)

Fig. 3.4 Transverse and oblique bellies of corrugator muscle. (Source: Chapter 2 The Central Forehead. In: Pessa J, Rohrich R, ed. Facial Topography: Clinical Anatomy of the Face. 1st Edition. Thieme; 2012.)

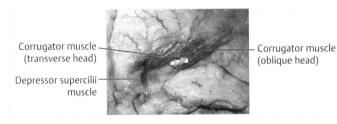

Corrugator muscle (transverse head)

Depressor supercilii muscle

Corrugator muscle (oblique head)

Fig. 3.5 Vertically oriented depressor supercilii muscle. (Source: Chapter 2 The Central Forehead. In: Pessa J, Rohrich R, ed. Facial Topography: Clinical Anatomy of the Face. 1st Edition. Thieme; 2012.)

bellies of the frontalis.[6] The procerus draws the medial angle of the eyebrow downward. The procerus is inferior to the corrugator supercilii.[6]

Innervation

The ophthalmic division of the trigeminal nerve (V1) gives off the supratrochlear and supraorbital branches and provides sensation to the forehead and scalp. The supraorbital nerve supplies sensation to the upper eyelid and forehead skin except for a midline vertical strip which is supplied by the supratrochlear nerve. The supraorbital nerve has two divisions: (1) a superficial (medial) division that passes within and over the frontalis, providing sensory supply to the forehead skin and the anterior margin of the hair baring scalp and (2) a deep (lateral) division that runs between 0.5 cm and 1.5 cm medial to the superior temporal line between the galea aponeurotica and the periosteum as a sensory nerve to the frontoparietal scalp.[3,9] The supraorbital nerve leaves the orbit via a notch in the supraorbital rim in approximately two-thirds of patients and through a foramen in one-third of patients (▶ Fig. 3.6).[3] The supratrochlear nerve exits the orbit by passing through the corrugator supercilii muscle.[3]

Vasculature

The internal carotid artery gives off the ophthalmic artery which gives off the supraorbital and supratrochlear arteries. The supraorbital and supratrochlear arteries, which travel with similarly named sensory nerves in a neurovascular bundle, are found deep to the corrugator muscle and frontalis muscle, until approximately 1 cm above the supraorbital rim where they pierce the frontalis to emerge superficially in the subcutaneous plane and supply the skin of the central forehead (▶ Fig. 3.7).[8] The central forehead artery is superficial in the glabella area and is likely responsible for vascular complications from superficial filler in the glabella (▶ Fig. 3.8).[8]

3.3.2 Temporal Fossa

Soft Tissue

The temporal fossa contains a complex layering of soft tissues. From superficial to deep, the outermost layers are the skin and subcutaneous tissue. Next is the temporoparietal fascia (superficial temporal fascia). This fascia consists of three distinct layers.[4] The temporoparietal fascia is continuous with the superficial musculoaponeurotic system (SMAS) in

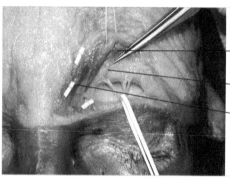

Oblique corrugator muscle

Supraorbital nerve

Transverse corrugator muscle

Fig. 3.6 Supraorbital nerve exiting the orbit. (Chapter 2 The Central Forehead. In: Pessa J, Rohrich R, ed. Facial Topography: Clinical Anatomy of the Face. 1st Edition. Thieme; 2012.)

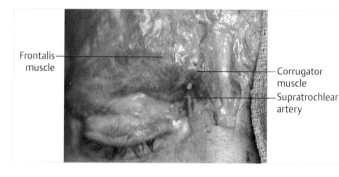

Frontalis muscle

Corrugator muscle

Supratrochlear artery

Fig. 3.7 Supratrochlear artery runs deep to the corrugator and frontalis muscles. (Source: Chapter 2 The Central Forehead. In: Pessa J, Rohrich R, ed. Facial Topography: Clinical Anatomy of the Face. 1st Edition. Thieme; 2012.)

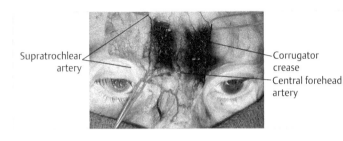

Supratrochlear artery

Corrugator crease

Central forehead artery

Fig. 3.8 Superficial central forehead artery. (Source: Chapter 2 The Central Forehead. In: Pessa J, Rohrich R, ed. Facial Topography: Clinical Anatomy of the Face. 1st Edition. Thieme; 2012.)

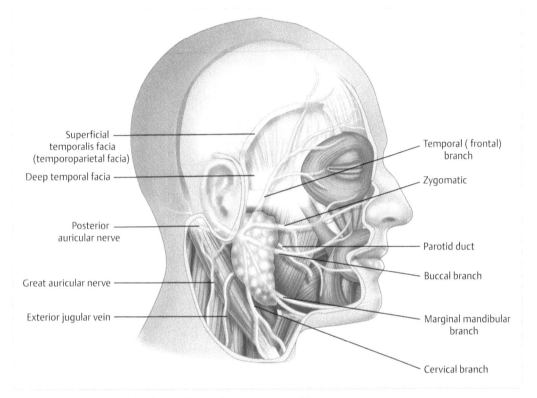

Superficial temporalis facia (temporoparietal facia)

Deep temporal facia

Posterior auricular nerve

Great auricular nerve

Exterior jugular vein

Temporal (frontal) branch

Zygomatic

Parotid duct

Buccal branch

Marginal mandibular branch

Cervical branch

Fig. 3.9 Frontal branch of facial nerve deep to the temporoparietal fascia.

the midface and merges in the central forehead with the galea.[10] The frontal branch of the facial nerve lies deep to the temporoparietal fascia (▶ Fig. 3.9). Next, the temporalis fascia is a dense layer of shiny white fascia that splits around the temporalis muscle, creating a superficial and deep layer.[4] The temporal line is the convergence of the deep and superficial layers of the temporalis fascia with the frontal periosteum. The temporal line meets the lateral margin of the galea to form the conjoint tendon.[10]

Muscle

The temporalis muscle sits in the temporalis fossa. It originates from the temporal fossa and inserts onto the coronoid process of the mandible, medial to the zygomatic arch. The temporalis is a muscle of mastication.

Fat Pads

The temporal fat pad is divided into a superficial and deep fat pad.[11] The superficial fat pad is immediately superior to the zygomatic arch between the superficial and deep layers of the temporalis fascia (▶ Fig. 3.10).[11] The deep fat pad is deep to the deep layer of the temporalis fascia and superficial to the temporalis muscle.[11] This fat pad is posterior to the zygomatic arch and is continuous with the buccal fat pad.[11]

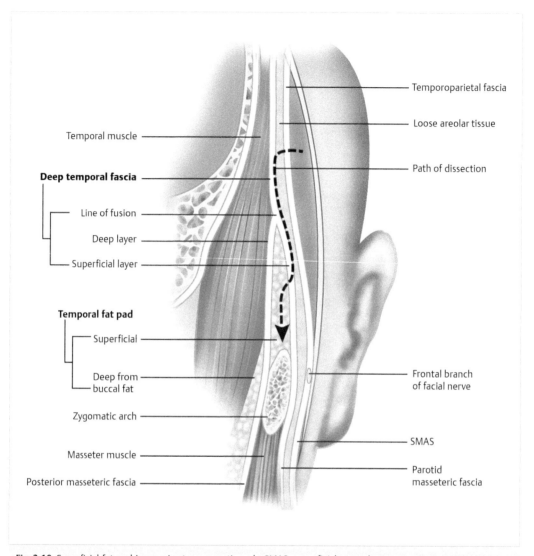

Fig. 3.10 Superficial fat pad is superior to zygomatic arch. SMAS, superficial musculoaponeurotic system.

Innervation

The maxillary division of the trigeminal nerve (V2) provides temporal sensation by the auriculotemporal and zygomaticotemporal branches.[10] Cranial nerve V innervates the temporalis muscle.

Vasculature

The superficial temporal artery and vein are found within the temporoparietal fascia. The sentinel vein is the key venous anatomy in browlifting. The sentinel vein runs superficial to the temporalis fascia near the region of the frontozygomatic suture.[10] The location of this vein is a marker for the frontal branch of the facial nerve which runs superficial to the sentinel vein.[10] Identification of this vein, particularly in endoscopic approaches indicates the inferior extent of dissection.

3.4 Periorbital Anatomy

3.4.1 Upper and Lower Eyelids

Topography

The palpebral opening in adults is 10–12 mm vertically and 28–30 mm horizontally.[6] The palpebral opening has a slight superior cant, with the lateral canthus about 2 mm superior to the medial canthus.[6] In adults, the upper eyelid covers 1–2 mm of the superior cornea and the apex of the upper lid margin is nasal to a vertical line drawn through the center of the pupil.[6] In Caucasians, the crease is 7–8 mm above the lid margin in men and 10–12 mm in women.[6] The lower eyelid margin sits at the inferior limbus of the cornea with a slight crease that is 2 mm below the lash line medially and 5 mm laterally.[6]

Soft Tissue

The upper and lower eyelids are divided into an anterior, middle, and posterior lamella. The anterior lamella is the eyelid skin and underlying orbicularis muscle. The middle lamella is the orbital septum. The orbital septum is an extension of the arcus marginalis, a band of thickened periosteum at the orbital rim. The posterior lamella includes the tarsal plate, eyelid retractors, and conjunctiva. The tarsal plate is a dense connective tissue structure along the margin of the upper and lower eyelid. The tarsal plate attaches to the periosteum of the orbital rim by the medial and lateral canthal tendons. Medially, the canthal tendon has a deep attachment to the posterior lacrimal crest and a superficial attachment to the anterior lacrimal crest.[6] Laterally, the canthal tendon has a deep attachment 3 mm posterior to the orbital rim at Whitnall tubercle.[6]

Muscles

The orbicularis oculi is a circular muscle that surrounds the eye. It is divided into an orbital, preseptal, and pretarsal section based on the anatomy beneath these sections. It functions to blink, squint, and forcefully close the eyelid, and its orbital component is a depressor of the forehead.[6] The orbital section arises from the medial canthal tendon, arches along the orbital rim, and meets laterally at the zygoma.[6] The orbital fibers of the orbicularis muscle interdigitate superiorly with the frontalis muscle fibers, pulling the skin of the forehead and eyelid downward, while elevating the cheek toward the eye, resulting in dynamic "crow's feet."[6] The preseptal fibers overlie the orbital septum. The pretarsal fibers are firmly adhered to the tarsus and travel in an elliptical path around the palpebral fissure.

Upper Eyelid Retractors

The upper eyelid retractors are responsible for elevation of the upper eyelid. The main retractor is the levator palpebrae superioris muscle. The levator arises from the orbital apex. The muscular portion is 40 mm in length with a terminal tendinous sheath that extends for 14–20 mm, called the levator aponeurosis.[12] The muscle transitions to the tendon at Whitnall ligament. The central portion of the levator aponeurosis joins the orbital septum and together they insert into the overlying eyelid skin and orbicularis forming the eyelid crease (▶ Fig. 3.11). The levator continues inferiorly and inserts onto the superior tarsal surface. The levator palpebrae superioris is innervated by CN III.[6]

Müller muscle is an accessory upper eyelid retractor. It is a smooth muscle that is posterior to the levator and firmly attached to the conjunctiva deep to it near the superior margin of the tarsus.[6] Unlike the levator palpebrae superioris, Müller muscle is sympathetically innervated.[6] It contributes about 2 mm to upper eyelid retraction.[6]

Lower Eyelid Retractors

The lower eyelid retractors are the capsulopalpebral fascia and the inferior tarsal muscle. They correspond to the levator aponeurosis and Müller muscle in the upper eyelid, respectively. The capsulopalpebral head originates from the fascia of the inferior rectus muscle and then envelopes the inferior oblique muscle to become the capsulopalpebral fascia, inserting on the inferior tarsal border with the orbital septum (▶ Fig. 3.12).[6] The inferior tarsal muscle has sympathetic innervation and is located posterior to the capsulopalpebral fascia.[6]

Fat Pads

Upper Eyelid

Two orbital fat pads are found posterior to the septum: the medial (nasal) fat pad and the central (preaponeurotic) fat pad (▶ Fig. 3.13). The medial fat pad is whiter than the yellow central fat pad. The central fat pad is just anterior to the levator aponeurosis. The lacrimal gland is found posterior to the septum in the lateral space. The central fat pad is encased in a thin membrane which harbors small blood vessels and is innervated by terminal branches of the supraorbital nerve.[13] The trochlea of the superior oblique muscle separates the medial and central fat pads (▶ Fig. 3.13).

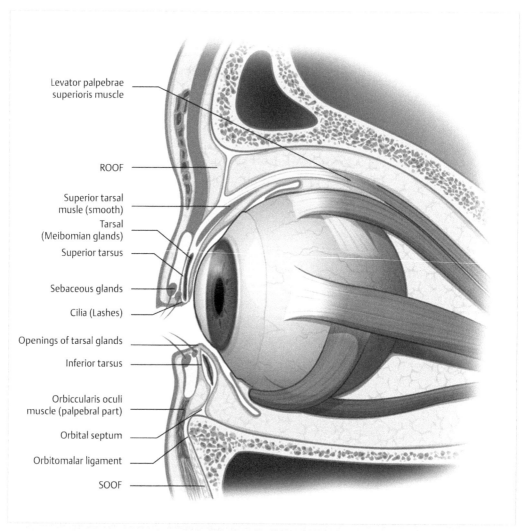

Levator palpebrae
superioris muscle

ROOF

Superior tarsal
musle (smooth)

Tarsal
(Meibomian glands)

Superior tarsus

Sebaceous glands

Cilia (Lashes)

Openings of tarsal glands

Inferior tarsus

Orbiccularis oculi
muscle (palpebral part)

Orbital septum

Orbitomalar ligament

SOOF

Fig. 3.11 Levator aponeurosis joins the orbital septum and then inserts into the overlying eyelid skin forming the eyelid crease. ROOF, retroorbicularis oculi fat pad; SOOF, suborbicularis oculi fat.

Lower Eyelid

There are three postseptal fat pads in the lower eyelid complex: medial, central, and lateral. The inferior oblique muscle divides the medial and central fat pads while its arcuate expansion divides the central and lateral fat pads (▶ Fig. 3.13).[14]

Innervation

Upper Eyelid

The upper eyelid is innervated by the supraorbital nerve and supratrochlear nerve (V1). The infratrochlear nerve, a terminal branch of the nasociliary nerve (V1) supplies the skin of the medial canthus.

Lower Eyelid

The lower eyelid is innervated by the palpebral branches of the infraorbital nerve (V2) and the zygomaticofacial nerve (V2).

Vasculature

Upper Eyelid

The upper eyelid is supplied by the marginal and peripheral arteries from the ophthalmic artery

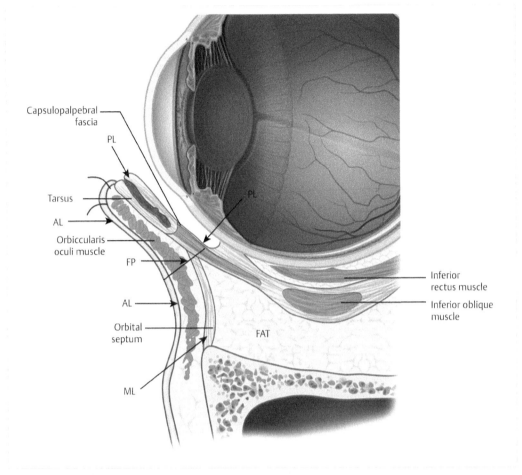

Capsulopalpebral fascia
PL
Tarsus
AL
Orbiccularis oculi muscle
FP
AL
Orbital septum
ML
PL
FAT
Inferior rectus muscle
Inferior oblique muscle

Fig. 3.12 Capsulopalpebral fascia joins the orbital septum and inserts onto the inferior tarsal border. AL, anterior lamella; FP, fusion point; ML, middle lamella; PL, posterior lamella.

(▶ Fig. 3.14).[6] Terminal branches of the facial artery supply the medial eyelid.

Lower Eyelid

The angular artery, the transverse facial artery, and the infraorbital artery supply the lower eyelid (▶ Fig. 3.14). Care must be taken when fat grafting or fillers are used in the periorbital area. Fat embolism into the arterial system can lead to blindness.

3.4.2 Eyebrows

Topography

In men, the ideal brow position is relatively horizontal at the level of the supraorbital rim. In women, the ideal brow position sits superior to the supraorbital rim with the arch at the lateral limbus. In a youthful eyebrow, the brow projects off of the supraorbital rim with volume and highlight over the brow bone inferior to the lateral brow.

Descent of eyebrows with aging does not occur uniformly. The lateral eyebrow segment descends earlier than the medial eyebrow. The soft tissue over the temporalis fascia lateral to the temporal fusion line is unsupported and subject to gravitational descent of the lateral brows. Pseudoexcess upper eyelid skin develops over the lateral upper eyelid as the eyebrow skin is displaced onto the orbital space.[4]

Soft Tissue

The orbicularis-retaining ligament is a fusion zone between the orbicularis fascia and the periosteum that is circumferential around the orbit

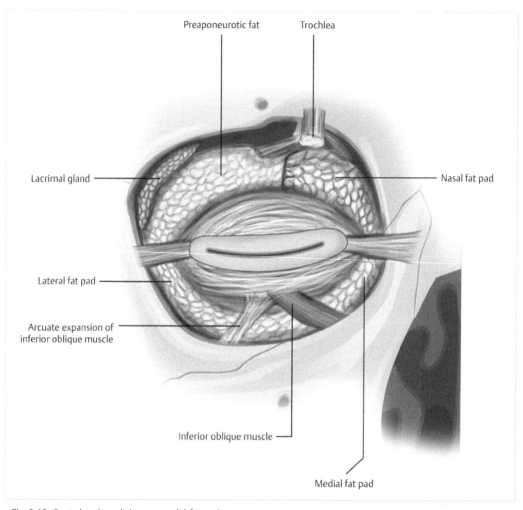

Fig. 3.13 Central and medial upper eyelid fat pads.

(▶ Fig. 3.15a, b).[15] The ligament is short medially and laterally where the orbicularis muscle is almost fused with the bone.[15]

Fat Pads

Deep to the interdigitation of the orbicularis and frontalis muscles is a fibrofatty layer, known as the eyebrow fat pad or retroorbicularis oculi fat pad (ROOF) between the orbital septum and orbicularis (▶ Fig. 3.11). The ROOF gives the eyebrow lateral support and projection from the superior orbital rim. The ROOF can be a significant factor in lateral lid hooding and puffiness. The ROOF is continuous with the posterior orbicularis fascia in the eyelid.[14]

3.5 Midface

3.5.1 Lid/Cheek Junction

Topography

Aging of the midface includes descent and deflation of soft tissues leading to demarcation of the orbitomalar sulcus at the lid/cheek junction. The orbitomalar sulcus has three parts: palpebromalar groove laterally, the nasojugal groove medially (tear trough deformity), and the midcheek or "v" groove inferiorly.[16]

Soft Tissue

There are conflicting reports on the cause of the tear trough deformity. Some reports say that it

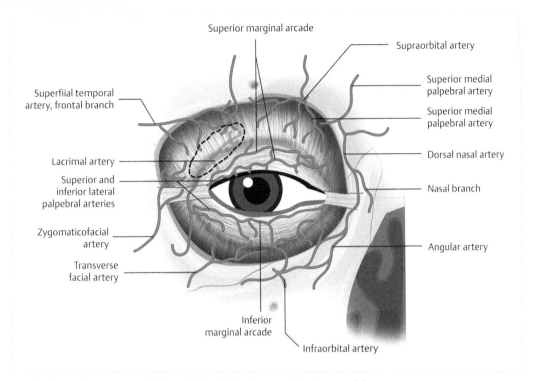

Superior marginal arcade

Supraorbital artery

Superior medial palpebral artery

Superior medial palpebral artery

Dorsal nasal artery

Nasal branch

Angular artery

Superfiial temporal artery, frontal branch

Lacrimal artery

Superior and inferior lateral palpebral arteries

Zygomaticofacial artery

Transverse facial artery

Inferior marginal arcade

Infraorbital artery

Fig. 3.14 Angular, transverse facial, and infraorbital artery supply the lower eyelid.

represents the cutaneous insertion of the orbicularis-retaining ligament. This is an osteocutaneous ligament that originates from the orbital rim periosteum, traverses the orbicularis oculi muscle, and inserts into the skin of the lid/cheek junction.[17] In the lateral canthal region, the orbicularis-retaining ligament merges with the lateral orbital thickening, which is a condensation of superficial and deep fascia that crosses the frontal process of the zygoma onto the deep temporal fascia.[18] The orbicularis-retaining ligament is thicker and less distensible in its lateral part.[18] Loosening of the orbital septum superior to the ligament and elongation of the preseptal segment of the orbicularis muscle and its fascia inferior to the ligament with the downward displacement of the lid/cheek junction leads to the typical "V" sign of lid/cheek junction aging.[18]

Muscles

An anatomic study by Haddock et al noted that there is a cleft between the palpebral and orbital portions of the orbicularis muscle precisely at the tear trough deformity.[19] They also noted that along the tear trough, there was no dissectible anatomical

plane deep to the orbicularis. In this location, it is rigidly attached to the maxilla where it takes origin. Laterally, however, along the lid/cheek junction, the attachment between the orbicularis muscle and the underlying bone was the orbicularis-retaining ligament. In this region, there was a dissectible plane deep to the orbicularis muscle. The distinction between the bony attachments of these muscular portion correlates with the palpebromalar and nasojugal grooves.[19]

Fat Pads

At the superior border of the malar region, on the deep surface of the orbicularis muscle, is the suborbicularis oculi fat (SOOF). The SOOF contributes to the shape and contour of the upper cheek and cheekbone. A thick lateral SOOF will show as prominent cheek bones. When there is little or thin SOOF, the surface of the zygoma becomes apparent.[20] The SOOF has two distinct areas, the lateral and medial SOOF (▶ Fig. 3.16a,b).[21] The lateral SOOF lies several millimeters below the rim, immediately on the orbital rim periosteum.[20] Inferior descent of the SOOF as well as the SMAS contributes to unmasking of the inferior orbital rim.

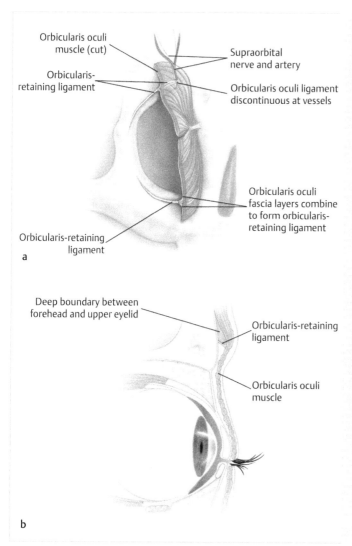

Orbicularis oculi
muscle (cut)

Orbicularis-
retaining ligament

Supraorbital
nerve and artery

Orbicularis oculi ligament
discontinuous at vessels

Orbicularis oculi
fascia layers combine
to form orbicularis-
retaining ligament

Orbicularis-retaining
ligament

a

Deep boundary between
forehead and upper eyelid

Orbicularis-retaining
ligament

Orbicularis oculi
muscle

b

Fig. 3.15 (a, b) Orbicularis-retaining ligaments. (Source: Chapter 2 The Central Forehead. In: Pessa J, Rohrich R, ed. Facial Topography: Clinical Anatomy of the Face. 1st Edition. Thieme; 2012.)

3.5.2 Cheek

Topography

The midface is characterized by distinct fat pads that behave independently. The deep medial fat pad, buccal fat pad, and SOOF fat pads can be seen on surface anatomy (▶ Fig. 3.17a,b).

Soft Tissue

The SMAS is a continuation of the platysma inferiorly and the temporoparietal fascia superiorly. The SMAS is firmly attached to the skin by retinacular cutis fibers within the subcutaneous tissue. The SMAS has only limited attachments to the underlying bony skeleton, contributing to its descent in midfacial/lower facial aging.[19]

Muscles

The zygomaticus muscles draw the mouth superolaterally when smiling. The zygomatic nerve courses deep to the plane of the zygomaticus major muscle.[6] The zygomaticus major is just medial to the buccal fat pad.

Fat Pads

The contour of the cheek is affected by superficial and deep fat pads. Deep medial cheek fat exists in the central cheek, extending from the lower eyelid

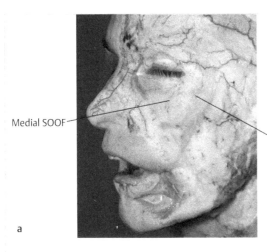

Fig. 3.16 (a) Lateral and medial suborbicularis oculi fat (SOOF) fat pads. (b) Lateral and medial SOOF fat pads underlying the orbicularis muscle. (Source: Chapter 3 The Cheek. In: Pessa J, Rohrich R, ed. Facial Topography: Clinical Anatomy of the Face. 1st Edition. Thieme; 2012.)

Medial SOOF

Lateral SOOF augments prominence of cheekbone

a

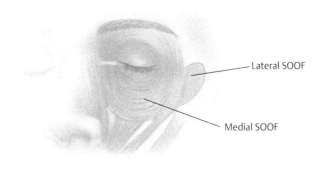

Lateral SOOF

Medial SOOF

b

to the cheek-lip crease (▶ Fig. 3.18). The deep medial fat pad contributes to the anterior projection of the cheek.[20]

Buccal fat lies immediately lateral to the deep medial cheek fat and has its own capsule. The territory of the buccal fat extends from the edge of the upper mandible into the temporal region (▶ Fig. 3.19).[20] The buccal fat can lie over the masseter muscle and can exist as multiple lobes. Each lobe is contained within a separate capsule. The inferior lobe is safe to manipulate because the parotid duct travels above this lobe between the middle and inferior lobe.[20] The inferior lobe also predicts the location of the facial artery, which always crosses the mandible below the inferior lobe. The inferior lobe contributes the most to lower cheek contour.[20]

When the nasojugal groove continues downward, it is called the midcheek furrow.[22] Between the midcheek furrow and the lateral palpebromalar groove is the malar bag or malar mound.[22] The infraorbital fat pad is a superficial fat pad also called the malar mound (▶ Fig. 3.20).[20] The shape of the malar mound, triangular with the apex medially, mirrors the underlying prezygomatic space.[22] The superior boundary is the orbicularis-retaining ligament and the lower boundary is the zygomatic ligament.[22] Laxity of tissue tone within the roof of the zygomatic space seems to explain the presence and degree of malar mounds.[22] The boundary between the eyelid and cheek is the superior boundary for the malar mound.[20] Above the orbit-cheek crease, the orbicularis oculi has little fat and is superficial.[20] Below the orbit-cheek crease, the orbicularis oculi dives below the malar mound.[20] The lateral SOOF is deep to the malar mound.[20] Manipulation of the infraorbital fat pad can lead to prolonged edema.[20]

Innervation

Sensory innervation to the skin overlying the malar region is from the maxillary branch (V2) of the trigeminal nerve. This nerve innervates the lower eyelid, cheek, side of the nose, nasal vestibule, and the skin/mucosa of the upper lip. The infraorbital

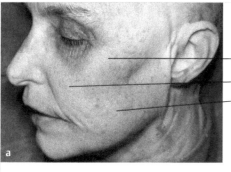

Suborbicularis oculi fat

Deep medial cheek fat

Buccal fat

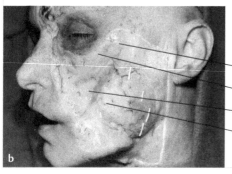

Suborbicularis oculi fat

Orbicularis oculi fat
(preorbital)

Deep medial cheek fat

Buccal fat

Fig. 3.17 (a) Surface anatomy showing deep medial fat pad, buccal fat pad, and suborbicularis oculi fat (SOOF) fat pad. (b) Underlying anatomy of the deep medial fat pad, buccal fat pad, and SOOF fat pad. (Source: Chapter 3 The Cheek. In: Pessa J, Rohrich R, ed. Facial Topography: Clinical Anatomy of the Face. 1st Edition. Thieme; 2012.)

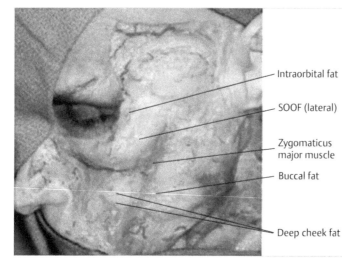

Intraorbital fat

SOOF (lateral)

Zygomaticus
major muscle

Buccal fat

Deep cheek fat

Fig. 3.18 Deep medial cheek fat. (Source: Chapter 3 The Cheek. In: Pessa J, Rohrich R, ed. Facial Topography: Clinical Anatomy of the Face. 1st Edition. Thieme; 2012.)

nerve supplies sensation to the skin and conjunctiva of the lower eyelid, the lateral aspect of the nose, the anterior cheek, and the upper lip.[23] The anterior superior alveolar nerve descends from the infraorbital nerve into or along the maxillary bone, supplying sensation to the anterior maxillary dentition and gingiva.[23] Damage to the anterior superior alveolar nerve from trauma or surgery can result in numbness to the ipsilateral anterior maxillary gingiva.[23]

Vasculature

The infraorbital neurovascular bundle travels through the infraorbital foramen in the midpupillary line on the anterior maxilla and runs through the medial SOOF or the deep medial fat. The zygomaticofacial artery and nerve travel through the lateral SOOF over the lateral zygoma (▶ Fig. 3.21).[20]

The lateral facelift flap is supplied by large fasciocutaneous perforating vessels from named

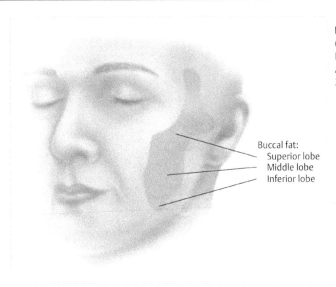

Fig. 3.19 Multiple lobes of buccal fat pad. (Source: Chapter 3 The Cheek. In: Pessa J, Rohrich R, ed. Facial Topography: Clinical Anatomy of the Face. 1st Edition. Thieme; 2012.)

Buccal fat:
Superior lobe
Middle lobe
Inferior lobe

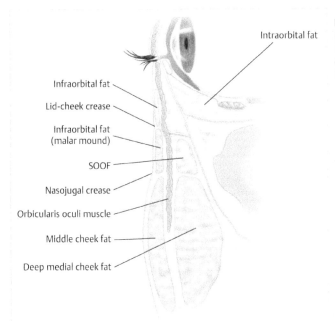

Intraorbital fat

Infraorbital fat

Lid-cheek crease

Infraorbital fat
(malar mound)

SOOF

Nasojugal crease

Orbicularis oculi muscle

Middle cheek fat

Deep medial cheek fat

Fig. 3.20 Infraorbital fat is a superficial fat pad (SOOF). (Source: Chapter 3 The Cheek. In: Pessa J, Rohrich R, ed. Facial Topography: Clinical Anatomy of the Face. 1st Edition. Thieme; 2012.)

vessels. The most significant contribution is from the transverse facial artery. Other major contributions come from the submental, facial, and superficial temporal arteries.[24]

Retaining Ligaments

Retaining ligaments of the face are strong, fibrous attachments that originate from the periosteum (osteocutaneous) or deep fascia (fasciocutaneous) and travel perpendicularly through facial layers to insert on the dermis.[17] Furnas was the first to describe the concept of a retaining ligament when he described the retaining ligaments of the cheek.[17,25]

Zygomatic Ligaments

The zygomatic ligaments are strong fibers that originate at the inferior border of the zygomatic arch and extend anteriorly to the junction of the arch and

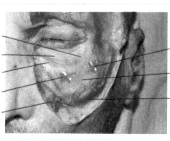

Lateral SOOF
Intraorbital fat
Medial SOOF
Infraorbital artery and nerve
Levator labii superioris muscle

Zygomaticofacial artery and nerve
SOOF (lateral)
Preorbital orbicularis oculi muscle

Fig. 3.21 Zygomaticofacial artery and nerve travel through the suborbicularis oculi fat (SOOF). (Source: Chapter 3 The Cheek. In: Pessa J, Rohrich R, ed. Facial Topography: Clinical Anatomy of the Face. 1st Edition. Thieme; 2012.)

body of the zygoma to attach to the dermis.[17] Mendelson et al also described zygomatic ligaments medial to the junction of the arch and body along the origins of the zygomaticus major/minor and levator labii superioris.[16] These ligaments are weaker and can often be disrupted by blunt finger dissection.

The zygomatic-retaining ligaments are landmarks for the zygomatic facial nerve branches.[17] Furnas was the first to show that a zygomatic branch passes in a deep plane just inferior to the zygomatic ligaments.[17,25] An anatomic study concluded that 1 cm inferior to the main zygomatic ligament is relatively safe except in 5 to 9% of cases in which the upper zygomatic nerve gives off a more superficial branch that travels superficial to the zygomaticus muscle.[26,27]

Masseteric Ligaments

The masseteric cutaneous ligaments arise from the masseteric fascia over the masseter muscle. The masseteric ligaments are landmarks for the buccal facial nerve branches.[17] The lower masseteric-retaining ligaments along the caudal border of the masseter form a fibrous attachment between the platysma and the skin.[28]

Mandibular Ligament

The mandibular ligament is an osteocutaneous ligament that arises from the anterior third of the mandible and inserts directly into the dermis.[17] Its fibers penetrate the inferior portion of the depressor anguli oris muscle. Langevin reported the mandibular ligament was 4.5 cm anterior to the angle of the mandible and found that the mandibular nerve runs just posterior to the mandibular ligament (▶ Fig. 3.22).[29]

3.6 Nasal Anatomy

3.6.1 Skin–Soft Tissue Envelope

Topography

The nose has nine surface aesthetic subunits based on light reflections and shadows: dorsum, paired

sidewalls, columella, paired ala, paired soft tissue triangles, and tip (▶ Fig. 3.23). Incisions are optimally camouflaged when oriented along aesthetic subunit boundaries.

Soft Tissue

Cadaver dissections performed by Toriumi et al revealed well-defined layers of tissue, including epidermis, dermis, subcutaneous fat, muscle and fascia (musculoaponeurotic layer), areolar tissue, and cartilage or bone.[30] The skin varies in thickness at the dorsum; it is thinner cephalically and thicker toward the tip.[31]

3.6.2 Deep

Osseocartilaginous Structures

Bony Vault

The bony vault or pyramid of the nose includes paired nasal bones, the osseous septum, and the ascending process of the maxilla. The nasal bones attach superiorly to the frontal bone and laterally to the nasal process of the maxilla.

Cartilaginous Vault

The cartilaginous vault or middle vault includes the upper lateral cartilages and the cartilaginous septum. Embryologically, the nasal bones are laid down over the upper lateral cartilages; thus, the nasal bones overlap the upper lateral cartilages.[32] The junction of the nasal bones with the perpendicular plate of the ethmoid bone and the upper lateral cartilages is the keystone area.[31] The upper lateral cartilages are fused with the cartilaginous septum to form a single cartilaginous vault.[32]

Nasal Tip

The nasal tip consists of the tip lobule, alar sidewalls, infratip lobule, and the columella. The structural component is the lower lateral cartilages. The

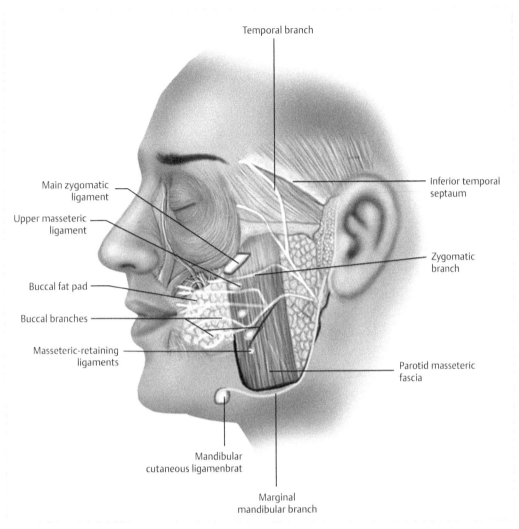

Temporal branch

Inferior temporal
septaum

Main zygomatic
ligament

Upper masseteric
ligament

Zygomatic
branch

Buccal fat pad

Buccal branches

Masseteric-retaining
ligaments

Parotid masseteric
fascia

Mandibular
cutaneous ligamenbrat

Marginal
mandibular branch

Fig. 3.22 Facial ligaments and nerve relationships.

lower lateral cartilages are comprised of a lateral crus, intermediate crus, and medial crus and are thought of structurally as a tripod. Most often, the lateral crus of the lower lateral cartilages overlaps the upper lateral cartilages in a "scroll" configuration.[32] The paired medial crura have a dense ligamentous adherence to one another as well as a tight skin envelope that lacks subcutaneous fat along the medial nostril walls. The medial crura footplates flare to accommodate the septum and overlap it for several millimeters. Marked muscular attachments are found on the medial crural footplates from the depressor septi nasalis.[32]

Septum

Posteriorly, the bony nasal septum is formed by the perpendicular plate of the ethmoid bone and the vomer.[33] Anteriorly, the quadrangular cartilage forms the cartilaginous septum.[33] Superiorly the cartilaginous septum is continuous with the upper lateral cartilages.[33]

Muscles

Tardy and Brown portrayed the muscles of the nose as encased and interconnected by the superficial musculoaponeurotic layer.[34] Nasal muscles are divided into dilators and compressors. Nasal

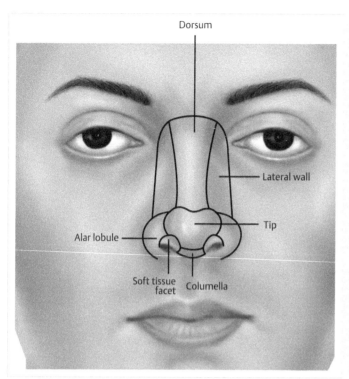

Dorsum

Lateral wall

Tip

Alar lobule

Soft tissue facet

Columella

Fig. 3.23 Subunits of nose.

dilators are the nasalis posterior and the nasalis anterior muscles.[33] Nasal compressors are the procerus, quadratus (levator labii and nasi superioris alaeque), nasalis (pars transversalis and pars alaris), and the depressor septi muscles.[33]

Innervation

The external nose is innervated by the ophthalmic (V1) and maxillary (V2) divisions of the trigeminal nerve. The dorsal nose is innervated by the infratrochlear nerve (V1) and the external branch of the anterior ethmoidal nerve (V1) (nasal skin from rhinion to tip). The nasal sidewall and inferior aspects of the nose are innervated by the infraorbital nerve (V2).[35]

Vasculature

There is significant variation in the vascular anatomy of the nose. Cadaver dissections performed by Toriumi et al identified a subcutaneous venous system above the muscular layer along the lateral wall, dorsum, and supratip regions of the nose.[30] Venous anatomy is variable but most vessels drain into the facial vein inferiorly and/or the angular vein as it courses toward the medial orbit.[30]

Toriumi et al. also found that, in most specimens, each side of the nose had an independent blood supply that could vary from one side to the other.[30] The arterial system is superficial to the musculoaponeurotic layer in the subcutaneous plane.[30] The dorsal nasal artery enters the nasal area from the medial orbit and courses over the dorsal surface of the nasal bones toward the nasal tip and contributes to the arterial arcade of the nasal tip.[30] Most noses have bilateral dorsal nasal arteries.[30]

The lateral nasal artery branches off the facial or angular artery (distal branch of the facial artery) and passes medially along the cephalic margin of the lateral crura (above the alar groove), giving off branches that course in a caudal direction over the lateral crura toward the nostril rim.[30] It moves medially to pass over the domes and down the columella (columellar artery) to the base of the nose (▶ Fig. 3.24).[30]

At the base of the nose, the columellar artery branches off the facial artery or the superior labial artery.[30] In most cases, the lateral nasal artery and the columellar artery meet over the domal region to form an alar arcade that runs along the cephalic margin of the lateral crura.[30]

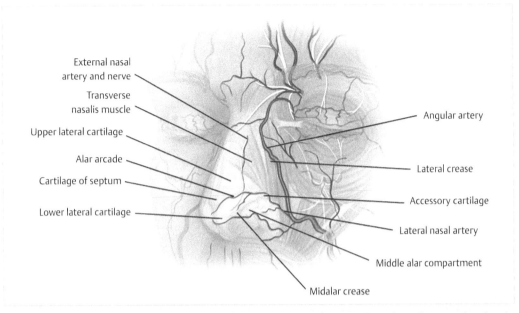

External nasal artery and nerve

Transverse nasalis muscle

Upper lateral cartilage

Alar arcade

Cartilage of septum

Lower lateral cartilage

Angular artery

Lateral crease

Accessory cartilage

Lateral nasal artery

Middle alar compartment

Midalar crease

Fig. 3.24 Vascular supply to the nose. (Source: Chapter 5 The Nose. In: Pessa J, Rohrich R, ed. Facial Topography: Clinical Anatomy of the Face. 1st Edition. Thieme; 2012.)

3.7 Facial Nerve Branches

The facial nerve has five terminal branches: frontal/temporal, zygomatic, buccal, mandibular, and cervical. In the midface, branches are deep to the SMAS and become superficial medial to the masseter muscle.

3.7.1 Frontal Branch

The frontal branch of the facial nerve exits the parotid gland deep to the SMAS and crosses the zygomatic arch as a plexus of three branches at the midpoint between the tragus and the lateral canthus.[3,36,37] The frontal branch is located just superficial to the zygomatic arch periosteum in the subdermal fat in the middle third, approximately 1.5 cm lateral to the orbital rim.[10] From here it travels just deep to the temporoparietal fascia to enter the undersurface of the frontalis muscle approximately 1 cm above the supraorbital rim.[10] The most inferior branch continues medially to innervate the transverse belly of the corrugator muscle and the depressor supercilii muscle.[3] The frontal branch innervates the superior fibers of the orbicularis oculi (upper eyelid).

3.7.2 Zygomatic Branch

The zygomatic branch of the facial nerve innervates the oblique head of the corrugator supercilii and the depressor supercilii muscle and the inferior fibers (lower eyelid) of the orbicularis oculi muscle.[3] The area at greatest risk for injury to the zygomatic branches is the region just inferior and lateral to the zygoma.[11] In this area, the zygomatic branches lie superficially and are adjacent to the high density of zygomatic and upper masseteric-retaining ligaments.[11]

3.7.3 Buccal Branch

Because of significant arborization, injuries to the buccal branch are typically temporary and less clinically significant than other branches. The buccal branches have many different branching patterns but have consistent decussations and interconnections contributing to spontaneous recovery.[11] The procerus is innervated by the buccal branch of the facial nerve.[6]

3.7.4 Marginal Branch

Similar to the frontal branch, the marginal mandibular branch lacks decussations with other facial nerve branches and has few rami.[11] Tzafetta and

Terzis found that decussations between the marginal mandibular nerve and buccal branch were common, in 50% of their dissections.[28] The marginal nerve exits the anterior caudal margin of the parotid and remains deep to the parotid masseteric fascia and deep cervical investing fascia. When the nerve runs inferior to the mandible, it runs across the surface of the posterior digastric muscle and submandibular gland. Staying deep to the platysma and deep fascia, it runs superficial to the facial artery as it rises above the mandibular border. Hazani et al have identified that, approximately 3 cm anterior to the mandibular tuberosity, the marginal mandibular nerve transitions over the facial vessels.[38]

3.7.5 Cervical Branch

The cervical branch of the facial nerve exits the caudal edge of the parotid gland just anterior to the angle of the mandible and, unlike the marginal mandibular branch, perforates the deep cervical fascia soon thereafter.[11] It then takes a superficial position in the fibroareolar connective tissue that attaches to the undersurface of the platysma.[11]

References

[1] Bennett RG. Anatomy and physiology of the skin. In: Papel ID, Frodel J, Holt GR, et al. Principles of Facial Plastic and Reconstructive Surgery. 2nd ed. New York, NY: Thieme;2002:3–14

[2] Bichakjian CK, Johnson TM. Anatomy of the skin. In: Baker SR, ed. Local Flaps in Facial Reconstruction. 2nd ed. Philadelphia, PA: Mosby;2007:3–13

[3] Ramirez OM, Robertson KM. Update in endoscopic forehead rejuvenation. Facial Plast Surg Clin North Am. 2002; 10(1):37–51

[4] Knize DM. An anatomically based study of the mechanism of eyebrow ptosis. Plast Reconstr Surg. 1996; 97(7):1321–1333

[5] Lemke BN, Stasior OG. The anatomy of eyebrow ptosis. Arch Ophthalmol. 1982; 100(6):981–986

[6] Tan KS, Oh S, Priel A, Korn BS, Kikkawa DO. Surgical anatomy of the forehead, eyelids, and midface of the aesthetic surgeon. In: Massry GG, Murphy MR, Azizzadeh B, eds. Master Techniques in Blepharoplasty and Periorbital Rejuvenation. New York, NY: Springer; 2011:11–24

[7] Macdonald MR, Spiegel JH, Raven RB, Kabaker SS, Maas CS. An anatomical approach to glabellar rhytids. Arch Otolaryngol Head Neck Surg. 1998; 124(12):1315–1320

[8] Pessa JE, Rohrich RJ. The central forehead. In: Pessa JE, Rohrich RJ, eds. Clinical Topography: Clinical Anatomy of the Face. St. Louis, MO: Quality Medical Publishers; 2012:13–46

[9] Knize DM. A study of the supraorbital nerve. Plast Reconstr Surg. 1995; 96(3):564–569

[10] Lighthall JG, Wang TD. Complications of forehead lift. Facial Plast Surg Clin North Am. 2013; 21(4):619–624

[11] Roostaeian J, Rohrich RJ, Stuzin JM. Anatomical considerations to prevent facial nerve injury. Plast Reconstr Surg. 2015; 135(5):1318–1327

[12] Most SP, Mobley SR, Larrabee WF, Jr. Anatomy of the eyelids. Facial Plast Surg Clin North Am. 2005; 13(4):487–492, v

[13] Persichetti P, Di Lella F, Delfino S, Scuderi N. Adipose compartments of the upper eyelid: anatomy applied to blepharoplasty. Plast Reconstr Surg. 2004; 113(1):373–378, discussion 379–380

[14] Putterman AM, Urist MJ. Surgical anatomy of the orbital septum. Ann Ophthalmol. 1974; 6(3):290–294

[15] Pessa JE, Rohrich RJ. The eyelids. In: Pessa JE, Rohrich RJ, eds. Clinical Topography: Clinical Anatomy of the Face. St. Louis, MO: Quality Medical Publishers; 2012:95–138

[16] Mendelson BC, Jacobson SR. Surgical anatomy of the midcheek: facial layers, spaces, and the midcheek segments. Clin Plast Surg. 2008; 35(3):395–404, discussion 393

[17] Alghoul M, Codner MA. Retaining ligaments of the face: review of anatomy and clinical applications. Aesthet Surg J. 2013; 33(6):769–782

[18] Muzaffar AR, Mendelson BC, Adams WP, Jr. Surgical anatomy of the ligamentous attachments of the lower lid and lateral canthus. Plast Reconstr Surg. 2002; 110(3):873–884, discussion 897–911

[19] Haddock NT, Saadeh PB, Boutros S, Thorne CH. The tear trough and lid/cheek junction: anatomy and implications for surgical correction. Plast Reconstr Surg. 2009; 123(4):1332–1340, discussion 1341–1342

[20] Pessa JE, Rohrich RJ. The cheek. In: Pessa JE, Rohrich RJ, eds. Clinical Topography: Clinical Anatomy of the Face. St. Louis, MO: Quality Medical Publishers; 2012:47–94

[21] Rohrich RJ, Arbique GM, Wong C, Brown S, Pessa JE. The anatomy of suborbicularis fat: implications for periorbital rejuvenation. Plast Reconstr Surg. 2009; 124(3):946–951

[22] Mendelson BC, Muzaffar AR, Adams WP, Jr. Surgical anatomy of the midcheek and malar mounds. Plast Reconstr Surg. 2002; 110(3):885–896, discussion 897–911

[23] Zide BM, Jelks GW. Surgical anatomy of the orbit. Plast Reconstr Surg. 1984; 74(2):301–305

[24] Whetzel TP, Mathes SJ. The arterial supply of the face lift flap. Plast Reconstr Surg. 1997; 100(2):480–486, discussion 487–488

[25] Furnas DW. The retaining ligaments of the cheek. Plast Reconstr Surg. 1989; 83(1):11–16

[26] Stuzin JM, Baker TJ, Gordon HL, Baker TM. Extended SMAS dissection as an approach to midface rejuvenation. Clin Plast Surg. 1995; 22(2):295–311

[27] Alghoul M, Bitik O, McBride J, Zins JE. Relationship of the zygomatic facial nerve to the retaining ligaments of the face: the Sub-SMAS danger zone. Plast Reconstr Surg. 2013; 131(2):245e–252e

[28] Tzafetta K, Terzis JK. Essays on the facial nerve: Part I. Microanatomy. Plast Reconstr Surg. 2010; 125(3):879–889

[29] Langevin CJ, Engel S, Zins JE. Mandibular ligament revisited. Paper presented at: Ohio Valley Society of Plastic Surgery Annual Meeting; May 17, 2008; Cleveland, OH

[30] Toriumi DM, Mueller RA, Grosch T, Bhattacharyya TK, Larrabee WF, Jr. Vascular anatomy of the nose and the external rhinoplasty approach. Arch Otolaryngol Head Neck Surg. 1996; 122(1):24–34

[31] Rohrich RJ, Muzaffar AR, Janis JE. Component dorsal hump reduction: the importance of maintaining dorsal aesthetic lines in rhinoplasty. Plast Reconstr Surg. 2004; 114(5):1298–1308, discussion 1309–1312

[32] Daniel RK, Letourneau A. Rhinoplasty: nasal anatomy. Ann Plast Surg. 1988; 20(1):5–13

[33] Gassner HG, Sherris DA, Friedman O. Rhinology in rhinoplasty. In: Baker SR, ed. Local Flaps in Facial Reconstruction. 2nd ed. Philadelphia: Mosby;2007:385–400

[34] Tardy ME Jr, Brown RJ. Surgical anatomy of the nose. New York: Raven Press, Ltd.; 1990:34

[35] Rozen T. Post-traumatic external nasal pain syndrome (a trigeminal based pain disorder). Headache. 2009; 49(8):1223–1228

[36] Furnas DW. Landmarks for the trunk and the temporo facial division of the temporal division of the facial nerve. Br J Plast Surg. 1965; 52:694

[37] Pitanguy I, Ramos AS. The frontal branch of the facial nerve: the importance of its variations in face lifting. Plast Reconstr Surg. 1966; 38(4):352–356

[38] Hazani R, Chowdhry S, Mowlavi A, Wilhelmi BJ. Bony anatomic landmarks to avoid injury to the marginal mandibular nerve. Aesthet Surg J. 2011; 31(3):286–289

4 Plumes, Laser/Cautery

Daniel A. Yanes and Mathew M. Avram

Summary

Laser plume and surgical smoke are consequential byproducts of minimally invasive surgery. The effects they have on those who inhale them are consequential, yet under appreciated. Protection from the harmful effects of the plume is essential for any who perform these procedures. This chapter reviews the contents of the plume and strategies to abate laser plume toxicity.

Keywords: laser, plume, cautery, smoke, ultrafine, UFP, ablative, nonablative, HPV, carcinogen, ventilation, evacuator, N95

4.1 Introduction

As lasers vaporize and coagulate tissue, the thermal interactions can produce an aerosolized mixture of vapor, particulate debris, and smoke that is known as "plume." The distinct odor is memorable to patients and those who use the lasers alike, and there are an increasing number of investigations into the laser plume and its impact on those who inhale it. In addition to inorganic irritating and mutagenic chemical matter, aerosolized organic particles (such as viral and bacterial matter) have been noted to be present in laser plume, depending upon the procedure. This chapter reviews the properties of laser plumes, their impact on human health, and protective strategies for those who perform and receive laser therapy.

Laser plumes are generated by laser treatments that ablate, vaporize, or heat their photothermolytic targets. Given their nature, ablative lasers such as CO_2 and Er:YAG will generate a plume as a consequence of direct tissue ablation. Nonablative lasers are also capable of creating laser plumes, depending on their therapeutic target and consequent generation of thermal energy.[1,2] Laser hair removal produces a plume as light is absorbed by melanin in the hair shaft and transformed into thermal energy, which results in the destruction of the follicular stem cells. The hair is consequently vaporized into plume as it combusts.

4.2 Inorganic Contents of the Plume

Studies of particulate matter within the laser plume closely followed after studies began to raise concerns about electrosurgical smoke. The majority of inorganic particulate matter in laser plume is composed of ultrafine particles (UFPs).[3] UFPs are defined as nanosized particulate matter less than 100 nm. As technology has become ubiquitous, so too have UFPs, which humans are exposed to in the environment regularly through driving, cooking, smoking, and operating household electrical devices.[4] Increased exposure to UFPs in particulate air pollution has been associated with increased mortality and cardiopulmonary disease.[5,6] The advent of modern technology has further brought about increased exposure to UFPs in activities of daily life, and nanotoxicological studies have highlighted the effects of UFPs on human health. When inhaled, UFPs are able to diffuse across respiratory and cutaneous epithelium, and their nanoscale size allows them to be taken up by a number of cells in the body, where they can exert oxidant and toxic effects.[7]

There are a number of factors that influence the content and concentration of laser plumes (▶ Table 4.1). Investigations have verified that the concentration of particulate matter in the air directly increases following laser procedures, and that the concentration of particulate matter decreases with time after the procedure and increased distance from the surgical site.[3,8] Compared to ambient concentrations, particulate concentrations in the procedure room increase during the procedure and remain elevated post-procedurally over an hour later.[9] UFP concentrations gradually drift back toward baseline levels as they diffuse into their sur-

Table 4.1 Factors associated with increased UFP concentration in laser hair removal[9]

Duration of treatment

Surface area of body part treated

Use of cryogen spray

Higher power

Lack of smoke evacuator

Lack of adequate ventilation

roundings, and their dissipation and peak concentration is heavily dependent on ventilation in the procedure room.[3,8,9] The duration of the procedure is the factor most closely associated with laser plumes.[9] Contact cooling with aqueous gel or lotion has been shown to reduce plume production when compared to cryogen devices for reasons that have not yet been elucidated.[9,10] It has been theorized that UFPs diffuse into and are retained by the coolant. In addition, the force of the cryogen spray as it is released is hypothesized to disperse UFPs. Increased laser energy has also predictably been linked to higher particulate concentrations.[3,9]

In vitro and in vivo studies of CO_2, Nd:YAG, and alexandrite lasers have characterized the gaseous particulate matter within the plume, which is composed of over 350 different identifiable compounds.[11]

The chemical contents of laser plumes have raised concerns about their carcinogenicity. As aforementioned, even ambient UFPs in the environment have been linked to carcinogenesis; in fact, particulate matter in outdoor pollution has been given a "1" rating by the International Agency for Research on Cancer, indicating a known carcinogen. Some of the chemicals found in higher concentrations within laser plumes include known carcinogens such as acetamide, acrylonitrile, benzene, butadiene, formaldehyde, naphthalene, propene, and styrene, among others.[11,12,13] In addition, some of the chemicals identified in plume have been linked to cancer, but without enough evidence for the International Agency for Research on Cancer to label the chemical a likely or known carcinogen. Taken together, the chemicals in the laser plume have been associated with a number of different malignancies. In particular, lung, urothelial, and hematologic malignancies seem to be quite common.[13] The close association with these malignancies in particular may likely be directly related to the small size of UFPs, as the chemicals are inhaled (where they contact respiratory mucosa), effectively enter endothelial cells as a result of their small size, spread to bone marrow, spleen, and lymph nodes, and are ultimately excreted into urine where they concentrate in the bladder.[7] It is unclear what the "safe" concentrations are for particulate matter. As an example, benzene, which is present in plume, has made its way to the public eye for its myelotoxicity and role in development of acute myeloid leukemia and acute nonlymphocytic leukemia.[13] Its extreme

carcinogenicity has led to the United States Environmental Agency setting a maximum permissible level of 5 parts-per-billion, with a goal of 0 parts-per-billion. While it is clear that no amount of benzene is safe, such regulations do not exist on every chemical within laser plume, making it difficult to know when particulate matter has exceeded a threshold of safety. Ultimately, although laser plume is composed of a number of carcinogenic compounds in various concentrations, there are no human studies investigating the long-term carcinogenic effect of plume itself. That being said, surgical smoke from electrocautery, which has a similar composition to laser plume, has been demonstrated to be mutagenic in several studies.[14] Clearly, further study is merited.

In addition to carcinogenicity, the inorganic contents of the laser plume have both direct and indirect effects on cardiopulmonary function. In animal models, exposure to Nd:YAG plume reproducibly and invariably induces significant emphysematous change.[1,15] This finding has been reproduced with exposure to CO_2 plume.[16] Many of the chemicals in laser plume are also found in cigarette smoke, albeit in lesser concentrations. In cigarette smokers, hydrogen cyanide is estimated to account for 89% of cardiovascular potency, whereas acrolein has been estimated to account for about 97% of respiratory potency.[17] Cyanides (i.e., acrylonitrile) and acrolein are found heavily within the plume, and potentially account for the cardiopulmonary impact observed in animal models, as they do in human cigarette smokers.[11] Cyanide toxicity leads to inhibition mitochondrial oxygen utilization, leading to cellular hypoxia.

Finally, an overwhelming number of chemicals in the plume are irritants to cutaneous, mucosal, and respiratory epithelium, and exposure to many can acutely cause malaise, dizziness, nausea, vomiting, and headache.[18] Outside of these acute mucocutaneous irritation and constitutional symptoms, there are no human studies that investigate the actual health effects of laser plume particulate matter.

4.3 Organic Contents of the Plume

In addition to harmful inorganic ultrafine particulate matter, there is aerosolized biologic material contained within laser plumes as well. Aerosolization of the human papilloma virus (HPV) is perhaps the most well-described biohazardous material within the laser plume. Early in-vitro and in-vivo studies of verrucae treated with CO_2 laser demonstrated that intact HPV DNA was readily detected in the plume of about 30 to 60% treated patients.[19,20] Aerosolization of the virus does not appear to be universal for every laser type, as HPV DNA has not been identified in the plume of patients with warts or papillomas treated with Er:YAG or KTP laser. While the virus is certainly detectable in the CO_2 laser plume, there have been a number of studies debating the true infectious potential of such aerosolized papillomavirus. This risk appears to increase when treating genital HPV, perhaps due to the propensity of the common causative HPV subtypes in genital warts (6 and 11) to also infect oropharyngeal mucosa.[21] CO_2 laser surgeons have a similar incidence of warts as the general population, yet have a higher incidence of anogenital, nasopharyngeal, and plantar warts.[21] There have been case reports of iatrogenic CO_2 laser-induced laryngeal papillomatosis, described in healthcare personnel who were extensively involved in treatment of anogenital condylomas.[22,23] In addition, there have been reports of HPV-positive tonsillar cancer occurring in laser surgeons without any other identifiable risk factors.[24] Taken altogether, the evidence appears to support a very low, albeit very real risk of infection from the liberalized virus.

Bacterial cultures of laser plume following CO_2 resurfacing demonstrated growth of skin flora including *Staphylococcus* and *Corynebacteria*,[25] implying that laser plume may contain viable bacteria. HIV proviral DNA has been detected in CO_2 laser plume; however, these findings have not been reproduced and simian immunodeficiency virus does not appear to be viable within plume.[26,27]

4.4 Protective Strategies

Given the mounting evidence that suggests actual and theoretical laser plume toxicity, it follows that protective strategies to minimize plume exposure are imperative.

As aforementioned, the peak concentration of UFPs and their rate of clearance are dependent on ventilation of the laser operating room. Dilution ventilation is a mode of ventilation that ventilates air from an entire building or area using exhaust fans. This is what many would consider to be standard ventilation for most office buildings. However, as previously mentioned, dilution ventilation is necessary, but not sufficient in removing

Table 4.2 Smoke evacuator properties associated with improved plume elimination[29]

Increased minimum airflow

Increased internal diameter of tubing

Increased suction strength and power

Decreased distance from source

Increased filtration efficiency

UFPs from the operating room.[9] Thus, local exhaust ventilation is necessary in eliminating laser plume. Local exhaust ventilation extracts the contaminant as it is generated, keeping it from being widely aerosolized. In the setting of laser surgery, local exhaust ventilation typically refers to the use of smoke evacuators. In light of a paucity of data, guidelines on laser plume exposure reduction are typically extrapolated from studies on surgical smoke. It has been repeatedly demonstrated that use of smoke evacuators significantly reduces but does not totally eliminate surgical smoke.[28] Guidelines often recommend keeping the smoke evacuator inlet nozzle within 2 inches of the site; however, keeping the inlet closer allows for more effective evacuation. In laser hair removal, the distance of the smoke evacuator from the source is directly proportional to the UFP concentration in the air.[9] Each smoke evacuator has inherent properties that impact its ability to remove UFPs from the air (▶ Table 4.2). It is important to select a smoke evacuator with high filtration efficiency. Ultralow-penetration air filters are preferable and characteristic of most modern smoke evacuators. These filters have an efficiency of 99.999% for particles 12 nm and smaller. As UFPs compose the majority of laser plume, a filter that captures these small particles is essential.[29] Guidelines for minimum airflow of electrocautery smoke have been described; however, it is important to note that the density of the laser plume is not necessarily comparable to that of electrocautery smoke, and so these guidelines cannot be effectively extrapolated to laser plumes. As would be expected, higher minimum airflow of the smoke capture device allows for improved capture of UFPs.[30] A capture of velocity of 100 to 150 feet per minute at the inlet nozzle is generally recommended for evacuation of laser plumes.

Given the previously discussed irritating effects of laser plumes on the ocular and respiratory mucosae, protective equipment is essential. Eye protection will prevent eye irritation from the UFPs in the plume. For the majority of laser procedures, laser safety goggles are required regardless to protect the eye from the laser beam. Masks are essential tools to prevent inhalation of the plume and its subsequent toxic effects. Not all masks have equivalent protective capability. The standard disposable surgical mask is capable of filtering 91.5% of particulate matter larger than 5,000 nm.[31] Given than UFPs (< 100 nm) make up the majority of the plume, the standard surgical mask provides insufficient respiratory protection. High-efficiency particulate air masks are capable of filtering particulate matter larger than 300 nm. The efficiency of the filtration masks is variable. Perhaps the most commonly used high-efficiency particulate air mask is the N95 respirator, named for its minimum 95% filtration efficiency. In actuality, the filtration efficiency of the N95 mask may be closer to 99.9%.[31] In face of the small particulate size characteristic of laser plume, the N95 mask or a similar high-efficiency particulate air mask is preferable to a standard mask. Proper fit of the mask is essential to its function. A mustache or beard can prevent proper fit. The mask should cover the nose and the mouth. So-called "laser masks" should be carefully examined for filtration efficiency and filtration size, as the name does not necessarily imply more respiratory protection.

As the properties and risks of the laser plume are further explored, further ways to prevent potential harm will likely be elucidated. As eluded to earlier in the chapter, contact cooling with aqueous gel appears to be a promising mechanism to suppressing laser plume. Until these methods are further developed, respirators, smoke evacuators, and effective ventilation systems remain the mainstay of laser plume hazard mitigation.

References

[1] Wenig BL, Stenson KM, Wenig BM, Tracey D. Effects of plume produced by the Nd:YAG laser and electrocautery on the respiratory system. Lasers Surg Med. 1993; 13(2): 242–245

[2] Dodhia S, Baxter PC, Ye F, Pitman MJ. Investigation of the presence of HPV on KTP laser fibers following KTP laser treatment of papilloma. Laryngoscope. 2018; 128(4): 926–928

[3] Lopez R, Lacey SE, Lippert JF, Liu LC, Esmen NA, Conroy LM. Characterization of size-specific particulate matter emission rates for a simulated medical laser procedure: a pilot study. Ann Occup Hyg. 2015; 59(4):514–524

[4] Wallace L, Ott W. Personal exposure to ultrafine particles. J Expo Sci Environ Epidemiol. 2011; 21(1):20–30

[5] Pope CA, III, Burnett RT, Thun MJ, et al. Lung cancer, cardiopulmonary mortality, and long-term exposure to fine particulate air pollution. JAMA. 2002; 287(9):1132–1141

[6] Pope CA, III, Thun MJ, Namboodiri MM, et al. Particulate air pollution as a predictor of mortality in a prospective study of U.S. adults. Am J Respir Crit Care Med. 1995; 151(3 Pt 1):669–674

[7] Oberdörster G, Oberdörster E, Oberdörster J. Nanotoxicology: an emerging discipline evolving from studies of ultrafine particles. Environ Health Perspect. 2005; 113(7):823–839

[8] Tanpowpong K, Koytong W. Suspended particulate matter in an office and laser smoke particles in an operating room. J Med Assoc Thai. 2002; 85(1):53–57

[9] Eshleman EJ, LeBlanc M, Rokoff LB, et al. Occupational exposures and determinants of ultrafine particle concentrations during laser hair removal procedures. Environ Health. 2017; 16(1):30

[10] Ross EV, Chuang GS, Ortiz AE, Davenport SA. Airborne particulate concentration during laser hair removal: a comparison between cold sapphire with aqueous gel and cryogen skin cooling. Lasers Surg Med. 2018; 50(4):280–283

[11] Chuang GS, Farinelli W, Christiani DC, Herrick RF, Lee NC, Avram MM. Gaseous and particulate content of laser hair removal plume. JAMA Dermatol. 2016; 152(12):1320–1326

[12] Kokosa JM, Eugene J. Chemical composition of laser-tissue interaction smoke plume. ICALEO. 1988; 1(1988)

[13] WHO. International Agency for Research on Cancer. IARC Monographs on the Evaluation of Carcinogenic Risks to Humans: Overall Evaluations of Carcinogenicity. An Updating of IARC Monographs 2008–03–06, Vols 1 to 42, Suppl. 7

[14] Lewin JM, Brauer JA, Ostad A. Surgical smoke and the dermatologist. J Am Acad Dermatol. 2011; 65(3):636–641

[15] Freitag L, Chapman GA, Sielczak M, Ahmed A, Russin D. Laser smoke effect on the bronchial system. Lasers Surg Med. 1987; 7(3):283–288

[16] Baggish MS, Elbakry M. The effects of laser smoke on the lungs of rats. Am J Obstet Gynecol. 1987; 156(5):1260–1265

[17] Laugesen M, Fowles J. Scope for regulation of cigarette smoke toxicity according to brand differences in published toxicant emissions. N Z Med J. 2005; 118(1213):U1401

[18] Katoch S, Mysore V. Surgical smoke in dermatology: its hazards and management. J Cutan Aesthet Surg. 2019; 12(1):1–7

[19] Sawchuk WS, Weber PJ, Lowy DR, Dzubow LM. Infectious papillomavirus in the vapor of warts treated with carbon dioxide laser or electrocoagulation: detection and protection. J Am Acad Dermatol. 1989; 21(1):41–49

[20] Garden JM, O'Banion MK, Shelnitz LS, et al. Papillomavirus in the vapor of carbon dioxide laser-treated verrucae. JAMA. 1988; 259(8):1199–1202

[21] Gloster HM, Jr, Roenigk RK. Risk of acquiring human papillomavirus from the plume produced by the carbon dioxide laser in the treatment of warts. J Am Acad Dermatol. 1995; 32(3):436–441

[22] Hallmo P, Naess O. Laryngeal papillomatosis with human papillomavirus DNA contracted by a laser surgeon. Eur Arch Otorhinolaryngol. 1991; 248(7):425–427

[23] Calero L, Brusis T. Laryngeal papillomatosis: first recognition in Germany as an occupational disease in an operating room nurse. Laryngorhinootologie. 2003; 82(11):790–793

[24] Rioux M, Garland A, Webster D, Reardon E. HPV positive tonsillar cancer in two laser surgeons: case reports. J Otolaryngol Head Neck Surg. 2013; 42:54

[25] Capizzi PJ, Clay RP, Battey MJ. Microbiologic activity in laser resurfacing plume and debris. Lasers Surg Med. 1998; 23(3): 172–174

[26] Starr JC, Kilmer SL, Wheeland RG. Analysis of the carbon dioxide laser plume for Simian immunodeficiency virus. J Dermatol Surg Oncol. 1992; 18(4):297–300

[27] Baggish MS, Poiesz BJ, Joret D, Williamson P, Refai A. Presence of human immunodeficiency virus DNA in laser smoke. Lasers Surg Med. 1991; 11(3):197–203

[28] Lee T, Soo JC, LeBouf RF, et al. Surgical smoke control with local exhaust ventilation: experimental study. J Occup Environ Hyg. 2018; 15(4):341–350

[29] Georgesen C, Lipner SR. Surgical smoke: risk assessment and mitigation strategies. J Am Acad Dermatol. 2018; 79(4): 746–755

[30] Hunter JG. Laser smoke evacuator: effective removal of mutagenic cautery smoke. Aesthetic Plast Surg. 1996; 20(2): 177–178

[31] Lu W, Zhu XC, Zhang XY, Chen YT, Chen WH. Respiratory protection provided by N95 filtering facepiece respirators and disposable medicine masks against airborne bacteria in different working environments. Zhonghua Lao Dong Wei Sheng Zhi Ye Bing Za Zhi. 2016; 34(9): 643–646

Section II

Injectables: Avoiding and Managing Complications

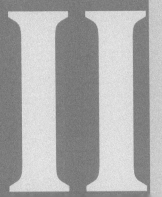

5 Fillers

Helen M. Moses, Louis M. DeJoseph, and Nikunj Rana

Summary

The use of cosmetic injectable fillers has become ever more prevalent. The physician's ability to safely produce consistent results relies on prevention and appropriate management of complications, should they arise. Knowledge of patient-, product-, and technique-related factors are all integral to being a complete injector. When the unfortunate complication does arise, having a systematic method for diagnosis of management of early and late complications can help facilitate recovery. Complications can occur for injectors of all skill level and experience and treatment protocols are constantly evolving. Constant review, understanding, and implementation of current treatment are paramount to high-quality patient care with fillers.

Keywords: vascular occlusion, nodule, granuloma, hyaluronidase

5.1 Introduction

Cosmetic, nonsurgical procedures such as injectable dermal fillers have the ability to produce consistent, effective, and safe results. In 2018, 810,240 dermal filler procedures were performed in the United States alone.[1] With increasing popularity and patient-driven demand, the clinician should be well versed in the prevention, identification, and management of complications. A recent global consensus statement from ASAPS declared that "optimal complication management is the largest unmet need with fillers." The safety profile of the numerous dermal filler agents has been widely established. However, there is constant evolution of injection paradigms and protocols. This includes the volume utilized, injection technique, development of new product classes, and indefinite number of repeated injections. These all mandate that the treating clinician remain vigilant to complications that may arise and practice in a manner capable of preventing and managing complications in a timely manner.[2] The focus of this chapter is to identify techniques for minimizing and managing complications secondary to dermal fillers and incorporating them into an injectable practice.

5.2 General Principles

A key tenet of complication management is prevention. The treating clinician for this diverse population must be aware of patient-, product-, and technique-related factors that can impact adverse reactions and the treatment of such complications.

5.2.1 Patient-Related Factors

Patient selection is key. Identifying both appropriate and inappropriate candidates for filler is the first step for avoidance and management of complications. Patient demographics, history and physical examination, and patient goals and desires are all considered. In addition to aesthetic patients, these may also include patients with prior facial trauma who desire improvement of facial disharmony. This population should heed caution as injecting over solid surgical implants could theoretically be a nidus of infection. Also of mention, while there has been no association established between use of fillers and autoimmune conditions, patients with uncontrolled immune deficiencies or patients with prior organ transplant may be affected by the filler injection or the condition may affect the behavior of the filler.[3] Immune suppression or depression is not an absolute contraindication but the presence of these medications or steroid use should yield a more discerning look into one's medical history.

A discussion of patient-related factors includes not only a relevant cosmetic surgical history and disclosure of previous complications but also assessing skin-related conditions and factors (quality, atrophy, etc.).[4] A history of prior surgeries and any complications with wound healing is helpful to note, but also a history of prior dental, facial surgery, or trauma as noted above requires caution.

This is important as there is potential for unusual vascular distribution due to neovascularization and the local soft tissue changes that can occur after trauma and healing.[5] Eliciting prior filler complications, significant allergies, and medical conditions is also imperative. Medical conditions that may heed caution include careful attention to any ongoing skin infections: particularly HSV, perioral HPV, Mollusca contagiosum, impetigo, or excessive amounts of *Propionibacterium acnes*. All of the aforementioned can make the patient an unsuitable candidate. In addition, active inflammatory dermatitis including atopic, allergic contact, or seborrheic dermatitis mandates caution but is at the discretion of the clinician. Patients should be counseled regarding the possibility of a rosacea flare secondary to the normal inflammatory effect on local tissue and mechanics of injection associated with filler placement. Active HSV infection should preclude treatment and prophylaxis should be prescribed (acyclovir, famciclovir, valacyclovir) for future injections in the perioral area specifically. There is also caution in performing dermal filler injections in patients with active sinusitis, periodontal disease, or other similar infections as these infections may subsequently involve areas where filler has been placed and induce a biofilm reaction.[6] A recent consensus guideline published in the *Journal of Clinical, Cosmetic and Investigative Dermatology* outlines a comprehensive list of preexisting conditions that may contraindicate or warrant caution in the use of dermal fillers and is worthy of review.

Medication review should focus on the use of immune modulators, anticoagulants, nonsteroidal anti-inflammatory medications, as well as vitamins and herbal supplements. As therapeutic anticoagulation is only a relative contraindication, injection technique can be modified by the clinician to still provide a safe, effective injection in this patient population. Technical modifications include the use of small needles, microcannulas, and immediate prolonged pressure.[2] Vitamin and herbal medications associated with anticoagulation include but are not limited to vitamin E, fish oil, krill oil, gingko, garlic, ginger, ginseng, and should ideally be discontinued 7 to 10 days prior to the procedure.[3] Also, worth mention is screening occupation/occupation factors that may increase the potential for facial skin microbial colonization, i.e., methicillin-resistant *Staphylococcus aureus* (MRSA) prevalence in health care workers and community-acquired staphylococcal microbes. While these numerous factors elicited above are not contraindications, front-end awareness allows for a timely diagnosis and treatment should a complication arise.

In a multifaceted approach to facial rejuvenation, adjunctive noninvasive or minimally invasive procedures are often combined with dermal filler. It is generally recommended that microdermabrasion, chemical peels, laser treatments, and intense pulsed light (IPL) should be carried out 1 to 2 weeks pre- or posttreatment in the same area to allow time for any erythema and edema to subside and the skin barrier

to reestablish.[4] From a more routine and practical standpoint as well, dental procedures should be performed at least 2 weeks pre- or posttreatment to minimize risk of hematogenous spread or biofilm formation, and makeup application is often avoided for the first 24 hours after injection.[6]

5.2.2 Product-Related Factors

Pertinent product-related factors include: concentration and flow properties of the filler, as well as the manufacturing and purification process. For hyaluronic acid (HA) fillers, having a working knowledge of these properties will aid in avoiding undesirable outcomes; an example being a higher resistance to deformation is desirable in volumizing in the supraperiosteal or subcutaneous planes, but not superficially where it is more visible.[3]

Factors such as G′ have been studied with HA fillers. G′ refers to the elasticity of the product or its ability to retain shape when pressure is applied. Lower G′ fillers spread more easily and are therefore better suited for more superficial placement. Of the non-HA dermal fillers, calcium hydroxylapatite (Radiesse, Merz Aesthetics) is a particulate suspension in methylcellulose gel and poly-L-lactic acid (Sculptra Aesthetic, Galderma) is a synthetic peptide polymer, both of which may stimulate collagen neogenesis and are considered by some to be semipermanent fillers.[7] A comprehensive review of the individual properties of the known dermal fillers is beyond the scope of this chapter, but an in-depth understanding of filler properties and filler selection will undoubtedly aid in avoiding and minimizing complications.

5.2.3 Technique-Related Factors

Multiple accepted injection techniques exist in the literature and are mostly dependent on the area being treated and the filler being utilized. However, there are several agreed upon principles that should be adhered to from a technique standpoint. While HA filler and non-HA fillers can be injected safely and effectively by microcannula or needle, the use of needles must be used with caution in areas prone to vascular complications. These distinct regions, such as the temple and glabella, may be better suited for blunt-tip microcannulas.[2] In addition, aspiration via needle or cannula is often heralded as imperative in these high-risk vascular areas but a negative aspiration should not be relied on in terms of avoiding a vascular complication. General technique principles include a slow injection with a low flow rate in small quantities at various points. Fast injections, aggressive fanning, and high-volume deposition should be avoided, to decrease the possibility of vasculature compression.

5.2.4 Pretreatment Prophylaxis

There is yet to be specific universal consensus guidelines outlining skin preparation prior to injectable soft tissue fillers. Given more recent awareness of risk of infection and possibility of a biofilm, the data for infection prevention for facial procedures is extrapolated from other surgical experiences of patients undergoing clean-contaminated surgery, which is similar to the wound classification during facial procedures. Selection of skin preparation should consider the risks of an adverse reaction vs. a possible small further decrease in the risk of infection. Skin cleansing with chlorhexidine-alcohol is more protective than povidone-iodine against superficial and deep incisional infections.[8] However, there is the greater possibility of significant allergic reaction and the risk of corneal ulceration. Some injectors favor the use of 2% chlorhexidine gluconate in 70% isopropyl alcohol on the facial skin with the exception of the periocular region, given the risk of keratitis and ocular injury.[2,9] Others believe that considering the increased associated risks with chlorhexidine skin prep it should not be used and only betadine should be used. Most physicians consider fillers similar to an injectable implant and therefore favor skin cleansing and prep prior to injection. There are currently prep solutions under review that may prove to be better than the current commonly used prep solutions.

5.3 Adverse Reactions and Complications

Complications have been categorized throughout the dermal filler literature in several different structural formats. A recent review in Facial Plastic Surgery grouped complications by type into three categories including injector-dependent adverse events (AEs), lumps and bumps, and ischemia and necrosis.[3] Secondarily, one of the most commonly used classification paradigms is based on timing of the complication for both identification and management, such as early and late, which is the format that is commonly used and one that our discussion will follow. Early complications, often within the first 14 days to 4 weeks, are often attributed to acute inflammation, acute infection, or ischemia. Late (14 d to 1 y) and delayed (up to 1 y)

are generally secondary to granuloma formation and possibility of biofilm development.[3]

5.4 Early Adverse Reactions and Management of Complications

5.4.1 Bruising

Bruising may be seen as a "normal" complication if performing filler treatments on the face, but to the patient this can be quite concerning on a social level. Bruising, bleeding, and edema may be prevented or decreased by using smaller gauge instruments and/or cannulas (discussed below), slow injection, smaller aliquot deposition, exercise avoidance, and manual or cold compression. Arnica by mouth (started 2 d prior to injectable procedure), arnica cream or gel, and topical vitamin K are adjuncts as well to managing these early limited AEs. For those who can tolerate it, eating pineapple for the anti-inflammatory benefits of the bromelain may help to reduce related inflammation. Some favor using an AccuVein device to identify veins not readily visible on the skin surface; however, most physicians do not routinely utilize this device.[10] Some physicians favor the option of trying to treat a bruise with a vascular laser to boost recovery. Fitzgerald et al reported that resolution can be rapid if the bruise is at a level reached by the laser. Issue is that frequently the bruise is deep in the dermis or even the soft tissue in which case lasering the skin surface is unlikely to affect the bruise.

5.4.2 Edema

Edema and swelling are expected components of all injectable fillers but may vary in severity and time of onset depending on the particular filler used and the location treated. Swelling is most common to the lips and periorbital regions. Onset is typically within the first few hours after injection and may subside within a few days with the use of compresses, antihistamines, or corticosteroids. Periorbital edema can be idiosyncratic, due to too much volume used in the tear trough or incorrect placement. However, patients with preexisting malar edema and malar festoons should be counseled regarding an increased risk for persistent edema following injection. This is due to obstruction at the level of the microlymphatic channels responsible for draining this area.

Avoiding use of certain more hydrophilic products in this area should be considered, such as some clinicians' preference to avoid Juvederm Ultra and Ultraplusperiorbitals.[3]

5.4.3 Placement Related: Inappropriate Placement and Depth, Overcorrection

Contour deformities, lumps, and asymmetries may be seen immediately or early following injection. The Tyndall effect (▶ Fig. 5.1), a bluish discoloration due to filler acting as an optical chamber, is a known occurrence with augmentation and too superficial placement within the thin skin of the infraorbital region and the nasolabial folds. This can be treated with hyaluronidase (HYAL) and gentle massage as superficial filler may last for long periods of time in these tissues. Incorrect placement in the retroseptal region or poor filler selection may yield a characteristic "sausage" appearance as it settles along the orbital rim adjacent to the orbital-retaining ligament.[3] Filler migration may occur due to injection technique (excessive volume or pressure) or placement in a plane that is subject to muscular contracture that mechanically pushes the filler to an area other than the initial injection site, which is commonly seen in perioral and periorbital areas due to the shape and function of the orbicularis in each location.

Lumps and contour irregularities as described above following treatment with an HA filler can be altered or adjusted with the use of HYAL. Its use is FDA-approved for drug dispersion, i.e., local anesthetics into soft tissues as it is a mucolytic enzyme that hydrolyzes natural and cross-linked HA fillers. The majority of its use in the aesthetic practice is an off-label use for dissolution of HA filler product that has been incorrectly placed or has generated a suboptimal cosmetic result as well as following the occurrence of any number of AEs. In light of the risk of possible allergic reactions, limited use is recommended and the Global Aesthetics Consensus panel set forward a specific schema for judicious use of HYAL: 10 to 20 U single injection for an area less than 2.5 mm, and for an area 2.5 to 1 cm, two to four injection points with 10 to 20 U per injection point. Considering the risk of allergic reactions to HYAL, when possible, some physicians favor an intradermal

skin test prior to injection. Clinical judgment is recommended in order to titrate the dosage to the desired effect as this depends on the volume placed and product itself as not all HA fillers respond similarly to HYAL.[2] The ability of HYAL to dissolve filler is dependent on multiple factors that are discussed later in the vascular compromises section of the chapter. In short, heavier products with higher cross-linking require increased amounts of HYAL to obtain the desired effect.

Paresthesias and hypesthesias are reported after filler injection. These complications can be related to filler placement and depth of injection, a localized inflammatory response, compression or direct trauma to the nerves. Symptoms include transient numbness or pain and may include facial nerve branches dependent on location and depth of injection. Other placement-related complications include parotid duct obstruction or injury and exacerbation of temporomandibular joint pain. Parotid-related issues may arise secondary to chemical dermatitis from saliva tracking into the facial soft tissues or direct obstruction/duct injury with symptoms consisting of edema, erythema, pain, and trismus. Treatment options consist of compresses to the affected side, antibiotics, oral steroids, and HYAL after 24 hours of antibiotic therapy.

5.4.4 A Tool for Management of Early Adverse Events: Use of Blunt-Tip Cannula

Some studies have advocated for the use of blunt-tip cannulas to reduce bruising. This push toward cannula injection comes from a safety perspective as it relates to vascular events, particularly intravascular injection.[2,3,7,11,12] In a recent study by Pavicic et al investigating precision and avoiding filler diffusion, "if precision in filler injection is defined as the filler material remaining in the plane of intended implantation, then using cannulas resulted in a more precise injection of material as compared to needles. Others disagree with this approach and favor precise injection with a needle.

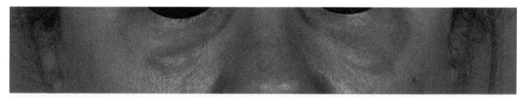

Fig. 5.1 Tyndall effect under eyes from hyaluronic acid injection.

Applications with needles resulted in the distribution of material into more superficial layers, which was not noted for cannulas." More importantly, this study also noted the similar ease of vessel wall penetration between 27 g needles and 27 g cannulas, thus suggesting the use of cannulas 25 g and larger when placing dermal filler.[13]

Hexel et al completed a double-blinded, randomized controlled trial to compare safety and efficacy between the use of metallic cannula vs. standard needle to augment the nasolabial folds. A total of 25 participants were included.This trial reported fewer side effects on the side injected with cannula for all parameters: pain, edema, erythema, and hematoma formation.[14]

5.5 Inflammatory Reactions

5.5.1 Allergic Reactions and HA Hypersensitivity

HA filler hypersensitivity treatment is a function of severity. With more purified and synthetic derivatives the rate of hypersensitivity reactions has decreased to about 0.02%.[7] Immediate hypersensitivity is often less severe and is more common in products with an anesthetic component. In the majority of cases it is self-limited and resolves with supportive measures within a few hours or days. If the patient's history suggests a more mast cell–mediated allergic profile the reaction may respond to antihistamines. Immediate substantial swelling and angioedema may occur, and rare anaphylactic reactions have been documented in the literature.[15,16] The authors recommend having an EpiPen on hand in the office to begin immediate treatment due to the possibility of impending airway compromise. Delayed hypersensitivity usually resolve without untoward consequences but may be treated with oral steroids depending on the severity of the reaction and the allergen should be removed if possible.

5.5.2 Acute Infection

Early infection is likely a function that may relate to inadequate skin preparation before injection and skin contamination. The diagnosis is made clinically and usually presents within the first few days after injection as an erythematous, warm, tender lump or as cellulitis. In this clinical situation, filler acts as a foreign body and therefore the bacterial load required for infection in this situation is markedly reduced. Often these infections are due to *Staphylococcus*species and with increasing frequency are MRSA-related infections. Returning to one of the key principles of complication management and prevention with appropriate skin preparation and also appropriate patient-related factors that may increase the propensity toward such an early acute infectious complication, including MRSA risk factors and prior HSV infection (which would warrant prophylaxis as injections can trigger a flare).

The Global Aesthetics Consensus panel on filler complication management has recommended a certain sequence for treatment of early acute infections: empiric antibiotics, consider HYAL, and then only once infection is ruled out or resolved, consider intralesional steroids for remaining inflammatory nodules. Empiric antibiotic therapy is based on clinical diagnosis of an acute bacterial infection and judgment. For both fluctuant and nonfluctuant infections, empiric coverage includes amoxicillin plus clavulanate or cephalexin; ciprofloxacin is an alternative for the penicillin-allergic patient. If methicillin-resistant staphylococcus aureus (MRSA) is a concern, both trimethoprim-sulfamethoxazole and rifampin may be considered. HYAL injection to prevent recurrence or hasten resolution by removing the offending agent should be weighed against the desire to save the aesthetic correction. HYAL injection should be performed only if antibiotic treatment has been initiated to avoid spreading the infected material into the adjacent soft tissue. If an abscess is present, it should be drained based on standard surgical principles.[17] If empiric therapy is unsuccessful, culture-directed therapy should be considered. In addition, the authors advocate that if the cause is uncertain and the clinical picture is less clear, a double-pronged approach with the use of antibiotics and antiviral agents may be considered, especially given the tolerability of antiviral formulations.

5.6 Vascular Events

Rightfully one of the most dreaded complications for the novice and experienced injector alike is a vascular event. Sequelae range from subtle skin changes that eventually resolve to areas of epidermolysis and necrosis to visual loss and permanent neurologic deficits. Carruthers et al analyzed the relative frequency of injection sites leading to vascular complications and while the glabella is the most high-risk area followed by the nasal region, the data shows virtually every location on the face has potential to yield vascular compromise.[18] ▸ Fig. 5.2 demonstrates anHA vascular injection into the lip treated with HYAL with complete resolution.

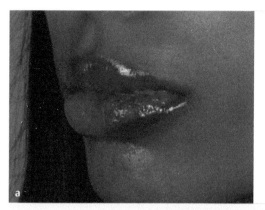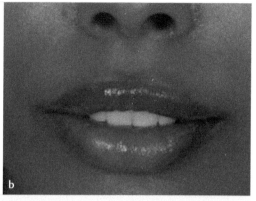

Fig. 5.2 (a, b) Preventing vascular events relies on a thorough understanding of the complex facial, orbital, cervical, and cranial anatomy and vasculature derived from both the internal and external carotid arterial systems. A noteworthy review and discussion of the anatomical implications can be found in a review published by Beleznay et al and is a strongly encouraged reading for the cosmetic injector.[19]

5.6.1 Anatomic Considerations and Mechanisms

For cases of blindness and central nervous system events, areas of the face are supplied directly by the internal carotid system, including the distal branches of the ophthalmic artery. These branches include vessels extending onto the forehead and nose as the supratrochlear, supraorbital, and dorsal nasal arteries and are most commonly involved in vascular events. The mechanism behind blindness and central nervous system (CNS) complications is retrograde flow – with penetration of one of these distal branches, the force of injection leads to expansion of the arteriole and retrograde flow ensues. Another mechanism to achieve retrograde flow is if the pressure applied during injection is greater than the systolic pressure in the artery, the filler is carried more proximally along the arterial system and upon release of the plunger moves more distally, obstructing the ophthalmic or retinal artery and its branches.[3,18] Worth mention is a supplementary theory regarding occlusion from perivascular swelling and resultant compression of vasculature. The hydrophilic nature of HA can lead to increased intratissue pressure and volume expansion, which, in turn, may result in decreased blood flow, ischemia, and necrosis.

The most common areas of vascular occlusion leading to tissue necrosis are areas or territories dependent on a singular blood supply, i.e., the nasolabial fold or nasal tip. As the filler material is propagated into increasingly smaller caliber vessels, the filler becomes lodged and occlusion blocks gas exchange and without collateral flow, ischemia occurs. Strategies to treat tissue damage from vascular compromise are thankfully more successful than those for blindness or CNS complications due in part to the level of hypoxia or ischemia that is better tolerated by the skin as opposed to the increased oxygen requirement by the eyes or brain to function properly.

5.6.2 Technique

In regards to injection technique and vascular compromise, there are key points to consider. These aspects include the use of blunt-tipped cannulas, minimal plunger pressure to avoid retrograde flow, use of smaller syringes with less volume, and constant movement of the needle or cannula. Some physicians favor needle injection while withdrawing the needle. The premise behind continual movement of the injection is to avoid delivering a high-volume intravascularly or if flow is obstructed secondary to compression. Injecting perpendicular and not parallel to facial creases is a factor to consider as these creases often develop over deep underlying arterial structures.[7,12,19] Deep tissue scars may stabilize and fix vessels in place, making them more susceptible to shearing or penetration. Tenting the skin is aimed at decreasing the probability of accidental cannulation as the vessel is theoretically less likely to be lifted up in the skin due to its fascial attachments. In addition, manual compression around the injection site to perhaps prevent filler migration into surrounding vasculature is a technique utilized by some injectors particularly in the glabellar region and for nonsurgical rhinoplasty. These latter two areas where vascular events are encountered more frequently can include dire consequences such as significant skin slough or blindness. In summary, individual injection techniques may vary but avoidance of high pressure injections is of supreme importance in avoiding dreaded vascular complications.

5.6.3 Identification

Early recognition of vascular compromise directly correlates with the severity and degree of damage incurred and potential resolution. Failure to recognize the impending vascular event and halt injection is a critical error. Symptoms vary widely and include: subtle to marked blanching lasting seconds to minutes, hyperemia, erythema, pain on injection or in the days following, pustule formation (▶ Fig. 5.3), livedo reticularis–like appearance (▶ Fig. 5.4) to the skin or skin changes resembling a herpetic outbreak. In addition, symptoms including immediate loss or change of vision, nasal obstruction, and more central neurologic findings such as peripheral weakness suggest a more ominous vascular complication.

The clinical presentation of arterial occlusion follows a predictable course from blanching to livedo-like pattern which may be faint yet is highly predictable of an intravascular event. The livedo-like pattern is then replaced by a bluish purple discoloration (▶ Fig. 5.5) and adjacent injured tissue may appear inflamed and show reactive hyperemia with slow capillary refill. The most affected tissue will then turn gray-white, lose capillary refill, and eventually blister. Skin breakdown ensues with varying degrees of epidermal or dermal loss and scarring may develop.

In a recent publication by Fitzgerald et al, special emphasis is made on the presence and recognition of the faint livedoreticularis–like pattern and the early blue-to-purple discoloration that may be either

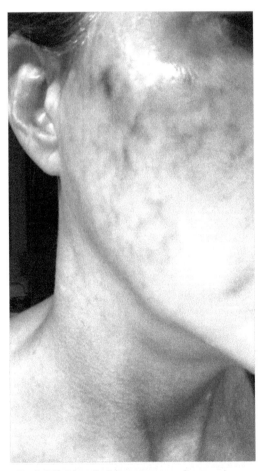

Fig. 5.4 Livedo reticularis appearance after vascular injection to cheek with hyaluronic acid.

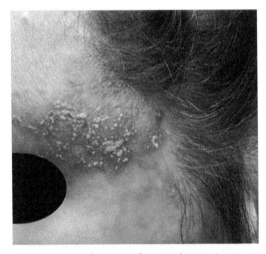

Fig. 5.3 Pustule formation after vascular injection to temple.

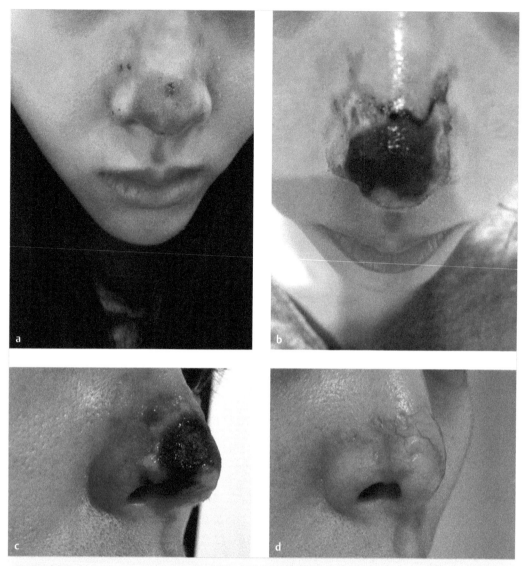

Fig. 5.5 **(a)** Hyaluronic acid intravascular injection to nasal tip with compromise, **(b, c)** tissue necrosis, **(d)** healed with hypertrophic scarring.

seen immediately or delayed.[3] Awareness represents a critical branch point in the management of vascular compromise. These subtle changes are often misinterpreted by physicians, injectors, office staff, and patients themselves as bruising. A differentiating factor between purpura vs. impending vascular compromise is blanching of the effected tissue. Purpura does not blanch whereas the ischemic areas that are violaceous, deeply erythematous, or overtly discolored may blanch. Another key element for early recognition is pain out of proportion to normal

injection-related discomfort. It is critical that not only the injector be aware of such "key indicators" but also that the office staff is properly educated regarding what type of patient complaint mandates prompt attention such as a painful bruise.

5.6.4 Treatment and Management of Vascular Compromise

In general, there exists a direct correlation between early intervention and the extent of permanent sequelae. The first principle in management is timely diagnosis and acknowledgment of what has occurred. Treatment of acute ischemic events centers around rapid restoration of circulation to the affected tissue. For both HA and non-HA fillers a "tool kit" should be immediately accessible with several critical items to help mitigate the impending cascade of complications.

Initial steps include immediate cessation of injection, HYAL injection, and massage with warm compresses. All of which should be accomplished simultaneously. The use of HYAL aids in dispersion and dissolution of the injectable HA and non-HA filler. This should be injected liberally into wherever the vasculature appears compromised in a "flood-the-field" technique.[2] The clinical endpoint for HYAL injection is resolution of ischemia, evidenced by clearing of the livedo pattern, blanching, or bluish discoloration that all herald tissue ischemia. Given the volume of HYAL that may be required to address areas of ischemia, ranging from small segments to a prolific watershed area, the authors advocate that each injector's office should keep at least four to six vials of HYAL readily available. Injection should be immediate and repeated daily in liberal doses where an indication of vascular compromise exists. The Global Aesthetic Consensus guidelines for dosing of HYAL for vascular complications include using doses 450 to 1,500 U over an entire area and along the course of the vessel occluded by serial puncture, continued massages, and heat. Subsequently, the patient should be assessed hourly to ensure capillary refill < 4 seconds. If unresolved, this process should be repeated hourly up to four cycles. The dosage required to alleviate a vascular incident is dependent on several factors.[20] These include whether the filler is particulate or not, amount of cross-linking present, and the concentration used. Studies have assessed how HYAL affects different types of HA degradation in a time- and dose-dependent manner with varying results. The most recent studies by Kim et al demonstrated that Belotero was fastest to dissolve as compared to higher cross-linked products such as Juvederm Ultra and Restylane Lyft.[5] The most important take away is that the literature offers a range of doses for filler dissolution. It is recommended to inject as much HYAL required to obtain the desired effect.[21] For completeness sake, with such high volumes of HYAL use, whether it be of animal origin or human recombinant HYAL, the risk of anaphylaxis is a rare but recognized risk of HYAL treatment, and it is advisable to have epinephrine available in the office, should this situation arise.

Other adjunctive strategies aimed at increasing circulation include aspirin 325 mg to be chewed by the patient, topical nitroglycerin paste (1%) applied to the area, and administration of vasodilators, such as sildenafil.[3] In addition, the use of systemic or topical steroids, and low-molecular-weight heparin have all been recommended with varying degrees of reported efficacy. The authors also advocate for the early use of empiric antibiotics, given the relationship between compromised vascularity in any wound and the propensity for development of infection.

Hyperbaric oxygen therapy has also been used with some frequency for management of vascular ischemic events secondary to HA and non-HA fillers. Hyperbaric's well-established role is for use in facilitating wound healing with compromised vascularity. The premise behind hyperbaric oxygen (HBO) is grounded in the ability to deliver oxygen at deeper levels in order to help sustain the viability of oxygen-dependent tissues. Promising case reports have been published and anecdotal experiences have been shared recently involving the use of HBO for treatment of occlusive events from calcium hydroxylapatite and poly-L-lactic acid (PLLA).[3,22] If available for use, the authors advocate early consideration of HBO therapy. This may take up to 6 weeks until reperfusion is established via neovascularization. The duration (number of dives) and frequency of therapy is again based on clinical gestalt, but if not prohibitively expensive or a major inconvenience, even for relatively small vascular complications its potential role should not be overlooked.

5.7 Specific Considerations

5.7.1 Blindness

Blindness, perhaps the most feared vascular complication, is reported in the literature with increasing frequency. This is due to the numerous anastomoses between the carotid circulations. Nearly every anatomic location on the face where filler is injected is a risk for blindness.[18] Approximately half of the cases of blindness involved autologous fat injection and were not reversible; the other half were due to dermal fillers. Majority of blindness cases reported are secondary to HA filler and are also rarely reversible. In 2015, the FDA issued a safety alert to consumers regarding the possibility of the occurrence of unintentional injection of soft tissue filler into blood vessels in the face, including the possibility of blindness and stroke. Due in part to the severity of the complication but also given the frequency of dermal filler injection treatments, a frank discussion regarding vascular complications including the risk of blindness and other vascular-related events should be part of both the written and verbal consent process undertaken between the injector and patient.

In the event of blindness secondary to dermal filler placement, vision loss or change and ocular pain are the most common presenting symptoms. Through mechanisms described above, the patient is also at risk of interval development of CNS complications if treatment is not immediate. Treatment strategies for ocular complications include immediate referral to an ophthalmologic specialist capable of retrobulbar injections of HYAL; ideally in an emergency room setting as opposed to outpatient clinics in the instance CNS disturbances develop (which may require neurointerventional procedures). Chesnut recently published a protocol for treating blindness secondary to HA injection.[23] Additional measurements to improve retinal perfusion described include ocular massage, topical timolol eye drops used to reduce pressure, diuretics (acetazolamide 500 mg PO or IV), and needle decompression of the anterior chamber. Should this rare, but real, devastating complication occur, one's individual practice protocol should be readily visible to all staff and listed in a central location near the treatment rooms as well as contact numbers for ophthalmologic referrals and the closest hospital with capabilities of treating these neurologic sequelae.

5.8 Delayed Adverse Reactions and Management of Complications

Nodules and granulomas are terms often used interchangeably but represent two distinct histopathologic entities. Noninflammatory nodules or papules represent an overabundance of product with scant foreign body giant cells on histology. Granulomas alternatively are true inflammatory lesions representing an overzealous host response to the product with an abundance of foreign body giant cells and inflammatory infiltrate on histology.

5.8.1 Noninflammatory Nodules

Noninflammatory nodules develop most commonly around the lips or eyes. Early nodules are due to incorrect filler placement and the main treatment strategy is prevention or the use of HYAL if the nodule has a delayed presentation (> 2 wk).

Fibrotic noninflammatory nodules occur days to weeks after injection with PLLA, calcium hydroxylapatite (CaHA), and polymethyl-methacrylate microspheres (PMMA) and occur less frequently with clinical experience. Preventative techniques include avoiding overcorrection, proper depth of placement, and avoiding highly mobile areas. These substances are thought to stimulate fibroplasia through a foreign body reaction and have characteristically little inflammation. Given that these nodules are due to an abundance of product, intralesional steroids or 5-fluorouracil/antimetabolite injections are not recommended. Surgical excision may be offered or one may elect to camouflage the asymmetries until the substance is metabolized.

5.8.2 Inflammatory Reactions Including Infection and Granuloma Formation

Late or delayed onset inflammatory reactions include infectious etiologies as well as granuloma formation.

Late onset infectious etiologies (greater than 2 wk) may be secondary to less common microbes including atypical mycobacterium. Specific late onset infectious complications and nodules from atypical mycobacterium are well-documented in the current surgical and nonsurgical cosmetic literature.[2,7,12] Rodriguez et al provide details of an experience with mycobacterial infections after HA dermal filler injections, which was ultimately traced back to ice cubes placed on the injection site from a compromised water supply at the clinical site.[24] Often the atypical mycobacterial infections will resolve with clarithromycin monotherapy, although some patterns of rapidly growing mycobacteria require multiple drug therapy.

One of the most common presentations of late and delayed reactions are granulomas which are a result of an exaggerated immune response to dermal filler. The exact trigger of this inappropriate immune response is widely unknown. Theories regarding antigenic stimulation as well as manufacturing specifics have been hypothesized yet not proven. A more recent theory is that of a low-grade infection that implicates biofilm formation in this delayed excessive immune response.

Nodules can appear weeks to years after dermal filler placement. It represents a systemic reaction and lesions may suddenly appear and at all treated sites. Regarding treatment, the first tenet is removal of the offending agent which is not always possible. With HA filler, HYAL can be used to dissolve product and may require multiple treatments. Caution is required with HYAL use in terms of avoidance of HYAL in the setting of active infection/cellulitis to prevent dispersion of infection into surrounding tissue. In terms of removal, fractional laser has also been utilized to allow product extrusion and egress. In longer lasting filler, treatment of granulomas with serial injection of low doses of triamcinolone plus 5-fluorouracil for a total of 1 mL injected at regular intervals (weekly × 2, every 2 weeks × 2, then monthly) has been successful.[25] In cases of repeated failure of other therapies, surgical excision is the treatment of choice for foreign-body granuloma.

Empiric antibiotic therapy has been recommended by a recent global consensus panel on management of complications due to dermal filler and the possible role of biofilms in the development of late and delayed complications.[2] Empiric therapy consists of clarithromycin 500 mg plus moxifloxacin 400 mg twice daily for 10 days, or ciprofloxacin 500 to 750 mg twice daily for 2 to 4 weeks, or minocycline 100 mg daily for 6 months.

A recently described treatment option for infectious or granulomatous lesions is the use of a minimally invasive laser technique (a 808-nm diode laser) that is capable of removing the foreign substance along with the inflammatory reaction. The laser is delivered intralesionally through a percutaneous insertion of a 200-μm laser into the lesion and drilling several small holes. Manual palpation confirms softening of the lesion, which is the clinical endpoint as the polymer is now more fluid. The liquefied material is then manually expressed through the skin entrance points of the probe and with removal of the implant it is presumed to be curative.[26]

References

[1] Cosmetic (Aesthetic) Surgery National Data Bank Statistics ASAPS. 2018. https://www.surgery.org/sites/default/files/ASAPS-Stats2018_0.pdf

[2] Signorini M, Liew S, Sundaram H, et al. Global Aesthetics Consensus Group. Global Aesthetics Consensus: avoidance and management of complications from hyaluronic acid fillers-evidence- and opinion-based review and consensus recommendations. Plast Reconstr Surg. 2016; 137(6):961e–971e

[3] Fitzgerald R, Bertucci V, Sykes JM, Duplechain JK. Adverse reactions to injectable fillers. Facial Plast Surg. 2016; 32(5):532–555

[4] De Boulle K, Heydenrych I, On behalf of the Consensus Group. Patient factors influencing dermal filler complications: prevention, assessment, and treatment. Clin CosmetInvestig Dermatol. 2015; 8:205–214

[5] Kim DW, Yoon ES, Ji YH, Park SH, Lee BI, Dhong ES. Vascular complications of hyaluronic acid fillers and the role of hyaluronidase in management. J Plast Reconstr Aesthet Surg. 2011; 64(12):1590–1595

[6] Narins RS, Coleman WP, Glogau RG. Recommendation and treatment options for nodules and other filler complications. DermatolSurg. 2009; 35 Suppl 2:1667–1671

[7] Dayan SH. Complications from toxins and fillers in the dermatology clinic: recognition, prevention, and treatment. Facial PlastSurgClin North Am. 2013; 21(4):663–673

[8] Darouiche RO, Wall MJ, Jr, Itani KM, et al. Chlorhexidine-alcohol versus povidone-iodine for surgical-site antisepsis. N Engl J Med. 2010; 362(1):18–26

[9] Bailey SH, Cohen JL, Kenkel JM. Etiology, prevention, and treatment of dermal filler complications. AesthetSurg J. 2011; 31(1):110–121

[10] Lee GS. Use of AccuVein™ for preventing complications from accidental venipuncture when administering dermal filler injections. J Cosmet Laser Ther. 2015; 17(1):55–56

[11] Zeichner JA, Cohen JL. Use of blunt tipped cannulas for soft tissue fillers. J Drugs Dermatol. 2012; 11(1):70–72

[12] Rohrich RJ, Bartlett EL, Dayan E. Practical approach and safety of hyaluronic acid fillers. PlastReconstrSurg Glob Open. 2019; 7(6):e2172

[13] Pavicic T, Frank K, Erlbacher K, et al. Precision in dermal filling: a comparison between needle and cannula when using soft tissue fillers. J Drugs Dermatol. 2017; 16(9):866–872

[14] Hexsel D, Soirefmann M, Porto MD, Siega C, Schilling-Souza J, Brum C. Double-blind, randomized, controlled clinical trial to compare safety and efficacy of a metallic cannula with that of a standard needle for soft tissue augmentation of the nasolabial folds. Dermatol Surg. 2012; 38(2):207–214

[15] Leonhardt JM, Lawrence N, Narins RS. Angioedema acute hypersensitivity reaction to injectable hyaluronic acid. Dermatol Surg. 2005; 31(5):577–579

[16] Lupton JR, Alster TS. Cutaneous hypersensitivity reaction to injectable hyaluronic acid gel. Dermatol Surg. 2000; 26(2):135–137

[17] DeLorenzi C. Complications of injectable fillers, part I. Aesthet Surg J. 2013; 33(4):561–575

[18] Carruthers JD, Fagien S, Rohrich RJ, Weinkle S, Carruthers A. Blindness caused by cosmetic filler injection: a review of cause and therapy. Plast Reconstr Surg. 2014; 134(6):1197–1201

[19] Beleznay K, Carruthers JDA, Humphrey S, Carruthers A, Jones D. Update on avoiding and treating blindness from fillers: a recent review of the world literature. Aesthet Surg J. 2019; 39(6):662–674

[20] King M, Convery C, Davies E. This month's guideline: the use of hyaluronidase in aesthetic practice (v2.4). J Clin Aesthet Dermatol. 2018; 11(6):E61–E68

[21] DeLorenzi C. Complications of injectable fillers, part 2: vascular complications. Aesthet Surg J. 2014; 34(4):584–600

[22] Darling MD, Peterson JD, Fabi SG. Impending necrosis after injection of hyaluronic acid and calcium hydroxylapatite fillers: report of 2 cases treated with hyperbaric oxygen therapy. Dermatol Surg. 2014; 40(9):1049–1052

[23] Chesnut C. Restoration of visual loss with retrobulbar hyaluronidase injection after hyaluronic acid filler. DermatolSurg. 2018; 44(3):435–437

[24] Rodriguez JM, et al. Mycobacterial infection following injection of dermal fillers. Aesthet Surg J. 2013; 33(20): 265–9

[25] Graivier MH, Bass LM, Lorenc ZP, Fitzgerald R, Goldberg DJ, Lemperle G. Differentiating nonpermanent injectable fillers: prevention and treatment of filler complications. AesthetSurg J. 2018; 38 Suppl_1:S29–40

[26] Cassuto D, Marangoni O, De Santis G, Christensen L. Advanced laser techniques for filler-induced complications. Dermatol Surg. 2009; 35 Suppl 2:1689–1695

6 Fat Transfers

Stephen E. Metzinger and Rebecca C. Metzinger

Summary

As with all cosmetic procedures, autologous fat grafting (AFG) or transfer (AFT) carries risks along with benefits. The benefits are well established and well documented; these include correcting facial imperfections and asymmetries, adding volume with the patient's own nonallergenic, autologous material and the benefits of adipose-derived stem cells. The ideal implant material is nonantigenic, durable, nontoxic, and resistant to infection. In terms of an injectable filler, fat comes closest to this ideal. It is important to consider the risks, benefits, potential complications, alternative treatments, and imponderables of fat transfer before electing to perform this procedure. As the benefits have been mentioned above and widely elucidated elsewhere, this chapter will focus on the description of possible risks and complications of facial fat transfer.

Keywords: fat transfer, complications blindness, CVA necrosis, atypical mycobacterium, embolism expectations

6.1 Introduction

Fat injection as a cosmetic treatment is natural, versatile, long-lasting, and safe. Fat transfer has become a preferred method of facial volume enhancement for patients who are allergic to traditional dermal fillers such as bovine-derived collagen, or simply prefer autologous material. One of the biggest benefits of volume enhancement via fat injection is that there is absolutely no chance of an adverse allergic reaction to the injected material. Another popular reason for choosing fat transfer/injection is the duration of benefit. Even though up to 50% of injected fat will be reabsorbed into the body within a few months of the fat injection, the remaining 50% will usually last for years. For longer lasting results, many patients choose to have several fat transfer sessions over the course of a few months. This approach helps with precision and seems to improve durability.

6.2 Risks and Complications

Fat transfer risks are few, rare, and usually minimal. Soreness and edema are the norms, but not experienced by every patient. The most significant downside of the procedure is that your face may simply reabsorb all or most of the injected fat. This may be technique dependent, but can happen in the most experienced of hands. The chances of this happening can't be predicted for a given individual, but it happens in up to 35% of all patients who receive fat injection treatments to the face.

Complications of fat transfer are uncommon but can include reaction to anesthesia, permanent or temporary discoloration caused by blood vessel injury at the treatment site, Tyndall effect, calcification, a distorted look if overcorrection is permanent, perioperative bleeding, a blood clot at the treatment or donor site, a blood-borne infection, venous thromboembolism, scar tissue, fat necrosis, and a fat embolism due to fat injection into a blood vessel which can cause necrosis, blindness, central nervous system (CNS) complications or even death.

Being disappointed with the results of a fat transfer procedure is also considered a risk; therefore, setting realistic expectations is a must. Discussion of all patient concerns and desires before undergoing a fat transfer procedure is mandatory and should be documented. The placement of the fat transfer may not be adequate, the patient may reject the transfer, or the duration of the effect may not be to the patient's expectation. It is possible, the patient's face or lips may not look exactly as they had envisioned. Lips can be challenging both due to potential trauma during the procedure and the constant motion of the orbicularis oris.

6.3 Vascular Occlusion

Visual loss is one of the most severe complications reported in patients undergoing facial filler procedures. In the majority of reported cases, visual deterioration was severe and irreversible[1,2,3] (▸ Fig. 6.1). Visual loss can be caused by ophthalmic artery occlusion (OAO), central retinal artery occlusion (CRAO), either localized or generalized posterior ciliary artery occlusion (PCAO) with sparing of the central retinal artery, branch retinal artery occlusion (BRAO) or posterior ischemic optic neuropathy (PION). Autologous fat injections are associated with the most severe visual impairment (CRAO or OAO).[1,2,4,5] Due to differences in particle size among the different types of facial fillers, patients with ocular symptoms following other types of fillers, such as hyaluronic acid injections, are more

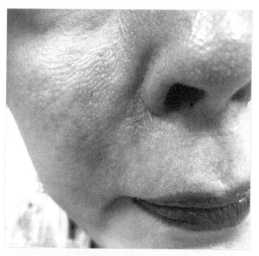

Fig. 6.1 POD #7 S/P fat grafting to the nasolabial folds. Patient with pain and tingling in the affected area. Treatment was with hyaluronidase, 325 mg aspirin, 1% nitroglycerine paste. No visual or central nervous system (CNS) changes.

likely to suffer from localized ocular occlusion with milder clinical manifestations and better visual prognosis than patients who received autologous fat injections.[2,4,5,6] Preventative strategies proposed in the literature to reduce the risk of vascular complications following fat injections include: using small-diameter nontraumatic blunt-tip cannulas instead of sharp cannulas and needles, limiting syringe size to 1 mL, aspirating before injection, injecting the filler slowly with minimal pressure, limiting the amount of filler to less than 0.1 mL with each pass, mixing the filler with vasoconstrictor, using a topical vasoconstrictor before injection, and moving the needle tip while injecting.[2,3,7,8] Avoiding injection at the sites of previous trauma, or at sites with chronic inflammation or scarring, is also advised. Facial filler injections should be performed with extra caution in patients who have previously undergone facial or plastic surgeries.[2,3,9]

According to the literature, no fully effective treatment for CRAO or OAO is available. Nevertheless, there are several papers presenting various treatment modalities that recover some degree of visual function for the patient. The aim of the treatment after facial fat or filler embolism is to restore the perfusion of the retina as soon as possible. The retina is very sensitive to hypoxia, and after 90 minutes damage due to retinal ischemia becomes permanent.[2,3,10,11,12] Most previously reported cases of vision loss secondary to fat

embolism have remained without any improvement. Therefore, no evidence-based treatment strategies are available. Slightly better outcomes have been reported in cases of vision loss following injection of fillers other than autologous fat.[2,3] From 23 cases of ocular complications following injections of hyaluronic acid into the facial area, permanent vision loss was observed in 9 cases, and in 6 cases some level of improvement in visual acuity was reported.[2] Early, immediate identification of arterial occlusion is key with treatment aimed at lowering intraocular pressure to boost retinal perfusion, dilating arteries to eliminate embolus or dislodging embolus to a more peripheral location, and reducing the inflammatory component of the injury. To decrease intraocular pressure, Diamox (PO, IV, or OS) or mannitol (IV) is immediately given if there are no contraindications, eye drops are administered (e.g., alpha agonists, B-blockers, carbonic anhydrase inhibitors), and ocular massage and anterior chamber paracentesis are performed. Carbon dioxide and oxygen inhalation or vasodilatory agents such as prostaglandin E1 provoke arterial dilation. Hyperbaric oxygen therapy and systemic corticosteroids decrease the inflammatory response.[1,2,9,10,11,12] ► Table 6.1 presents the currently recommended treatments and their underlying mechanism of action.

The crucial factor in the management strategy is the immediate assessment and referral to the ophthalmologist or retina specialist, to start the proper treatment within the 90-minute time span after which the damage to the retina is irreversible.[6,12] Loh et al[12] have proposed a treatment algorithm for managing vision loss following filler injections. When a patient presents the first symptoms of vascular compromise in the retina, filler injection should be instantly stopped and the patient should be laid in a supine position. Immediate treatment (including topical instillation of timolol, and/or oral acetazolamide and ocular massage) should be administered by a nonophthalmologist injector before arranging and transferring the patient to a specialist for a definitive therapy, which consists of further medical administration and—when indicated—anterior chamber paracentesis. In cases of hyaluronic acid–induced vision loss, hyaluronidase may be used to dissolve hyaluronic acid emboli.[1,2,3,4,5,6,7,8,9,10,11,12,13,14] Unfortunately, there is no effect on fat. After these acute measures have been taken, additional supportive therapy (corticosteroids, hyperbaric oxygen therapy, anticoagulants) should be introduced to protect retinal cells.

Table 6.1 Currently recommended treatments for vision loss following autologous fat injections into facial area

Treatment	Mechanism of action
Timolol 0.5% drop administered topically	Lowers intraocular pressure and dislodges the embolus to a more peripheral downstream location[2,3,5]
Acetazolamide 500 mg per os or intravenously	Reduces intraocular pressure that may increase blood flow in the retina[3]
Nitroglycerin 2% paste or sublingual isosorbide dinitrate or systemic pentoxifylline	Dilates the retinal arteries[3,13]
Intravenous infusion of mannitol 20% (100 mL over 30 min)	Lowers intraocular pressure and dislodges the embolus to a more peripheral downstream location[3,5]
Ocular massage—performed digitally or using a Goldmann fundus contact lens[5]	Decreases intraocular pressure and increases blood flow in the arterioles, potentially dislodging the embolus[3,5,14]
Anterior chamber paracentesis	Rapidly reduces intraocular pressure and encourages blood flow in the retina[2,3]
Systemic and topical corticosteroids	Decreases retinal edema and inflammatory reaction[3,9]
Hyperbaric oxygen therapy	Reverses any salvageable retinal damage[5,9]
Inhalation of carbogen (95% oxygen with 5% carbon dioxide)	Dilates the retinal arteries and increases delivery of oxygen[2,3]
Intravenous prostaglandin E1	Causes vasodilatation and increases blood flow in the retina, decreases activation of thrombocytes, improves cell metabolism by increasing oxygenation, decreases activation of neutrophils and the release of their toxic metabolites, helping to reduce tissue damage from inflammation and possibly from hypoxia[2,3,9]
Anticoagulation with oral acetylsalicylic acid or low-molecular-weight heparin	Prevents further thrombosis[3,5]

In previously reported cases, the treatment provided has usually been incomplete, since the majority of patients suffering from ocular complications received at most a 3-step therapy.[3,9] As noted by Chen et al,[3] combination therapy may contribute to the recovery of visual symptoms. In addition to commonly used treatment options such as ocular massage, acetazolamide, mannitol, and corticosteroids, alprostadil and vinpocetine have been successfully used in the treatment regimen. Alprostadil is a synthetic variant of prostaglandin E1. It causes vasodilatation through directly affecting the vascular smooth muscles and increases blood flow in the retina. Alprostadil also decreases thrombocyte activation, improves cell metabolism by increasing oxygen supply to the tissues, and decreases neutrophil activation and the release of their toxic metabolites, helping to reduce tissue damage caused by inflammation and possibly by hypoxia. The use of prostaglandin E1 as a part of comprehensive therapy for visual loss following hyaluronic acid injection was also reported by Chen et al.[3] This resulted in improvement in visual acuity, extraocular movement, and visual field defects. Vinpocetine, chemically known as ethyl apovincamine, is a vinca alkaloid that increases cerebral blood flow and has neuroprotective effects.[15] This drug is used in the treatment of ischemic cerebrovascular diseases and vascular dementia. Vinpocetine may help to increase retinal perfusion (▶ Table 6.1).

6.4 Atypical Infections

The differential diagnoses of delayed nodule formation after autologous fat grafting (AFG) include fat necrosis and atypical infection. Atypical infections reported include nontuberculous mycobacteria (NTM) infection after AFG for facial augmentation. In these reported cases, multiple flesh-colored and erythematous nodules and tumors developed 6 weeks after the initial procedure. Tissue cultures yielded *Mycobacterium abscessus*, *Mycobacterium chelonae*, *Mycobacterium fortuitum*, and *Mycobacterium avium-intracellulare*. Some presented with concurrent sinus tracts and fistulas.

Cases of chronic infection have been reported in patients who received a cryopreserved facial fat graft. A 22-year-old female patient presented with multiple abscesses of her face. Four months prior, she received a second fat graft with the fat harvested at a previous surgery which was cryopreserved for 2 months. On examination, she had tender erythematous nodules on both cheeks. A computed tomography scan of her neck showed multiple peripheral enhancing nodular lesions. In an open pus fungus culture, *Aspergillus fumigatus* growth was observed. On the mycobacterium other than tuberculosis identification polymerase chain reaction (PCR), *M. fortuitum* was found. She was treated with levofloxacin, clarithromycin, and minocycline for 11 months, and finally, the symptoms subsided. To avoid infection after the fat graft, cryopreserved fat should not be used. In cases of persistent infection, or in cases where the infection waxes and wanes after drainage of pus and short-term antibiotics therapy, atypical *Mycobacterium* or *Aspergillus* should be suspected and a PCR for them should be carried out.

Mycobacterium conceptionense is a nonpigmented member of the rapidly growing mycobacteria (RGM) that was first described as a novel species belonging to the *M. fortuitum* group in 2006 after isolation from the wound samples of a patient with posttraumatic osteitis.[16] The bacterium was later reported as causing a subcutaneous abscess in an immunocompetent patient.[17] Another case of *M. conceptionense* infection in a patient following aesthetic surgery with fat grafting has been reported. This subspecies is very difficult to treat and may only respond to surgical excision. In all cases of atypical infection whether they be mycobacterium or fungal we recommend infectious disease consultation.

6.5 Fat Necrosis

Fat necrosis resulting from AFG performed for facial augmentation has been less extensively reported and is noteworthy of recognition especially due to the potential for permanent scarring.

There may be several factors relevant to the causation of fat necrosis post AFG, which include preoperative patient selection, intraoperative and postoperative risk factors. Special consideration must be given to the identification of any underlying inflammatory dermatoses prior to the performance of AFG and ensuring correct patient selection for this procedure. An underlying active inflammatory dermatosis may accelerate lipolysis of the transferred fat due to the body's inherent defense response to areas of infection or inflammation.

AFG as a procedure requires operator skill as well as practice and precision. This sets this procedure apart from other intradermal fillers as a high level of skill is involved in the harvesting, the preparation, and the injection of the fat. Factors that have been reported to improve graft survival include:
1. Low vascularity of the donor site.
2. High vascularity of the recipient site.
3. A low-pressure technique used to aspirate the fat.
4. Skillful washing and preparation of fat.
5. A sufficiently large cannula.
6. The use of a multilayered approach to replace the fat.
7. Do not overfill the defect as this may also impair graft survival depending on the blood supply.

It is possible that a delayed hypersensitivity response to the prepared fat may also be a cause for graft failure. This may be compounded if the fat is not replaced in its pure form, i.e., after washing off any residual blood and tumescent anesthesia collected at the time of harvesting. An autologous fat transfer may lead to complications other than fat necrosis. The early recognition and treatment of these complications enhance a clinician's procedure prowess.

Some other complications include rapid absorption of the replaced fat. This is exacerbated by the presence of blood, damaged fat cells, and high-pressure technique. Infection presenting pre-, intra-, or postoperatively may affect graft survival. Viral infections or warty growths have also been reported at the site of cannula entry. Cyst formation is more common when a large amount of fat is transferred. Calcification of fat posttransfer has been reported particularly when used for breast augmentation and may present as breast lumps.[2] Calcification may lead to ossification over time. This can be seen in the face as well. Skin necrosis and sinus formation may result from overfilling or overaugmentation of the desired site (▶ Fig. 6.2, ▶ Fig. 6.3, ▶ Fig. 6.4, ▶ Fig. 6.5). Compression atrophy may result from overaugmentation with associated avascular necrosis due to excessive pressure on vasculature which can result in arterial or venous thrombosis. Hematoma (▶ Fig. 6.6) or seroma formation may occur more commonly if blunt cannulae are not used and when the patient is on other anticoagulant medication or supplements providing an anticoagulant effect. Iatrogenic injury to the nerves and blood vessels of the face may also be seen.

Transferred fat often behaves as it would at the donor site. This includes a rare but recognized side effect that can be seen if fat is transferred from areas such as the buffalo hump to the face in the form of facial fat hypertrophy or "Hamster syndrome" due to the resultant swollen facial appearance resembling a hamster.

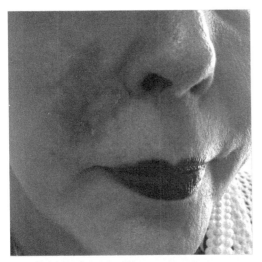

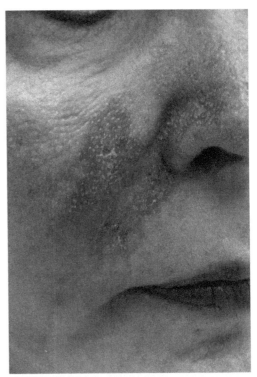

Fig. 6.2 POD # 15 S/P fat grafting to nasolabial fold and treatment with hyaluronidase, aspirin and nitro past. After one week added dimethyl sulfoxide (DMSO). Notice blisters and skin slough. The contralateral side is within normal limits. No visual or central nervous system (CNS) symptoms.

Fig. 6.3 POD #22 S/P fat grafting to nasolabial fold. Treatment with hyaluronidase, acetylsalicylic acid (ASA or commonly called Aspirin), nitro paste, and dimethyl sulfoxide (DMSO). Skin slough spreading to the nose. Added hyperbaric oxygen therapy. Notice the redness and blisters continue to progress.

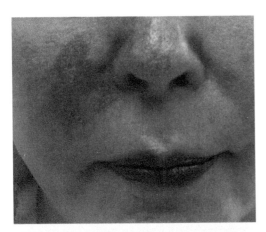

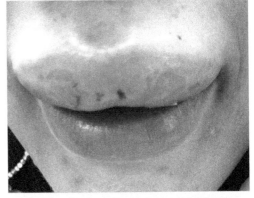

Fig. 6.4 POD # 25 after 3 hyperbaric oxygen (HBO) dives with hyaluronidase, acetylsalicylic acid (ASA or commonly called Aspirin), nitropaste, dimethyl sulfoxide (DMSO) the spread has finally stopped and the skin is beginning to heal. The patient also on day #14 of doxycycline 100 mg PO every 12 hours and topical bactroban two times a day.

Fig. 6.5 POD #2 S/P upper and lower lip fat grafting. Large hematoma deep in the upper lip with pain, blister, and distortion. Treatment was with Bromelain 500 mg three times a day, Valtrex 1 g PO q day, arnica gel to lips three times a day, and Keflex 500 mg PO three times a day for 5 days. Caution with herbal remedies both preop and postop.

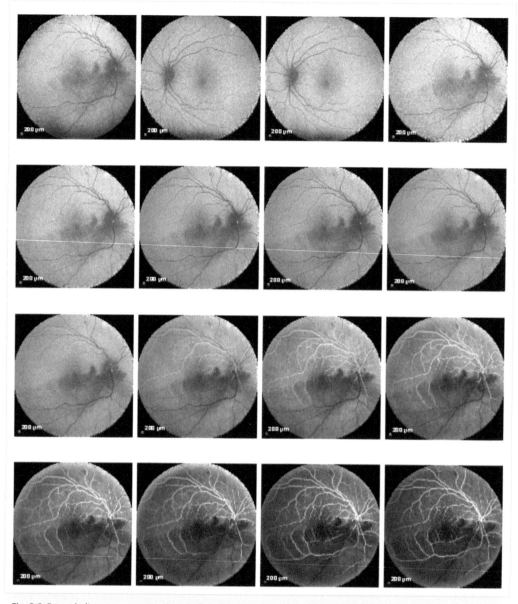

Fig. 6.6 Fat embolism on retina view (IVFA) after glabellar injection. Visual loss with progressive loss of vascularity from the central retinal artery. There was no recovery of vision despite maximal treatment including carbogen and retrobulbar hyaluronidase. Carotid duplex and computed tomography angiography (CTA) confirmed no carotid disease.

6.6 Treatment of Facial Fat Necrosis

An area of fat necrosis can resolve without any treatment. Massaging the area firmly can help resolve some of the firmness. However, if an area or areas of fat necrosis are particularly bothersome to a person, a surgeon can perform several removal options:

Injection with dilute corticosteroid, plus or minus dilute 5-FU: This must be done judiciously and may require more than one treatment. In this situation, less is more when paired with massage.

Needle aspiration: This procedure involves inserting a thin, hollow needle into the area of fat necrosis to drain the oily contents. This will usually cause the lump to disappear. Massage after aspiration is also helpful.

Surgical removal: If the lump is larger or in a difficult place to access with a needle aspiration procedure, the lump may be removed surgically.

6.7 Conclusion

The common use of facial injections, most often performed in aesthetic medicine, has resulted in an increased number of ocular and CNS complications. Immediate ophthalmological intervention and comprehensive therapy potentially including prostaglandins and vinpocetine may make it possible to restore retinal perfusion and achieve better recovery of visual acuity. However, most reported episodes have resulted in permanent sequelae.

Awareness of iatrogenic artery occlusions associated with facial fat grafting and the need for immediate treatment should be popularized among injectors to prevent devastating consequences such as permanent vision loss and stroke. Strict aseptic technique should always be used at both donor and recipient sites. If nodules appear, consider atypical mycobacterium, fungal infections, and fat necrosis. Early and appropriate treatment is key to success.

References

[1] Park SW, Woo SJ, Park KH, Huh JW, Jung C, Kwon OK. Iatrogenic retinal artery occlusion caused by cosmetic facial filler injections. Am J Ophthalmol. 2012; 154(4):653–662.e1

[2] Beleznay K, Carruthers JD, Humphrey S, Jones D. Avoiding and treating blindness from fillers: a review of the world literature. Dermatol Surg. 2015; 41(10):1097–1117

[3] Chen W, Wu L, Jian XL, et al. Retinal branch artery embolization following hyaluronic acid injection: a case report. Aesthet Surg J. 2016; 36(7):NP219–NP224

[4] Park KH, Kim YK, Woo SJ, et al. Korean Retina Society. Iatrogenic occlusion of the ophthalmic artery after cosmetic facial filler injections: a national survey by the Korean Retina Society. JAMA Ophthalmol. 2014; 132(6):714–723

[5] Carruthers JD, Fagien S, Rohrich RJ, Weinkle S, Carruthers A. Blindness caused by cosmetic filler injection: a review of cause and therapy. Plast Reconstr Surg. 2014; 134(6):1197–1201

[6] Chen CS, Lee AW. Management of acute central retinal artery occlusion. Nat Clin Pract Neurol. 2008; 4(7):376–383

[7] Coleman SR. Avoidance of arterial occlusion from injection of soft tissue fillers. Aesthet Surg J. 2002; 22(6):555–557

[8] Yoshimura K, Coleman SR. Complications of fat grafting how they occur and how to find, avoid, and treat them. Clin Plast Surg. 2015; 42(3):383–388, ix

[9] Lazzeri D, Agostini T, Figus M, Nardi M, Pantaloni M, Lazzeri S. Blindness following cosmetic injections of the face. Plast Reconstr Surg. 2012; 129(4):995–1012

[10] Hwang CJ. Periorbital injectables: understanding and avoiding complications. J Cutan Aesthet Surg. 2016; 9(2):73–79

[11] DeLorenzi C. Complications of injectable fillers, part 2: vascular complications. Aesthet Surg J. 2014; 34(4):584–600

[12] Loh KT, Chua JJ, Lee HM, et al. Prevention and management of vision loss relating to facial filler injections. Singapore Med J. 2016; 57(8):438–443

[13] Rumelt S, Dorenboim Y, Rehany U. Aggressive systematic treatment for central retinal artery occlusion. Am J Ophthalmol. 1999; 128(6):733–738

[14] Li X, Du L, Lu JJ. A novel hypothesis of visual loss secondary to cosmetic facial filler injection. Ann Plast Surg. 2015; 75(3):258–260

[15] Patyar S, Prakash A, Modi M, Medhi B. Role of vinpocetine in cerebrovascular diseases. Pharmacol Rep. 2011; 63(3):618–628

[16] Adékambi, T., A. Stein, J. Carvajal, et al. Description of Mycobacterium conceptionense sp. nov., a Mycobacterium fortuitum group organism isolated from a post-traumatic osteitis. J Clin Microbiol. 2006; 44:1268–1273

[17] Chun-Hsing Liao CH, Lai CC, Huang YT, et al. Subcutaneous abscess caused by Mycobacterium conceptionense in an immunocompetent patient. J Infect. 2009; 58(4), 308–309

7 Neuromodulators for Muscle Induced Wrinkles

Timothy M. Greco, Lisa Coppa-Breslauer, and Jason E. Cohn

Summary

This chapter describes the use of neuromodulators for rejuvenation in the face and neck. Neuromodulators have now been expanded to improve facial shaping, correct facial asymmetry, and even improve skin texture and tone. The different FDA-approved neuromodulators include onabotulinum (Ona), abobotulinum (Abo), and incobotulinum (Inco). The clinical approach can be broken down into four anatomical regions: the upper face, midface, lower face, and neck. The key muscles of the upper face include frontalis, orbital and pretarsal orbicularis oculi, corrugator supercilii, and procerus. The muscles in the midface that are discussed include the nasalis, zygomaticus major, zygomaticus minor, levator anguli oris, levator labii superioris, levator labii superioris alaeque nasi, and depressor septi nasi. Treatment of the lower face focuses on the orbicularis oris, depressor anguli oris (DAO), depressor labii inferioris (DLI), mentalis, and masseter muscles. Finally, treatment of the neck region is reviewed with emphasis on platysmal bands and necklace lines as well as the Nefertiti lift. Pearls are emphasized in order to demonstrate safe and effective treatment of these regions as well as the avoidance and treatment of complications.

Keywords: facial rejuvenation, neuromodulator, botulinum, facial plastic surgery, cosmetic surgery, aesthetic surgery, dermatology, avoidance and treatment of complications

7.1 Introduction

Neuromodulators for the treatment of muscle-induced wrinkles of the head and neck have become the most popular procedure in aesthetic medicine. Due to an increase in the interest of patients looking younger without undergoing more invasive procedures with extended recovery periods, neuromodulators have become an important tool in the armamentarium to the aesthetic physician. The interest in neuromodulators and their success has sparked an increase in a better understanding of the muscles of facial expression. There has been a renewed interest in cadaver dissections, which has resulted in a better understanding of the origin, insertions, actions, and aesthetic implications of the muscles of facial expression. In addition, these dissections may have helped decrease the complications of neuromodulator injections in the face and neck. It should be noted that neuromodulators initially were used to treat wrinkles of the face but now have been expanded to improve facial shaping, correct facial asymmetry, and even improve skin texture and tone. It is important that when injecting the facial musculature that one has a firm grasp of the differences between the FDA-approved neuromodulators, which include Botox™ (onabotulinum), Xeomin™ (incobotulnum), and Dysport™ (abobotulinum). Throughout this chapter, the face is discussed in regions as da Vinci has described. However, there are no boundaries between regions, instead a continuum that exists from the frontalis muscle to the platysma, which is important in understanding the effects of the muscles of facial expression on adjacent and distant areas when aesthetic neuromodulator treatments are applied to the face. It is not only important to understand the anatomy of the muscles but also the dilution of the product (▶ Table 7.1, ▶ Table 7.2, ▶ Table 7.3, ▶ Table 7.4), the characteristics of needle used for placement (length and gauge), and the angle, force, and depth of injection. All of these factors are critical to the final result and help to avoid complications.

7.2 Upper Face

Neuromodulators are commonly used in the upper face to minimize wrinkles due to muscular contraction. The muscles that benefit the most from neuromodulators in this anatomic area are the frontalis, procerus, corrugator supercilii, and orbicularis oculi (▶ Fig. 7.1). These injections help to minimize the appearance of facial lines including vertical glabellar rhytids (corrugator supercilii), horizontal glabellar rhytids (procerus), horizontal forehead rhytids (frontalis), and crow's feet (orbicularis oculi). Neuromodulators are central to cosmetic practitioners. Successful use of these agents depends not only on improving individual lines but on improving facial symmetry. It is advisable to use the smallest effective dose in the upper-third of the face to try to avoid unwanted outcomes such as asymmetry, brow or lid ptosis, and mouth asymmetry. An important consideration when choosing which neuromodulator to use

Table 7.1 Neuromodulators in the upper face

Muscle	Onabotulinum	Incobotulinum	Abobotulinum
Orbicularis oculi (lateral Crow'sfeet)	6–12U	6–12U	18–36U
Orbicularis oculi (jellyroll)	1–2U	1–2U	3–6U
Glabellar complex (women)	15–25U	15–25U	45–75U
Glabellar complex (men)	25–40U	25–40U	75–125U
Frontalis (women)	5–12U	5–12U	15–36U
Frontalis (men)	12–20U	12–20U	36–60U

Abbreviation: U, units.

Table 7.2 Neuromodulators in the midface

Muscle	Onabotulinum	Incobotulinum	Abobotulinum
Zygomaticus major	2U	2U	3–6U
Levator labii superioris	1–4U	1–4U	3–12U
Levator labii superioris alaeque nasi	1–2U	1–2U	3–6U
Depressor septi nasi (midline)	3–6U	3–6U	9–18U
Dilators of nares	2–6U	2–6U	6–18U

Abbreviation: U, units.

Table 7.3 Neuromodulators in the lower face

Muscle	Onabotulinum	Incobotulinum	Abobotulinum
Orbicularis oris (upper)	3–4U	3–4U	9–12U
Orbicularis oris (lower)	2U	2U	6U
Depressor anguli oris	3–5U	3–5U	9–15U
Depressor labii inferioris	3–4U	3–4U	9–12U
Mentalis	4–10U	4–10U	12–30U
Masseter (each side)	10–40U	10–40U	30–120U

Abbreviation: U, units.

Table 7.4 Neuromodulators in the neck

Muscle	Onabotulinum	Incobotulinum	Abobotulinum
Platysma[a]	2.5U	2.5U	7.5U
Necklace lines[b]	1U	1U	3U

Abbreviation: U, units.
[a]Every 1.5 cm along vertical bands (do not exceed 50 U/50 U/150U).
[b]Every 1 cm along flexion crease.

in each anatomic location is the spread of effect. Onabotulinum and incobotulinum have comparable spread, while abobotulinum has a greater spread of effect. Unwanted spread into untargeted muscle groups can lead to undesirable clinical effects. A neuromodulator with a low and predictable spread would be preferable for treating the glabellar muscle complex and a larger spread of effect could optimize treatments for the forehead lines and crow's feet. Particularly in the lower one-third of the face, injection sites are very close to untargeted muscles; therefore, it is important that the neuromodulator does not spread. A rough estimate of 1U onabotulinum or incobotulinum corresponds to 2.5 to 3U of abobotulinum.[1,2]

Before discussing the musculature of the upper-third of the face and injection techniques, it is important to understand the ideal positioning of the anatomic landmarks, especially the brow. The aesthetic importance of the brow has been highlighted for centuries. It is considered to be of primary importance in facial expression and beauty. The brows create a characteristic appearance to the face and are critical in expressing emotion. The shape and position of the brow also contributes to sexual dimorphism. The eyebrows form the superior aesthetic

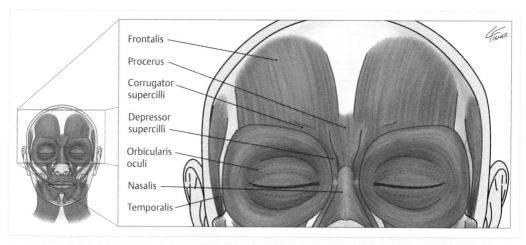

Frontalis
Procerus
Corrugator supercilli
Depressor supercilli
Orbicularis oculi
Nasalis
Temporalis

Fig. 7.1 Anatomy of the muscles of the upper face.

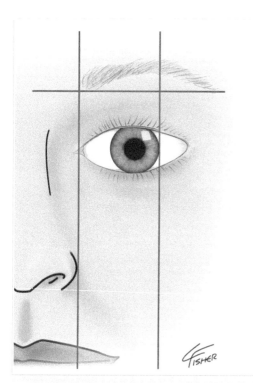

Fig. 7.2 Brow position in relation to surrounding anatomical structures.

frame of the eyes. They can impart a range of emotions through the patient's expression in addition to a youthful or aged appearance. The ideal shape of the brow begins with alignment of the brow head with the lateral nostril margin. The medial and lateral ends of the brow lie approximately at the same

horizontal level. The apex of the brow lies on a vertical line directly above the lateral limbus (▶ Fig. 7.2). The brow should lie at the orbital rim in males and be several millimeters above the rim in females. Over elevation creates an unnatural, surprised, or unintelligent look. Superior displacement of the medial brow can create an undesirable quizzical appearance. Furthermore, a low medial brow with a high lateral peak creates an angry look.[3,4]

The muscles of the upper-third of the face can be divided into eyebrow elevators and eyebrow depressors. The frontalis is the sole muscle responsible for elevation of the eyebrows. The corrugator supercilii, procerus, and the orbital portion of the orbicularis oculi are primarily responsible for depression of the eyebrow.

The frontalis is the only muscle responsible for elevation of the brows. It originates from the galea aponeurotica and inserts into the skin of the lower forehead. It is frequently a fan-shaped, bifurcated muscle that lies in a superficial plane. The frontalis interdigitates with the brow depressors. It is this interdigitation that allows the frontalis to determine the position and shape of the eyebrow. Contraction of the frontalis is what creates horizontal forehead rhytids and brow elevation. The location, size, and use of the muscles vary markedly among individuals. It is the lower 2.5 to 4 cm of the frontalis that moves the brows. Therefore, it is recommended to inject the muscle 3 to 4 cm above the orbital rim to maintain expression. Treatment of horizontal forehead lines associated with frontalis activity is FDA-approved for onabotulinum only; however, other neuromodulators are used for the same purpose off-label.[5]

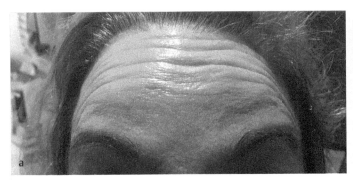

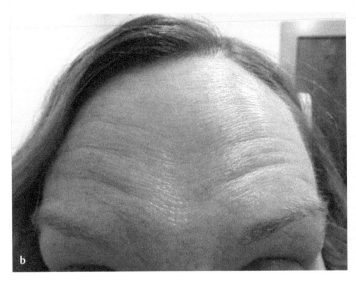

Fig. 7.3 (a) Continuous band of frontalis muscle. (b) Midline dehiscence of frontalis muscle.

Patient selection and treatment parameters cannot be formulaic. Patients will have a difference in the anatomy of their frontalis, whether it is a continuous band (▶ Fig. 7.3a) or if it has a midline dehiscence which is indicative of dual muscular components (▶ Fig. 7.3b).

It is important to remember that the frontalis is the only brow elevator and overtreatment of it can result in brow depression from unopposed action of the depressor muscles. A treatment plan should be based upon careful assessment of the action of brow elevators and depressors, overall forehead shape and size, pattern of rhytids upon contraction and evaluation of any preexisting eyebrow or eyelid ptosis. For example, the patient in ▶ Fig. 7.4 has a very low, horizontal brow position which would be made worse if the frontalis was injected below the midline of the forehead.

Contraction of the frontalis causes dynamic lines to form which may or may not be present at rest. Repetitive contraction of the frontalis eventually leads to formation of static lines which are visible even upon relaxation of the muscle. Neuromodulators yield the best result when dynamic lines with little to no static component are being treated. Because the bulk of the muscle lies above the medial two-thirds of the brow, facial aging results in the descent of the less supported lateral-third containing the tail of the brow. This is due to a loss of soft tissue and bony support and the downward force of the lateral orbital orbicularis oculi.

The evaluation should take into consideration the goals of the patient. The trend in clinical practice over the past few years has been to have a more refreshed and rested look as opposed to complete muscle inhibition that can be perceived as frozen or overdone by patients. The shape as well as the position of the brow in relation to the orbital rim needs to be assessed. The medial and lateral ends of the brow should fall in horizontal alignment and a subtle downward cant of the lateral brow should be present. Any preexisting brow ptosis should be evaluated. If there is a question as to how much the patient is recruiting the frontalis to maintain an elevated position of the brow, there is a simple way to make this determination. Have the patient look forward with their head in a neutral position (▶ Fig. 7.5a). The patient should close their eyes and relax their forehead. Place one finger above both brows holding the frontalis in position without unnaturally forcing it downward and have the patient open their eyes (▶ Fig. 7.5b). The initial position upon opening is where the brow will be after treatment. Acquired ptosis of the eyelid can be evaluated in a similar fashion.

The frontalis extends from the hairline superiorly to the supraorbital ridge and the nasal root inferiorly. It extends laterally to a boundary known as the temporal fusion line. In some people, this line may be shifted laterally and suspensory muscle fibers may continue into the lateral forehead region extending to the temporal hairline. The recommendation is

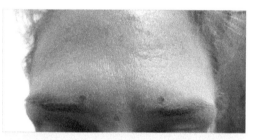

Fig. 7.4 Patient with a very low, horizontal brow position which would be made worse if the frontalis muscle was injected below the midline of the forehead.

four to nine injection points spaced at least 1 cm apart. The muscle typically requires 5 to 20 U of onabotulinum or incobotulinum, or 15 to 60 U of abobotulinum. If the lateral fibers of the frontalis muscle are not injected, patients may develop a Mephisto or Jack Nicholson appearance. If the lateral aspect is injected too low or with too many units, it may cause the brow to droop or sag giving a tired or heavy look. Injection technique for the brow may vary by injector, with some placing four to six depots of neuromodulator in the main body of the frontalis. Others prefer smaller doses with more injection sites throughout the muscle. Each of these techniques is dependent on multiple factors including the neuromodulator dilution, depth of injection, and physical characteristics of the forehead.[6] For those patients with high foreheads, two separate lines of injection may be required to prevent excessive hairline rhytids postinjection due to frontalis recruitment.

Suprabrow lateral forehead lines or commas are a source of cosmetic dissatisfaction for many patients. Inhibiting the muscle laterally especially in a patient with mild lateral brow ptosis can easily lead to an unsatisfying cosmetic outcome. One way to circumvent this problem is to use 1 to 2 U of neuromodulator reconstituted with 2 mL preservative saline. Draw it into a 31-gauge, 8-mm (5/16") length 0.3 mL insulin syringe then add an additional 0.2 to 0.4 mL of preservative saline, resulting in a double dilution. This can then be injected in several small, equal aliquots over the lateral brow (▶ Fig. 7.6). In addition, a low-viscosity filler can be used to treat the static aspect of these lines.

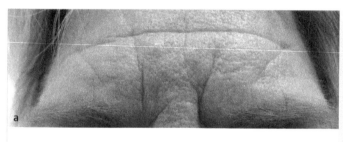

Fig. 7.5 (a) Evaluating preexisting brow ptosis by having the patient look forward with their head in a neutral position. **(b)** Evaluating preexisting brow ptosis by placing one finger above both brows holding the frontalis in position without unnaturally forcing it downward and have the patient open their eyes.

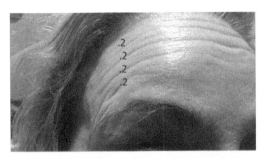

Fig. 7.6 Lateral forehead or comma lines addressed using reconstituted neuromodulator in four equal aliquots.

Lateral brow descent is also partially caused by the downward pull of the orbital orbicularis oculi muscle. Paresis of the lateral portion of the orbicularis oculi allows for an elevation of the tail of the brow because of the remaining pull of the frontalis. Brow descent can be prevented through a detailed examination, noting the preprocedural brow position. A balance must then be achieved between the postinjection muscular forces of the frontalis, orbicularis oculi, and glabellar complex to maintain an aesthetically pleasing brow position and shape.

In patients who have a significant amount of bony or soft tissue loss, as well as acquired lid ptosis or in patients who have very deep static forehead rhytids, a neuromodulator alone is not going to give an optimal outcome and will likely have a higher incidence of side effects. In these patients it is best to consider ablative laser resurfacing or the use of soft tissue fillers to mitigate the depth of the rhytids without affecting brow elevation. All neuromodulators are best injected in the superficial aspect of the frontalis muscle creating small blebs. It is prudent to use a conservative amount of units and reassess a patient in 7 to 10 days than to overinject and cause an unwanted result for 3 to 4 months.

A form of reshaping of the forehead with neuromodulators can be accomplished with treatment of temporalis muscle hypertrophy. Although this muscle is not one of facial expression and is a muscle of mastication (innervated by the trigeminal nerve), hypertrophy can create an unusual-shaped forehead as seen in ▶ Fig. 7.7. This patient benefited from injection of anterior hypertrophy of the temporalis to create a smooth, fresher, and rested appearance with a softer shape to her forehead. This can be accomplished by injecting 4 U of onabotulinum or incobotulinum, or 12 U of abobotulinum into three injection points on each side

(▶ Fig. 7.7a—before resting, ▶ Fig. 7.7b—before clenching, ▶ Fig. 7.7c—injection technique, ▶ Fig. 7.7d—after resting, ▶ Fig. 7.7e—after clenching).

A simple technique for lateral brow elevation involves an injection of 1 to 3 U of onabotulinum or incobotulinum, or 3 to 9 U of abobotulinum at a single point into the lateral brow depressor (superolateral orbital orbicularis oculi) which weakens it. It is advisable to palpate the superolateral portion of the orbicularis oculi in animation (smiling) to identify the point at which neuromodulator should be injected because eyebrow position varies considerably, especially in women who tweeze their brows as well as patients who have tattooed brows.[7]

The glabellar complex comprises the medial brow depressors: procerus, corrugator supercilii, depressor supercilii, and the orbicularis oculi muscles. Understanding the depth of the glabellar musculature is important to treat those muscles needed for the desired effect while avoiding unnecessary paralysis of the frontalis. The procerus originates at the junction of the nasal bones, running superiorly, and inserts into the skin just above the glabella. Contraction of the procerus produces horizontal lines overlying the glabella.

The corrugator supercilii originates medially and deep along the nasofrontal suture, traveling laterally and superiorly above the orbital rim. As the corrugator supercilii travels laterally, it becomes more superficial, interdigitating with the frontalis. Neuromodulators injected medially should be placed in a deep plane just above bone, injecting more superficially along the course of the muscle laterally. Knowledge of the depth of muscle and its location is critical to achieving optimal results when injecting neuromodulator.

The final depressors of the brow are the orbicularis oculi and depressor supercilii muscles. Although some consider the depressor supercilii to be a portion of the orbicularis oculi, most aesthetic physicians recognize it as a distinct muscle with an origin on the medial orbital rim near the lacrimal bone and an insertion onto the medial portion of the brow just inferior to the insertion of the corrugator supercilii.

Careful placement at the correct depth is critical for consistent aesthetic result. Injection of the procerus should include one injection site above and below the horizontal rhytids in the region of the radix. The injection should be superficial since the muscle runs immediately subcutaneously and is usually 3 to 6 U of onabotulinum or incobotulinum, or 9 to 18 U of abobotulinum.

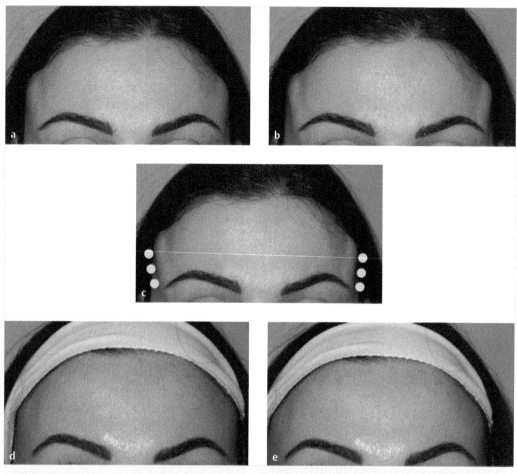

Fig. 7.7 (a) Appearance of anterior temporalis muscle hypertrophy before treatment (resting). **(b)** Appearance of anterior temporalis muscle hypertrophy before treatment (clenching). **(c)** Injection technique for temporalis muscle hypertrophy accomplished by injecting neuromodulator into three injection points on each side. **(d)** Improvement of anterior temporalis muscle hypertrophy after treatment (resting). **(e)** Improvement of anterior temporalis muscle hypertrophy after treatment (clenching).

The injection of the corrugator supercilii is more complex. Treating this muscle close to the origin requires a deeper injection to capture its medial portion and the depressor supercilii muscle. Laterally, the injection of the corrugator supercilii should be slightly more superficial as the muscle approaches the dermis. The corrugator supercilii typically require 16 to 20 U of onabotulinum or incobotulinum, or 48 to 60 U of abobotulinum. The glabellar complex typically requires 20 to 25 U of onabotulinum or incobotulinum, or 60 to 75 U of abobotulinum with one injection site into the body of the procerus and one to two injection sites (on each side) for the corrugators. Higher doses of neuromodulator in the glabellar complex are required

in the male population due to a more robust glabellar complex. Onabotulinum, incobotulinum, and abobotulinum have all received FDA approval for treatment of moderate-to-severe glabellar lines due to procerus and corrugator supercilii muscle activity (▶ Fig. 7.8).[8]

As discussed previously, dynamic facial lines respond better to neuromodulators than do deep static lines. Deeper, etched-in static lines may need to have a combination approach including neuromodulation, laser resurfacing, and soft tissue fillers. The glabellar complex when contracted can often times convey a sense of worry or anger. Patients are often more likely to want significant inhibition of this muscle group as this results in a

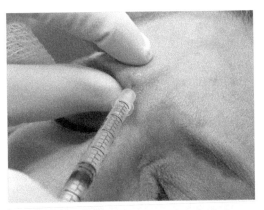

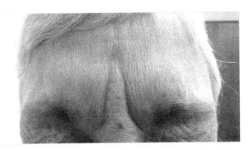

Fig. 7.9 Lateral corrugator supercilii injection medial to its dermal insertion point and medial to the midpupillary line.

Fig. 7.8 Neuromodulator treatment of moderate-to-severe glabellar lines due to procerus and corrugator supercilii muscle activity.

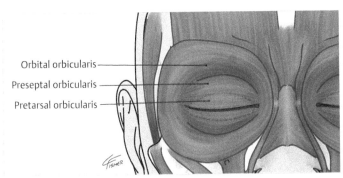

Orbital orbicularis

Preseptal orbicularis

Pretarsal orbicularis

Fig. 7.10 Anatomy of the orbicularis oculi muscle divided into pretarsal, preseptal, and orbital portions.

relaxed, happier look. Treatment of the frontalis should result in some mobility to impart a natural look. The degree of muscle inhibition needs to be clearly defined with the patient prior to treatment.

As outlined before, the frontalis at its inferior border interdigitates with the brow depressors. As a result of this interdigitation, there can be some spread of neuromodulator to the frontalis when the depressor complex is injected. For this reason, it is prudent to use a concentrated neuromodulator (1 to 2 mL reconstitution) and to inject low on the procerus and medial belly of the corrugators. The lateral aspect of the corrugator supercilii should be injected just medial to its dermal insertion point and in the region of the midpupillary line (▶ Fig. 7.9). This technique prevents spread to the medial inferior frontalis, thus preventing medial brow ptosis.

The next muscle to be discussed will be the pretarsal orbicularis oculi. The orbicularis oculi muscle is divided into pretarsal, preseptal, and orbital portions (▶ Fig. 7.10). The pretarsal portion of the muscle lies on the tarsal plate. This muscle is responsible for maintaining the contact of the upper and lower ciliary margins of the eyelids with the globe.[9]

The orbital orbicularis oculi is responsible for the forceful closure of the palpebral fissure which is a conscious protective mechanism for the eye. In contrast, the pretarsal and preseptal portions are responsible for the natural blink reflex. The pretarsal portion is in intimate contact with the lower eyelid skin. It is the contraction of this muscle with smiling that creates several unappealing aesthetic facial features. The relative closure of the palpebral fissure can be seen in the before picture of this patient (▶ Fig. 7.11a). This patient has a relative hypertonicity of her pretarsal orbicularis oculi of both the left upper and lower eyelid. The contraction of this muscle is creating ptosis to the upper eyelid and elevation of the lower lid. Therefore, the preinjection marginal reflex distance-1 (MRD-1) (the distance from the light reflex of the pupil and the upper ciliary margin) and MRD-2 (the distance

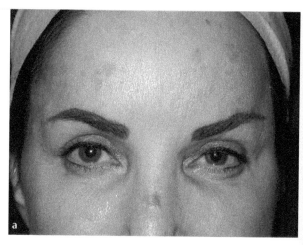

Fig. 7.11 (a) Relative closure of the palpebral fissure due to contraction of the orbital orbicularis oculi muscle with smiling, creating unappealing ptosis to the upper eyelid and elevation of the lower eyelid. (b) Contraction of the pretarsal orbicularis oculi creating ptosis to the upper eyelid and elevation of the lower lid resulting in a decreased marginal reflex distance-1 (MRD-1) and marginal reflex distance-2 (MRD-2). (c) Favorable improvement in MRD-1 and MRD-2 by applying neuromodulator to the upper eyelid pretarsal orbicularis oculi muscle medially and in the lower pretarsal muscle laterally.

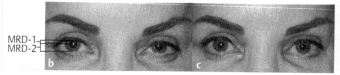

MRD-1
MRD-2

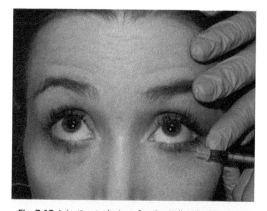

Fig. 7.12 Injection technique for the "jellyroll" deformity.

During smiling and animation, contraction of the pretarsal orbicularis oculi diminishes the palpebral aperture. This can produce a "jellyroll" deformity where the contracted muscle produces a subciliary bulge. It can be treated by injecting 2 U of incobotulinum or onabotulinum, or 6 U of abobotulinum, 3 mm below the midpupillary line immediately subcutaneous. When injecting, the needle is oriented parallel to the ciliary margin and not perpendicular to it. Lateral tension is placed on the skin with the opposite hand, and the tip of the needle is placed just below the skin creating a wheal (▶ Fig. 7.12). Using a cotton-tipped applicator the wheal is then rolled lateral to medial allowing for even distribution of neuromodulator throughout the muscle. A similar technique is used for the upper eyelid. All three neuromodulators can be used on the jellyroll; however, onabotulinum or incobotulinum are better alternatives to be used when correcting upper eyelid ptosis. In contrast, abobotulinum may lead to complications in this area due to a greater spread of effect. This treatment can assist in reducing the muscle bulge as well as open up the palpebral aperture (distance between the upper and lower lids) at rest and when smiling, producing a more wide-eyed, alert appearance.

It is important for one to evaluate the patient's vector of the midface when contemplating an inferior pretarsal orbicularis oculi injection. The

of the light reflex of the pupil and the lower ciliary margin) are decreased (▶ Fig. 7.11b). In this particular patient, a favorable result was achieved by injecting 0.5 U of onabotulinum to the upper eyelid pretarsal orbicularis oculi muscle medially and laterally and 2 U midpupillary in the lower pretarsal muscle (▶ Fig. 7.11c). These injections involve subcutaneous placement with the tip of the needle just encroaching the surface of the skin of the upper eyelid. Placing tension on the upper eyelid skin and applying gentle traction with the noninjecting hand with the patient looking downward allows for a safe and accurate injection.

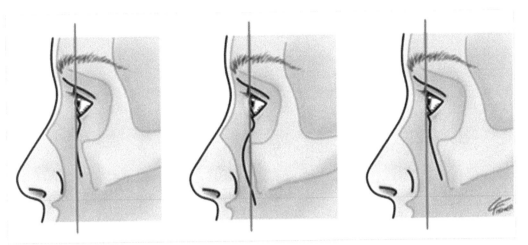

Fig. 7.13 Midface vectors drawing a line from the cornea to the malar eminence (left-to-right: Normal-Positive-Negative).

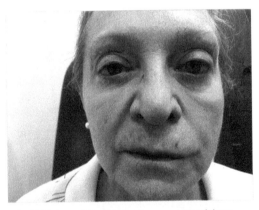

Fig. 7.14 Lower lid ectropion from neuromodulator treatment after decreasing the muscle function of an already compromised lower eyelid.

patient with a negative vector is defined as a line drawn perpendicular from the cornea and extending inferiorly and falling anterior to the malar eminence. These patients may experience an increase in the MRD-2 with injection of this muscle, creating a lid retraction. Normal and positive vector patients should tolerate this injection well (▶ Fig. 7.13). The last situation to consider for injection of the jellyroll is the preexistence of scleral show (increase in MRD-2 on preinjection photographs on normal gaze). These patients may be prone to worsening of this condition with this injection.

Caution must be used when treating this area, especially by the novice injector. Overtreatment can affect the ability to close the eye and result in keratoconjunctivitis sicca (dry eye syndrome). Therefore, a thorough history should be taken including previous lower eyelid surgery, history of dry eye syndrome, and a history of Bell's palsy. When evaluating for this kind of injection, a simple physical exam is helpful to determine if the patient is a candidate for such an injection. A snap test is merely a downward traction on the lower eyelid with the index finger and observing how quickly the lower eyelid returns to its normal position. The distraction test involves pulling the eyelid directly anterior from the orbit. If the lower eyelid distracts more than a centimeter from the orbit, this may indicate medial and/or lateral canthal tendon laxity and this patient may not be an ideal candidate for this injection.[10] Neuromodulator treatment should be carried out with caution in patients who have had a cosmetic procedure which may have affected the anterior lamella or created lid retraction. Lower-lid skin or skin-muscle excision or aggressive laser resurfacing can decrease the vertical height of the anterior lamella predisposing the patient to ectropion (▶ Fig. 7.14).

When treating the crow's feet, it is important to understand the contraction of the orbital fibers of the orbicularis oculi. This very large muscle extends beyond the orbital rim and creates the crow's feet. It is important to explain carefully to the patient while they are smiling that the zygomatic cheek lines cannot entirely be treated with a neuromodulator. You can only relax the areas lateral to the orbit that are created by contraction of the orbicularis oculi.

The injection of the crow's feet occurs at or lateral to the orbital rim. Bright light along with tensing the skin helps to identify periorbital veins, thus avoiding bruising. A 0.3-mL, 5/16" 31-gauge needle should be used, and injection is performed by directing the needle away from the globe and creating a small wheal either intradermal or immediately subcutaneous. The medial injections involved with treatment of the crow's feet should not extend more medial than the extent of the orbital rim. Injections placed medial to this critical anatomic landmark can result in diplopia and/or strabismus from paralysis of the lateral rectus muscle. Treatment of the crow's feet typically requires 6 to 12 U of onabotulinum or incobotulinum, or 18 to 36 U of abobotulinum (per side) are injected evenly in three to four sites within the muscle.[8]

Another major side effect of using neuromodulators in the upper-third of the face is eyelid ptosis. The incidence of ptosis after such injections initially was reported to be approximately 5%, but recent studies have shown a reduced incidence of this complication.[11,12] Ptosis can occur up to 2 weeks after injections. Ptosis results from migration of the neuromodulator to the levator palpebrae superioris muscle. The levator is the only muscle responsible for opening the eyelid. To avoid ptosis, injections should occur at least 1 cm above the superior orbital rim and should not cross the midpupillary line. Apraclonidine 0.5% (Iopidine™) eye drops are recommended for treating neuromodulator-induced ptosis. Apraclonidine is an α2-adrenergic agonist, which causes Müller muscles to contract, quickly elevating the upper eyelid 1 to 3 mm.[13] Another eye preparation which can be used for ptosis is Naphcon-A, which contains naphazolin which is also an α2-adrenergic agonist. Acquired ptosis may be compensated for by an overactive frontalis muscle. Overtreatment of the frontalis usually unmasks this form of ptosis.

When trying to treat lines in the lower crow's feet region that occur after the injection of neuromodulator, it is important that the patient understand that we have now created an interaction between an adynamic area and a dynamic area of the face. The adynamic area is created by relaxation of the vertical fibers of the orbital portion of the orbicularis oculi muscle. The dynamic area is that portion of the face that elevates when the patient smiles. So the junction between the dynamic and adynamic areas creates single or multiple lines that the patient will express concern about after they have been treated with a neuromodulator. It should be explained to the patient that these lines can be treated with a flexible low G' hyaluronic acid injection to create increased turgor to the skin which then decreases the static and dynamic rhytids in this particular situation. This is best demonstrated in the before and after photos of the patient in ▶ Fig. 7.15a, b.

The orbital portion of the orbicularis oculi muscle is an accessory muscle to smiling. There is an intricate relationship between the lateral inferior orbicularis oculi and the zygomaticus major. These muscles are critical in creating the elevation of the oral commissure with smiling along with levator anguli oris. When this muscle is weakened, there is a relative ptosis of the oral commissure seen with smiling when compared to the opposite unaffected side. A way to prevent this is to make sure that the application of your neuromodulator is above the Frankfort horizontal line (▶ Fig. 7.16).[14] Extending your

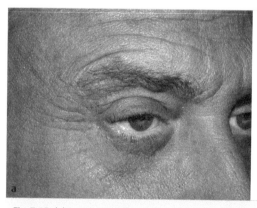
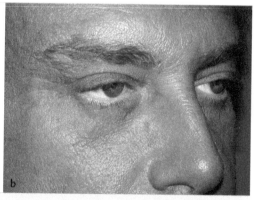

Fig. 7.15 (a) Lower crow's feet static and dynamic rhytids before treatment. (b) Lower crow's feet after treatment with a flexible low G' hyaluronic acid injection to create increased turgor to the skin.

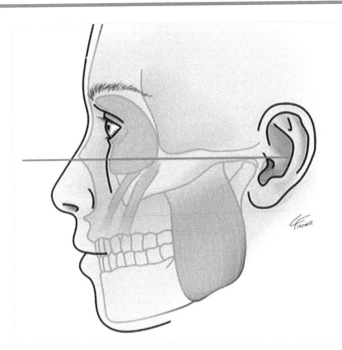

Fig. 7.16 Frankfort horizontal line used as a guide for injection placement.

neuromodulator injection below this line can affect the zygomaticus major resulting in this complication. In addition, lowering the number of units injected in this region is prudent.

Pain with neuromodulator injection is usually minimal but patient satisfaction is dependent upon providing a comfortable and relaxing experience. The reconstitution of neurotoxin with preserved saline results in less pain on injection than with preservative-free saline.[15] Preservative saline contains benzyl alcohol, which can serve as an anesthetic during injection.

Precise toxin deposition and correct dose is essential for optimizing treatment outcomes with neuromodulators. The Ultra-Fine II which is an 8-mm (5/16"), silicone-coated 31-gauge short needle with a .3-mL insulin syringe is the optimal method for accurately delivering a specific number of units of neuromodulator to the underlying musculature. There is minimal waste of product because there is no dead space in the needle hub. A sharp and precise design allows for accurate and more comfortable injection. The needle will stay sharp for four to six injections. Therefore, the amount of the neuromodulator should be divided among multiple syringes to avoid exceeding these number of injections with the same needle.[16]

Lastly, the gate theory hypothesizes that nonpainful input closes the nerve gates to painful input. This can be utilized by gently massaging an area proximal to the injection point to minimize the pain of percutaneous puncture.

Treatment of the upper face with neuromodulators is best summarized in ▶ Table 7.1.

7.3 Midface

The midface, which is essentially defined as the region from the zygomatic arch and malar eminence to the nasolabial fold, is primarily an aesthetic region of the face enhanced by fillers. However, neuromodulators have begun to play an increasingly important role in the aesthetic enhancement in this region. It is critical that there is an understanding of the muscular anatomy in the midface, which includes the origin and insertion (▶ Fig. 7.17). In addition, understanding rhytid formation, facial expression, and dynamic asymmetry that occur with contraction is crucial. Unique to facial musculature is the fact that they essentially all originate on the facial skeleton and insert onto the dermis of the face.

The muscles in the midface to be discussed include the nasalis, depressor septi nasi, and upper lip elevators. The lip elevators proceeding lateral to medial include the zygomaticus major, zygomaticus minor, levator anguli oris, levator labii superioris, and levator labii superioris alaeque nasi (▶ Fig. 7.17). The zygomaticus major originates on the lateral inferior surface of the malar eminence of the zygoma and

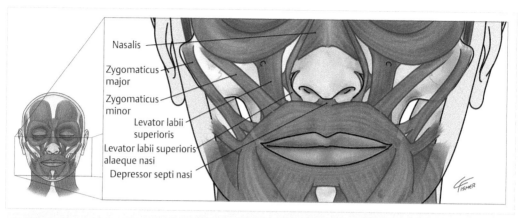

Fig. 7.17 Anatomy of the muscles of the midface including the lip elevators.

proceeds inferiorly and medially to insert on the modiolus. The modiolus is the structure that is found just lateral to the oral commissure and is a small collection of fibromuscular tissue acting as an insertion for multiple muscles of facial expression that controls the fate of the position of the oral commissure. One reason for injecting this muscle may be to create symmetry when asymmetry of the oral commissures occurs with smiling. The major muscles that elevate the oral commissure are the zygomaticus major and levator anguli oris (a deep muscle found in the midface). The major depressor muscle for the oral commissure is the depressor anguli oris (DAO). Treatment of the zygomaticus major muscle involves injecting 2 U of onabotulinum or incobotulinum, or 3 to 6 U of abobotulinum. This injection is usually done just below the lateral malar eminence in the region of the origin of the zygomaticus major. The zygomaticus minor originates medial to the zygomaticus major and inserts on the lateral upper lip complex. It is partially responsible for creating the gummy smile.

The next muscle moving lateral to medial is the levator anguli oris. It originates on the canine fossa and inserts on the modiolus. This muscle is involved with elevating the oral commissure. It is not a muscle usually treated in the midface for aesthetic purposes.

Moving further medially, the levator labii superioris originates on the orbital rim and runs over the orbital foramen inserting onto the orbicularis oris as well as the skin and mucosa of the upper lip. This muscle is a major elevator of the upper lip. Injection in the region of the infraorbital foramen is a safe way of injecting this muscle as well as inferiorly just lateral to the nasal ala. This muscle can be

primarily injected with 1 to 4 U of onabotulinum or incobotulinum, or 3 to 12 units of abobotulinum in a concentrated form to prevent increased spread of effect. The purpose of injecting this muscle is primarily for the gummy smile.

Rubin described three types of smiles that appear most commonly in patients.[17] The first is the "Mona Lisa" smile where the zygomaticus major has the greatest effect and the oral commissures are found above the level of the central portion of the upper lip. The next smile is known as the "canine smile" or "gummy" smile, and this is caused by increased tone of the levator labii superioris and levator labii superioris alaeque nasi. These muscles are responsible for elevating the central portion of the lip in relation to the oral commissures, and this results in the gummy smile. The third smile, which is the least common, involves contraction of both the upper lip elevators and lower lip depressors, which then allows for full view of the dentition, thus known as the "full denture" smile.

In evaluating a patient with a gummy smile, it is important to understand that the muscles most likely responsible are the levator labii superioris and levator labii superioris alaeque nasi with a minor component of the zygomaticus minor. The levator labii superioris alaque nasi muscle originates on the medial maxilla and inserts onto the medial aspect of the orbicularis oris as well as the skin and mucosa of the medial upper lip. It also sends a slip of muscle along the alar rim which serves the purpose of dilating the nares. The injection point for this muscle is at the apex of the nasolabial fat compartment approximately 2 mm lateral to the nasal alar groove. Another injection can be placed 2 mm lateral to this injection point to capture the levator labii superioris. Hwang et al described another injection point for the gummy smile known as the Yonsei point. It is located in the center of a triangle formed by the muscle vectors of levator labii superioris, levator labii superioris alaeque nasi, and zygomaticus minor. It is usually located 1 cm lateral to the nasal ala and 3 cm directly inferior and perpendicular to the aforementioned point.[18] The dosage for the levator labii superioris alaeque nasi is 1 to 2 U of onabotulinum or incobotulinum, or 3 to 6 U of concentrated abobotulinum. The dose to the levator labii superioris is 2 to 4 U of onabotulinum or incobotulinum, or 6 to 12 U of concentrated abobotulinum.

Patients with deep nasolabial folds can be treated with filler as well as a careful injection to the levator labii superioris alaeque nasi.[19] This muscle is extremely sensitive to neuromodulators and it is important that an accurate injection is given with an appropriate dosage. The effect on this muscle from neuromodulators can last up to 6 months. An injection here involves between 1 and 2 U of onabotulinum or incobotulinum, or 3 to 6 U of abobotulinum in a concentrated form.

The asymmetric smile can also be treated with a neuromodulator to restore balance. As seen in this patient, the hypertonicity of the levator labii superioris alaeque nasi not only creates an asymmetry of the upper lip with smiling but there is also an increase in the depth of the nasolabial fold and elevated posture to the alar lobule accentuated with smiling. It is important to understand the subtleties that exist in the midface, particularly with this muscle. A single injection can result in subtle but important changes in the face. In this patient, when the patient smiles before her treatment we can see the three specific issues occurring (▶ Fig. 7.18a). After one single injection, correction of a unilateral gummy smile, improvement in the depth of the left nasolabial fold, and lowering

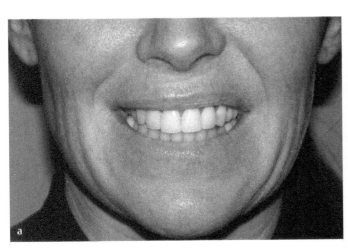
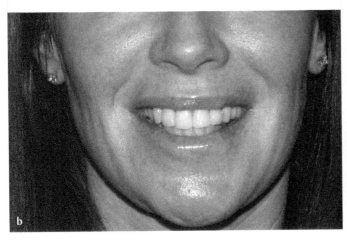

Fig. 7.18 (a) Asymmetry of the upper lip, increase in the depth of the nasolabial fold, and elevated posture to the nostril accentuated with smiling due to left levator labii superioris alaeque nasi hypertonicity. (b) Improvement in upper lip asymmetry, nasolabial fold depth, and posture to the nostril after treatment of levator labii superioris alaeque nasi hypertonicity with neuromodulator.

of the left nostril position to provide symmetry is accomplished (▶ Fig. 7.18b).

With aging of the midface, there are characteristic wrinkles that occur in the superior medial cheek with smiling. These are created by the zygomaticus major and minor, buccinators and risorious. Injection of these muscles is very difficult without creating an irregular smile. Treatment of these dynamic superficial rhytids can be accomplished with mesotherapy. This involves a dilute form of neuromodulator injected superficially during microneedling.[20]

The final muscle to be discussed in this region is the depressor septi nasi. This muscle creates ptosis of the nasal tip with smiling (animation ptosis), as well as shortening of the upper lip. The action of this muscle can also create a troublesome horizontal wrinkle that can occur in the midportion of the upper lip which unfortunately runs perpendicular to the perioral rhytids in this region. This muscle usually originates on the orbicularis oris and inserts onto the feet of the medial crura.[21] Patients can be injected for animation ptosis by using 3 to 6 U of onabotulinum or incobotulinum, or 9 to 18 U of abobotulinum. The injection is placed at the base of the anterior nasal spine at the columellar-labial junction in the midline. Further improvement of this horizontal rhytid occurs with filler placement. The results of this injection can be improved with a lateral injection found in the region of the alar portion of the nasalis and the levator labii superioris alaeque nasi muscles. This lateral injection is accomplished with 2 to 6 U of onabotulinum or incobotulinum, or 6 to 18 U of concentrated abobotulinum.[19] Improvement of animation ptosis can be seen in this patient who received neuromodulator to the depressor septi nasi, alar portion of the nasalis and the levator labii superioris alaeque nasi (▶ Fig. 7.19a—frontal view before, ▶ Fig. 7.19b—lateral view before, ▶ Fig. 7.19c—injection technique, ▶ Fig. 7.19d—frontal view after, ▶ Fig. 7.19e— lateral view after).

Another unique application for neuromodulator in the nose is to address nasal flaring. This occurs in individuals who unconsciously flare their nostrils under stress. This imparts subliminal anger, fear, exhaustion, concern, or distress. This is caused by alar nasalis and the medial alar portion of levator labii superioris alaeque nasi. Treatment involves 4 to 10 U of onabotulinum or incobotulinum, or 12 to 30 U of abobotulinum in the center of each alar rim. Best results are seen in those patients who can actively dilate their nostrils as

demonstrated in the before and after photo of this patient (▶ Fig. 7.20a, b).

Treatment of the midface with neuromodulators is best summarized in ▶ Table 7.2.

7.4 Lower Face

The lower face has become a popular and challenging region for neuromodulator therapy. It is an area that benefits primarily from volume replacement and rhytid effacement, with neuromodulators playing an increasing role in its rejuvenation. It is imperative to understand the complexity and intricacy of the muscles in the region of the lower face, which are responsible for the multiple expressions found in the perioral region (▶ Fig. 7.21). Due to the complexity of the muscles in the lower face, misplacement of neuromodulators is not tolerated as it is in the upper-third of the face. It is critical to understand the origin, insertions, and actions of the muscles of the lower face as well as the selection, application, and concentration of the neuromodulator to obtain the desired outcome. Patients are becoming extremely in-tuned to their smiles, particularly with the "Selfie generation." Any alteration or subtle aberrancy seen in these pictures that occurs after an injection is scrutinized intensely by the patient and their peers.

The central portion of the lower face is dominated by the orbicularis oris. This sphincteric muscle, which creates a centripetal action, allows for puckering and protrusion of the lips, and closure of the mouth. This muscle has a superficial portion, which originates and inserts on itself and is firmly attached to the dermis of the glabrous skin of the lips. This is responsible for the creation of rhytids seen in this region. Repetitive actions, such as puckering, smoking, and drinking through a straw, result in the forces created by the superficial portion of the muscle being transmitted to the overlying skin. Actinic damage, loss of soft tissue volume, and maxillary and mandibular resorption ultimately contribute to aging characteristics found in the perioral region.

An effective adjuvant therapy for treating perioral lines involves the application of neuromodulator. The technique involves the use of 3 to 4 U of onabotulinum or incobotulinum, or 9 to 12 U of abobotulinum in the upper lip, and 2 U of onabotulinum or incobotulinum, or 6 U of abobotulinum in the lower lip. The injection is made 1 mm above and below the vermilion borders, creating a superficial wheal with the injection. Four injections are performed in the upper lip, two on each side of

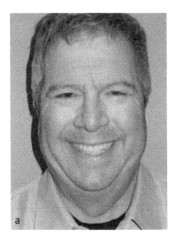
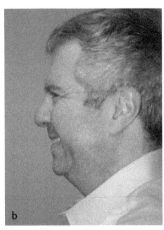

Fig. 7.19 **(a)** Ptosis of the nasal tip and shortening of the upper lip with smiling due to depressor septi muscle hypertonicity (frontal view). **(b)** Ptosis of the nasal tip and shortening of the upper lip with smiling due to depressor septi muscle hypertonicity (lateral view). **(c)** Injection technique for depressor septi muscle—neuromodulator placed at the base of the anterior nasal spine at the columellar-labial junction in the midline and lateral injection into the alar portion of the nasalis and the levator labii superioris alaeque nasi muscles. **(d)** Improvement of animation ptosis with treatment of depressor septi muscle (frontal view). **(e)** Improvement of animation ptosis with treatment of depressor septi muscle (lateral view).

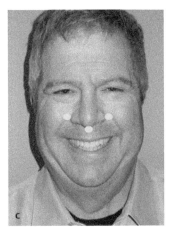

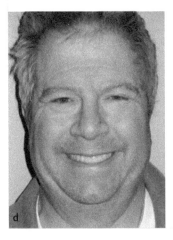
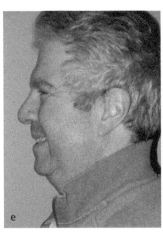

Cupid's bow, and two injections in the lower lip, one on either side of the midline just below the tubercles (▶ Fig. 7.22).

The purpose of injecting both the upper and lower lips is to maintain a relative symmetry with puckering. Injecting the upper lip alone can result in a flat upper lip and a contracted lower lip with puckering, which can be disturbing to the patient. It is also important when injecting the perioral lip region that the injection is made very superficial,

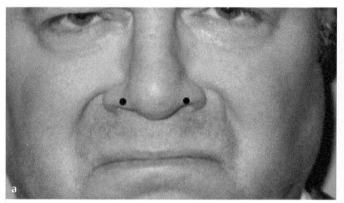

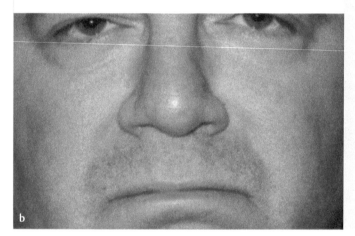

Fig. 7.20 **(a)** Nasal flaring caused by alar nasalis and the medial alar portion of levator labii superioris alaeque nasi muscles. **(b)** Improvement of nasal flaring with placement of neuromodulator into the center of each alar rim.

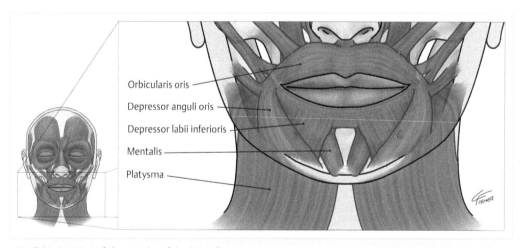

Orbicularis oris

Depressor anguli oris

Depressor labii inferioris

Mentalis

Platysma

Fig. 7.21 Anatomy of the muscles of the lower face.

and that injections are not placed deep into the orbicularis oris. This can create weakening of the muscle with resultant oral incompetence. When injecting the upper lip, one should avoid Cupid's bow. Injecting this area may lead to unappealing flattening of this attractive portion of the upper lip. Avoiding injections closer than 1 cm to the oral commissure will prevent spread to the upper lip

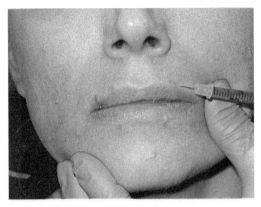

Fig. 7.22 Perioral injection technique—four injections in the upper lip, two on each side of Cupid's bow, and two injections in the lower lip, one on either side of the midline just below the tubercles.

elevators, thus preventing subsequent ptosis of the oral commissure.

Another aesthetic benefit to injecting the perioral region is a subtle eversion that occurs when relaxing the superficial fibers of the orbicularis oris which creates a more desirable increase in vermilion show. The positive results of using neuromodulator for perioral rhytids can be seen in the before and after pictures of the patient in ▶ Fig. 7.23a, b.

Along with the upper lip elevators, the lower lip depressors create a centrifugal force, which opposes the sphincteric action of the orbicularis oris. It is this precision between the opposing muscle forces which allows for the plethora of expressions seen in the perioral region, as described earlier. The depressors of the lower lip that will be discussed will be the DAO, depressor labii inferioris (DLI), and mentalis muscles as well as the platysma muscle which will be discussed in the Neck section (▶ Fig. 7.21).

The DAO is a unique muscle that originates along the oblique line of the mandible between the canine and first molar, and inserts on the modiolus. It is responsible for the downward pull of the oral commissure, thus creating several unaesthetic aging characteristics to the lower face. These include enhancement of the marionette fold, rhytids or parentheses below the corner of the mouth and a constant downturning of the oral commissures creating a ubiquitous frown to the perioral region. Treating this muscle with neuromodulator can be seen in the before and after pictures of this patient both in repose and frowning (▶ Fig. 7.24a—repose

before, ▶ Fig. 7.24b—frowning before, ▶ Fig. 7.24c—injection technique, ▶ Fig. 7.24d—repose after, ▶ Fig. 7.24e—frowning after).

Injection of the DAO can occur in multiple areas. First, a single injection can be performed 1 cm directly lateral to the oral commissure then proceeding 1 cm directly perpendicular, which will result in placement of the injection in the body of the muscle (▶ Fig. 7.25a). The second place for injection is found by extending a line from the nasolabial fold to the inferior margin of the mandible. The intersection of these two lines, which is usually 5 to 10 mm in front of the anterior border of the Masseter, is the preferred injection point (▶ Fig. 7.25b). For this muscle, 3 to 5 U of onabotulinum or incobotulinum, or 9 to 15 U of abobotulinum is used. Placement here is intended to capture the central and lateral fibers of the DAO at the origin of the muscle, thus creating the desired effect. It is prudent to avoid medial placement of neuromodulator in this region to prevent weakening of the DLI. This will result in an asymmetric smile similar to a unilateral marginal mandibular paresis. If this occurs, the opposite DLI can be injected with 3 to 4 U of onabotulinum or incobotulinum, or 9 to 12 U of abobotulinum. This injection should occur about 1 cm inferior to the lower lip tubercle of the unaffected side. The reason for injecting in this region of the lower lip is that the DLI inserts onto the tubercle, and is responsible for the downward displacement of the lower lip. The use of abobotulinum in the lower-third of the face is effective, but should be done judiciously because of its increased spread of effect. Concentrated dilutions are suggested. Filler placed in the marionette fold can improve not only the contour of the marionette fold, but also the posture of the downturned oral commissure.

It should be mentioned that when injecting the DAO and DLI, if necessary, the injection is accomplished by pinching the skin between your thumb and forefinger, thus creating a cushioned area in which to introduce the needle to the hub (▶ Fig. 7.25a, b). This prevents deep placement of neuromodulator into the orbicularis oris and potential oral incompetence.

The next area in the lower face frequently injected for aesthetic purposes is the mentalis. This muscle may be a single sheet, or consist of two bellies, which then results in the formation of a central dimple of the chin. The muscle originates on the anterior mandible in the region of the incisors and inserts on the inferior aspect of the chin. It is the major protruder of the lower lip. It creates

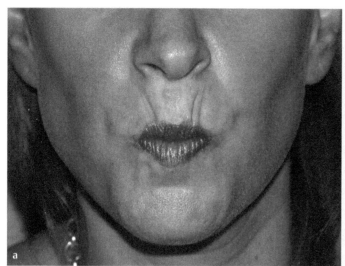

Fig. 7.23 (a) Perioral rhytids exaggerated with puckering due to superficial portions of the orbicularis oris muscle being transmitted to the overlying skin. (b) Positive results of using neuromodulator for perioral rhytids producing subtle eversion that occurs when relaxing the superficial fibers of the orbicularis oris which creates a more desirable increase in vermilion show as well as a decrease in the severity of perioral rhytids seen with animation.

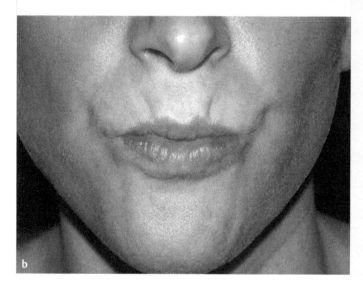

dimpling of the skin with elevation (cobblestoning or peau d'orange) as well as a prominent mental crease, which produces an unappealing appearance. The best way to have the patient produce this action is to have them push their lower lip against their upper lip. Injection of this muscle is best accomplished with one injection in the midline. In addition, two injections can be placed corresponding to lines drawn through each apex of the Cupid's bow, extending perpendicular to either side of the midpoint of the mentum (▶ Fig. 7.26).

Usually, a single injection in the midline of 4 to 10 U of onabotulinum or incobotulinum, or 12 to 30 U of abobotulinum can be performed. If one chooses to inject bilaterally on either side of the midline in the areas shown in ▶ Fig. 7.26, two injections can be performed with either 4 to 5 U per injection site with onabotulinum or incobotulinum, or 12 to 15 U of abobotulinum lateral to the midpoint, as described. The injection should be placed down to the bone in the region of the insertion of the mentalis. Injections made superior and lateral to these points may result in DLI compromise, causing an undesirable asymmetric smile. The skin of the mental region may also exhibit undesirable changes at rest, such as scarring from previous acne and loss of mental fat, which can be exacerbated by contractions of the mentalis. These surface changes can be treated with multimodality therapy with fillers and neuromodulators (▶ Fig. 7.27a, b).

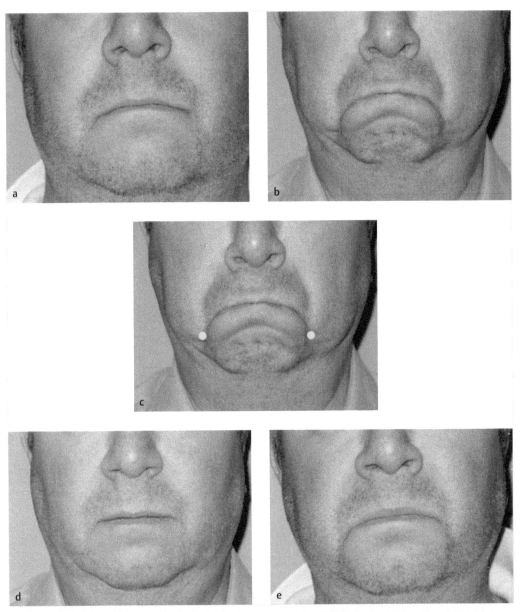

Fig. 7.24 **(a)** Depressor anguli oris creating an undesirable downward pull of the oral commissure seen in repose. **(b)** Depressor anguli oris creating unaesthetic aging characteristics including enhancement of the marionette fold, rhytids, and parentheses below the corner of the mouth and downturning of the oral commissures with frowning. **(c)** Injection technique for depressor anguli oris hypertonicity—1 cm directly lateral to the oral commissure then proceeding 1 cm directly perpendicular. **(d)** Improved position of the oral commissure in repose after treatment of depressor anguli oris with neuromodulator. **(e)** Improved marionette fold, rhytids, and parentheses below the corner of the mouth and downturning of the oral commissures after treatment of depressor anguli oris with neuromodulator.

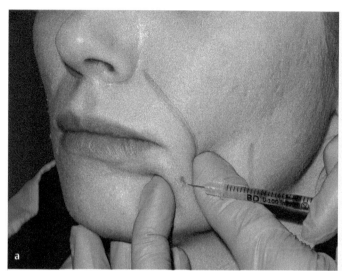

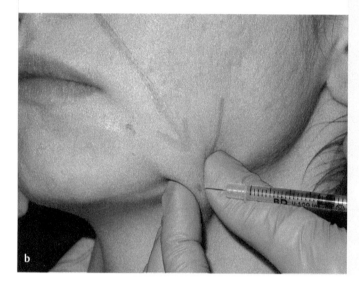

Fig. 7.25 **(a)** First depressor anguli oris (DAO) injection performed 1 cm directly lateral to the oral commissure proceeding 1 cm directly perpendicular. **(b)** Second DAO injection found by extending a line from the nasolabial fold to the inferior margin of the mandible; where these two lines intersect, which is usually 5 to 10 mm in front of the anterior border of the masseter muscle, is the preferred injection point.

The next muscle to be discussed in the lower one-third of face is the masseter. This muscle is found at the lateral aspect of the lower face and hypertrophy can create a masculine appearance in women. A softer, oval appearance to the lower face is the aesthetic goal. The masseter muscle is a primary muscle of mastication, and extends from its origin on the zygomatic arch to its insertion on the lateral angle and body of the ramus (▶ Fig. 7.28). Treatment in this region is an example of the powerful effect of facial reshaping with neuromodulators.

Hypertrophy may be associated with malocclusion, temporomandibular joint dysfunction, or bruxism, and may be unilateral or bilateral. This boxy look to the lower one-third of the face creating this masculine appearance can be seen in any ethnic background; however, it is more prevalent in Korean women.

Injection of this muscle involves its proper identification. With the patient biting down, the anterior, posterior, and inferior borders can be marked. The superior limit is determined by a line drawn from the attachment of the ear lobe to the oral commissure. This creates a square, in which three to four injections can be placed, based on the bulk of the muscle. This method is illustrated in a diagram and a patient in ▶ Fig. 7.28 and ▶ Fig. 7.29, respectively.

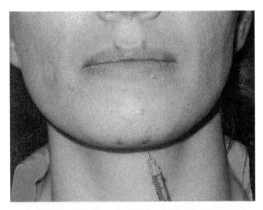

Fig. 7.26 Mentalis injection technique placing two injections corresponding to lines drawn through each apex of the Cupid's bow, extending perpendicular to either side of the midpoint of the mentum.

Injections should not be placed outside of this square. Using the previously described 0.3-mL insulin syringe, the patient is asked to bite down, creating a firm muscle mass allowing for ease of injection by pressing the hub to the skin. Anywhere between 10 and 40 U of onabotulinum or incobotulinum, or 30 to 120 U of abobotulinum are placed in sites determined by the preinjection drawing. Frequently, patients are seen several weeks later to determine if further injection is necessary. Atrophy can last 6 to 9 months if adequate dosing is applied. Patients who have temporomandibular joint (TMJ) symptoms along with masseter hypertrophy often express relief of their symptoms. Injecting in front of the anterior border of the masseter can result in weakness of the risorius with an asymmetric

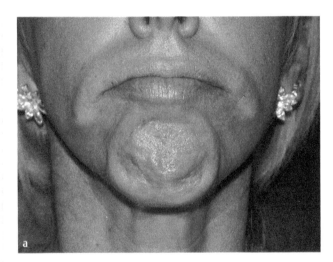

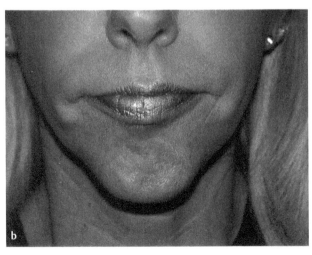

Fig. 7.27 **(a)** Pretreatment picture of a patient with dimpling of the skin with elevation (cobblestoning or peau d'orange) as well as a prominent mental crease, which produces an unappealing appearance. **(b)** Significant improvements of undesirable surface changes after treatment of mentalis muscle with neuromodulator.

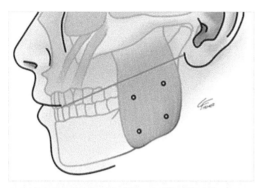

Fig. 7.28 Diagram illustrating masseter muscle extending from its origin on the zygomatic arch to its insertion on the lateral angle and body of the ramus creating a square area to inject into the bulk of the muscle.

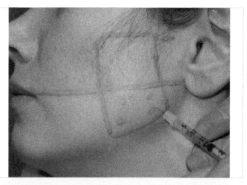

Fig. 7.29 Injection points marked out on a patient depicting a safe square region to place neuromodulator.

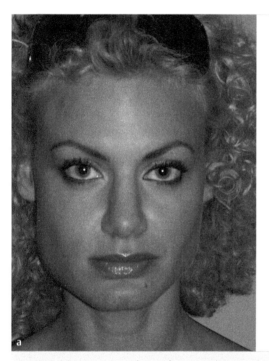

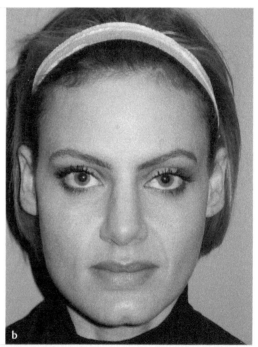

Fig. 7.30 (a) Pretreatment photos of masseter hypertrophy giving a boxy look to the lower one-third of the face creating a masculine appearance. (b) Improvement in the jawline and facial contour after treatment of masseter hypertrophy with neuromodulator.

smile, and should be avoided. Successful treatment is demonstrated in the before and after picture of this patient (▶ Fig. 7.30a, b).

Treatment of the lower face with neuromodulators is best summarized in ▶ Table 7.3.

7.5 Neck

The primary muscle of the neck is the platysma. The anatomy of the platysma, especially its insertions, has evolved and become more clear with the advent

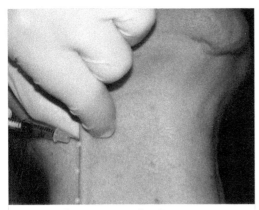

⬤ = 2.5 units, onabotulinum

Fig. 7.31 Platysma injection technique placing neuro-modulator every 2 cm along the vertical bands of the muscle, which is best performed by grasping the contracted band between thumb and index finger and injecting tangentially to the surface of the skin, thus preventing the spread of neuromodulator to the deeper neck muscles.

of careful cadaver dissections and intraoperative observations particularly during facelifting. It acts as a major depressor of the lower lip. It creates a downward vector pull on the soft tissues overlying the mandible. This results in obscuring or washing out of the margin of the mandible. The origin of the muscle is the fascia of the deltoid and pectoral muscles. Medially, it courses superiorly to insert onto the mandible. Moving laterally, it then inserts onto the DAO, DLI, and lower orbicularis oris. Finally, the most lateral extent of the platysma muscle inserts onto the superficial musculoaponeurotic system (SMAS) and has a significant component that extends into the midface.[20] This anatomy is different from what was originally considered for the platysma which was inserted primarily along the inferior border of the mandible. This newer understanding of the insertion of the platysma, particularly the lateral platysma, helps to define the success and strategy behind the Nefertiti lift.[22] By injecting the vertical platysmal band, which courses superiorly into the jowl while simultaneously injecting along the shadow of the mandible, the downward vector of the soft tissue overlying the mandible is negated. A net upward vector is then created by the lateral facial extent of the platysma muscle and the midface

elevators, thus providing better definition of the jawline. The dosage can be 2.5 U of onabotulinum or incobotulinum, or 7.5 U of abobotulinum every 1.5 cm along the vertical bands of the platysma (▶ Fig. 7.31). Usually multiple bands are found with contraction and these can be identified and treated. The Nefertiti lift is performed by identifying the important contractile band of the platysma extending into the jowl along with selected injections along the mandible. A benefit of injecting the medial vertical bands of the platysma muscle is that one can create a sharper cervicomental angle which can be blunted by the presence of these bands.

When injecting the platysmal bands, it is best to grasp the contracted band between thumb and index finger and inject tangentially to the surface of the skin, thus preventing the spread of neuromodulator to the deeper neck muscles (▶ Fig. 7.31). Improper injection technique and/or excessive dosing of neuromodulator (greater than 50 U of onabotulinum or incobotulinum, or 150 U of abobotulinum) in this region may create dysphagia and dysphonia. Proper placement of neuromodulator along the border of the mandible involves three injection sites 1.5 cm apart staying lateral to the extended nasolabial fold line previously described for the DAO injection. The successful treatment of platysmal bands with neuromodulator can be seen in the before and after photos of this patient (▶ Fig. 7.32a, b).

Iatrogenic formation of platysma bands may result after treatment of the neck. Liposuction and facelifting as well as the use of deoxycholic acid (Kybella™) may cause exposure of the bands after removal of pre-platysmal fat in the neck. Patients should be seen two weeks after the platysma has been treated to rule out formation of new bands due to recruitment of untreated platysma muscle.

Necklace lines (tech lines) are difficult lines to treat with one modality. These lines run horizontally across the neck and are found in flexion creases. These are best treated with neuromodulators and a low-viscosity hyaluronic acid. Conservative resurfacing techniques may also be helpful. Injection of 1 U of onabotulinum or incobotulinum, or 3 U of abobotulinum separated 1 cm along the necklace line starting at the midline of the neck and extending to the medial border of the sternocleidomastoid (SCM) is complemented by filler injection.

Treatment of the neck with neuromodulators is best summarized in ▶ Table 7.4.

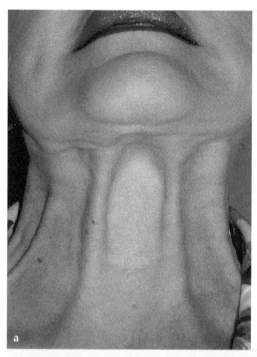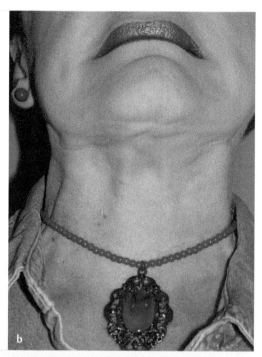

Fig. 7.32 (a) Pretreatment photo of platysmal bands. **(b)** Improvement of platysmal bands after injection with neuromodulator.

Acknowledgment

We would like to acknowledge Casey Fisher, DO for the diagrams illustrated for this chapter.

References

[1] Kerscher M, Roll S, Becker A, Wigger-Alberti W. Comparison of the spread of three botulinum toxin type A preparations. Arch Dermatol Res. 2012; 304(2):155–161

[2] Bentivoglio AR, Del Grande A, Petracca M, Ialongo T, Ricciardi L. Clinical differences between botulinum neurotoxin type A and B. Toxicon. 2015; 107(Pt A):77–84

[3] Yalçınkaya E, Cingi C, Söken H, Ulusoy S, Muluk NB. Aesthetic analysis of the ideal eyebrow shape and position. Eur Arch Otorhinolaryngol. 2016; 273(2):305–310

[4] Cohen JL, Ozog DM, Porto DA. Botulinum toxins: cosmetic and clinical applications. Hoboken: John Wiley & Son; 2017

[5] https://www.accessdata.fda.gov/drugsatfda_docs/label/2017/103000s5302lbl.pdf

[6] Alam M, Dover JS, Klein AW, Arndt KA. Botulinum a exotoxin for hyperfunctional facial lines: where not to inject. Arch Dermatol. 2002; 138(9):1180–1185

[7] Sundaram H. Brow-Shaping Enhancement with Botulinum Neurotoxin Type A. Medscape Education Dermatology. https://www.medscape.org/viewarticle/738431

[8] Beer JI, Sieber DA, Scheuer JF, 3rd, Greco TM. Three-dimensional facial anatomy: structure and function as it relates to injectable neuromodulators and soft tissue fillers. Plast Reconstr Surg

Glob Open. 2016; 4 12 Suppl Anatomy and Safety in Cosmetic Medicine: Cosmetic Bootcamp:e1175

[9] Tong J, Patel BC. Anatomy, head and neck, eye orbicularis oculi muscle. In: StatPearls. Treasure Island (FL): StatPearls Publishing; 2018,https://www.ncbi.nlm.nih.gov/books/NBK441907/

[10] McClellan WT, Seckel BR. Non-surgical rejuvenation of the aging face. In: Weinzweig J, ed. Plastic Surgery Secrets Plus. 2nd ed. Mosby, 2010, pp. 579–584,http://www.sciencedirect.com/science/article/pii/B9780323034708000892

[11] Redaelli A, Forte R. How to avoid brow ptosis after forehead treatment with botulinum toxin. J Cosmet Laser Ther. 2003; 5(3–4):220–222

[12] Klein AW. Contraindications and complications with the use of botulinum toxin. Clin Dermatol. 2004; 22(1):66–75

[13] Scheinfeld N. The use of apraclonidine eyedrops to treat ptosis after the administration of botulinum toxin to the upper face. Dermatol Online J. 2005; 11(1):9

[14] Matarasso SL, Matarasso A. Treatment guidelines for botulinum toxin type A for the periocular region and a report on partial upper lip ptosis following injections to the lateral canthal rhytids. Plast Reconstr Surg. 2001; 108(1):208–214, discussion 215–217

[15] Allen SB, Goldenberg NA. Pain difference associated with injection of abobotulinumtoxinA reconstituted with preserved saline and preservative-free saline: a prospective, randomized, side-by-side, double-blind study. Dermatol Surg. 2012; 38(6):867–870

[16] Flynn TC, Carruthers A, Carruthers J. Surgical pearl: the use of the Ultra-Fine II short needle 0.3-cc insulin syringe for botulinum toxin injections. J Am Acad Dermatol. 2002; 46(6): 931–933

[17] Rubin LR. The anatomy of a smile: its importance in the treatment of facial paralysis. Plast Reconstr Surg. 1974; 53(4): 384–387

[18] Hwang WS, Hur MS, Hu KS, et al. Surface anatomy of the lip elevator muscles for the treatment of gummy smile using botulinum toxin. Angle Orthod. 2009; 79(1):70–77

[19] Kane MA. The effect of botulinum toxin injections on the nasolabial fold. Plast Reconstr Surg. 2003; 112(5) Suppl:66S–72S, discussion 73S–74S

[20] Atamoros FP. Botulinum toxin in the lower one third of the face. Clin Dermatol. 2003; 21(6):505–512

[21] Rohrich RJ, Huynh B, Muzaffar AR, Adams WP, Jr, Robinson JB, Jr. Importance of the depressor septi nasi muscle in rhinoplasty: anatomic study and clinical application. Plast Reconstr Surg. 2000; 105(1):376–383, discussion 384–388

[22] Levy PM. The 'Nefertiti lift': a new technique for specific recontouring of the jawline. J Cosmet Laser Ther. 2007; 9(4): 249–252

8 Deoxycholic Acid

Aubriana M. McEvoy, Basia Michalski, and Rachel L. Kyllo

Summary

Deoxycholic acid, an adipocytolic agent, is the first injectable therapy approved by the US Food and Drug Administration (FDA) to treat submental fullness (SMF). Excessive SMF contributes to facial aging, which influences social behaviors, confidence, and overall sense of attractiveness. The safety profile and efficacy of synthetic deoxycholic acid (ATX-101) were studied in five phase III double-blinded clinical trials. Injection site reactions like pain, swelling, and bruising are common side effects, managed traditionally with ice and NSAIDs. More serious complications like marginal mandibular nerve injury or dysphagia can occur rarely and are minimized with thorough preprocedure assessment and proper injection technique.

Keywords: deoxycholic acid, submental fullness, submental fat, lipolysis, marginal mandibular nerve injury

8.1 Description of Technology/Procedures

8.1.1 Introduction

Excess submental fullness (SMF) and blunting of the cervicomental angle contribute to the aging face, influencing social behaviors, confidence, and overall sense of attractiveness.[1,2] SMF is not necessarily due to excess body weight, but rather age-related fat distribution, and decreased skin and soft tissue elasticity.[2] Because SMF is multifactorial, it is difficult to target with diet and exercise routines alone.[2,3] Surgical procedures aimed to reduce SMF include liposuction and submentoplasty. However, these invasive methods are associated with long recovery times and the potential for complications including postoperative bleeding, hematoma, pain, and infection.[4] In 2015, the Food and Drug Administration (FDA) approved synthetic deoxycholic acid (ATX-101) as the first injectable therapy to treat SMF.[5,6,7] In five phase III double-blinded clinical trials conducted in North America and Europe, deoxycholic acid was injected into the submental fat and reduced SMF compared to placebo.[8,9,10,11,12,13] Patients and physicians reported subjective and objective improvement in SMF following treatment.[8,9,10,11,12,13,14]

8.1.2 Mechanism of Action

Deoxycholic acid is a bile acid produced by gut bacteria that emulsifies fat in the intestine.[15] ATX-101 is a synthetic deoxycholic acid formulated for subcutaneous injection that injures fat cell membranes, leading to adipocytolysis or fat cell destruction.[16] After injection into the submental fat, a local inflammatory response clears fragmented cells, recruits fibroblasts, and improves collagen deposition, leading to soft tissue tightening and improvement in the submental angle.[16,17,18,19,20] Given the inflammatory mechanism of this subcutaneous injection, patients may develop panniculitis with significant edema and discomfort.[21]

8.2 Optimizing Use and Avoiding Complications

8.2.1 Clinical Trials

Injection of deoxycholic acid for the treatment of SMF has been studied in multiple phase III clinical trials, including REFINE-1 and REFINE-2 conducted in North America (ClinicalTrials.gov identifiers: NCT01542034, NCT01546142). In those trials, deoxycholic acid resulted in statistically significant and clinically meaningful improvements in submental fat severity based on clinician-assessed scales, patient-reported outcomes, and objective assessments such as magnetic resonance imaging and caliper measurements. Representative results are pictured in ▶ Fig. 8.1. Three-year follow-up data from the REFINE trials indicated that most results, namely 25% reduction in submental thickness and unchanged or improved skin laxity in 75% of patients, were maintained. There were no unexpected safety concerns reported.[14]

8.2.2 Determination of Ideal Patient

It is important to select the ideal patient for this procedure to minimize complications and optimize the results. On examination, this assessment includes evaluating the submental region from multiple different planes of view. An issue is determining the amount of preplatysmal fat, subplatysmal fat, and skin laxity.[22,23] Patients with excessive

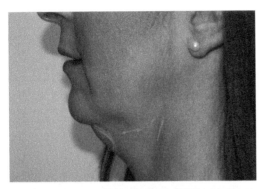

Fig. 8.1 Representative results from clinical trials. In randomized, double-blinded clinical trials, deoxycholic acid injections resulted in significant reduction in submental fullness and sharpening of the cervicomental angle. (This image is provided courtesy of Dr Paul J. Carniol.)

skin laxity, or strong platysmal bands are not good candidates, as the removal of submental fat in these patients may exacerbate their skin laxity or the prominence of their platysmal bands, leading to less aesthetically undesirable results.[5,24] Furthermore, it is important to identify any significant subplatysmal fat component as this should not be treated with deoxycholic acid.

Once a patient is deemed a good candidate for deoxycholic acid, they should be educated on the treatment course.

8.2.3 Assessing Preplatysmal Fat

Prior to injection of deoxycholic acid, the preplatysmal fat must be assessed. Adequate adiposity (as opposed to excessive skin laxity or other causes of SMF) will minimize the risk of injury to surrounding structures such as nerves, salivary glands, and muscle, as well as increase the likelihood for a desirable aesthetic result. Some individuals may have submental fat deep to the platysmal muscle which should not be treated with deoxycholic acid.[25]

Techniques have been identified to assess preplatysmal fat prior to deoxycholic acid injection. The physician should observe the patient while upright and supine (▸ Table 8.1). If SMF and blunting of the cervicomental angle is due to submental fat, the profile should appear consistent in both positions. In contrast, skin laxity would cause blunting of the cervicomental angle while upright, which could change significantly when the patient

is supine (▸ Fig. 8.2). To activate the platysmal muscle and best identify the preplatysmal component of submental fat, the physician can pinch the submental fat while the patient "grimaces" or while swallowing.[26]

8.2.4 Proper Injection Technique

In order to decrease the risk of complications, the region of preplatysmal fat should be identified and marked. The preplatysmal fat is bordered superiorly by the mandible, laterally by the sternocleidomastoid muscles, and inferiorly by the hyoid bone (▸ Fig. 8.3, ▸ Fig. 8.4).[23] Importantly, a "no treatment zone" must be marked to avoid injury to the marginal mandibular nerve. The "no treatment zone" includes the space from the angle of the mandible to the mentum.[23] Deoxycholic acid should not be injected within a region defined by a 1 to 1.5 cm line below the inferior border of the mandible, or above the inferior border of the mandible.[27]

Prior to injection, a temporary grid tattoo or skin markings can help identify the planned treatment area. In the area to be treated, the skin should be mobile and separated from underlying structures. Aliquots of deoxycholic acid are injected, 1 cm apart into each grid space within the planned treatment area.[23] Injections should be administered with the needle perpendicular to the skin. Injection in the mid-subcutaneous space is critical to avoid nerves along the deep surface of the platysma.[30] If there is any resistance noted upon injection, it may indicate infiltration of the muscle (injection too deep) or the dermis (injection too superficial). The physician should withdraw the needle, and try again. Furthermore, before injection, aspiration is recommended to minimize the risk of intra-arterial injection.[31]

Multiple treatments may be necessary to achieve a perceptible reduction in submental fat. Sessions should be at least 4 weeks apart, with a maximum of 50 injections (10 mL) per session.[5] In our experience, several physicians use less injection volume and less injections. Many physicians undertreat SMF with an insufficient amount of deoxycholic acid or insufficient number of treatment sessions. However, if injection site firmness/induration occurs after injection, subsequent injections should be delayed.

8.2.5 Common Complications

The most common reported complications (>5–10% of patients) have been pain (53.3–84.6% of

Table 8.1 Preprocedure assessment techniques to maximize deoxycholic acid injection success

Preprocedure assessment	Technique	Purpose
Sufficient preplatysmal fat	Pinch and palpate the submental area and then ask the patient to tense the platysmal muscles or "grimace".[27] These actions allow the physician to assess the targeted subcutaneous fat between the dermis and platysma.[23]	Insufficient preplatysmal fat may increase the risk of injury to surrounding structures, including the marginal mandibular nerve, and may lead to undesirable cosmetic results. Some individuals may also have submental fat deep to the platysmal muscle, which should not be treated with deoxycholic acid.[25]
Skin laxity	Clinical trials utilized the submental skin laxity grading (SMSLG) scale (1 = none, 4 = severe).[9,12,13] Exclusion criteria include (1) grade 4 on the SMSLG scale or (2) the presence of the following anatomic features: predominant postplatysmal fat, loose skin in the neck or chin area, prominent platysmal bands.[12]	Patients with severe skin laxity were excluded from deoxycholic acid clinical trials given the increased risk of undesirable cosmetic results.
Thyromegaly	Examine the thyroid gland. The normal thyroid gland is inferior to the thyroid cartilage on the anterolateral portion of the trachea. An enlarging thyroid usually grows outward, and may contribute to submental fullness.[28]	Screen patients for other potential causes of submental convexity and fullness, as not all convexity is amenable to deoxycholic injections.[27]
Cervical lymphadenopathy	Examine the submental, submandibular, and cervical lymph nodes for enlarged or tender nodes.	Screen patients for other potential causes of submental convexity/fullness.[27] To avoid tissue damage, deoxycholic acid should not be injected into or in close proximity (1 to 1.5 cm) to salivary glands, lymph nodes, and muscles.
Anticoagulation	Greater than 10 d prior to procedure, collect complete past medical history, prescriptions, and supplement use including aspirin, chronic NSAIDs (except COX-2 inhibitors), vitamin E, fish oil, and herbal medications such as ginkgo biloba, St John wort, and ginseng.[29]	Excessive bleeding or bruising in the treatment area may occur.[27]
Previous neck or face procedures	Collect a complete history of invasive procedures or trauma to the head and neck which may alter the underlying anatomy within the treatment area.	Altered anatomy may increase risk of injury to surrounding structures.
Dysphagia	Collect complete past medical history to assess for current or prior history of dysphagia.	Subjects with current or prior history of dysphagia were excluded from deoxycholic acid clinical trials, as deoxycholic acid may exacerbate the condition.[9,12,13,27]
Age	Patient should be between 18- and 65-y-old.	Safety and effectiveness in patients below the age of 18 y, or greater than 65-y-old have not been established.[27]
Infection	Examine the face, head, and neck for signs of infection.	Injection is contraindicated in the presence of infection at the injection sites.[27]
Pregnancy or breastfeeding	Collect a complete history.	There are no adequate and well-controlled studies of deoxycholic acid injection in pregnant or breastfeeding women to inform the drug-associated risk.[27]

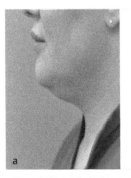 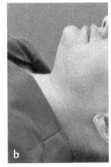 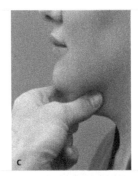 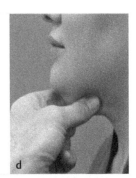

Fig. 8.2 Techniques for assessing preplatysmal submental fat. Prior to deoxycholic acid injection, the physician should observe the patient while upright and supine. Submental fat will contribute to visible submental fullness in both positions. To best identify the preplatysmal component of submental fat, the physician can pinch the submental fat while the patient "grimaces" or while swallowing. (Photo credit: Marc Pacifico 2019.)

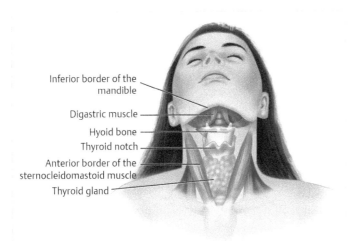

Inferior border of the mandible

Digastric muscle

Hyoid bone

Thyroid notch

Anterior border of the sternocleidomastoid muscle

Thyroid gland

Fig. 8.3 Landmarks for deoxycholic acid injection. The preplatysmal fat in the submental space is bordered superiorly by the mandible, laterally by the sternocleidomastoid muscles and inferiorly by the hyoid bone.

patients), hematoma (70.0–72.9% of patients), edema/swelling (37.4–67.8% of patients), anesthesia (47.9–66.9% of patients), erythema (6.5–40.5% of patients), induration or nodule (10.0–28.3% of patients), pruritus (8.6–16.3% of patients), and paresthesias (0–14.7% of patients). These adverse events were more common in the treatment groups than placebo groups.[8,9,10,11,12,13] Most injection site reactions were short-lived (< 30 d), but some reactions were longer lasting: anesthesia (occurring up to a median of 62 d) and nodule formation (occurring up to a median of 101 d).[13] When adverse events were stratified by mild SMF versus severe SMF, bruising, edema, anesthesia, swelling, pruritus, nodule, and erythema occurred at a higher rate in patients with more severe SMF.[13] Since FDA-approval of deoxycholic acid injections for SMF, few publications have addressed approaches to minimizing injection site reactions. Premedication with ibuprofen or pretreatment injection with epinephrine and buffered lidocaine can reduce pain and bruising. Following injection of each grid site in the treatment area, ice should be applied to reduce swelling.[29,32,33]

8.2.6 Complications: Nerve injury

In clinical trials of deoxycholic acid injection, temporary nerve injury events occurred in 0.9 to 4.3% of subjects, and resolved without sequelae within

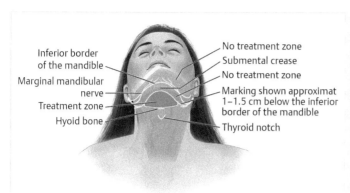

Fig. 8.4 Treatment area. Landmarks are helpful for identifying the treatment area. Deoxycholic acid should not be injected within a region defined by a 1 to 1.5 cm line below the inferior border of the mandible, or above the inferior border of the mandible (the "no treatment zone").

a range of 4 to 115 days.[9,12,13] Marginal mandibular nerve injury and "pseudomarginal mandibular nerve injury" have been reported. The course of this nerve varies. It can lie anteriorly above the inferior border of the mandible. In approximately one in five patients, however, the nerve courses 1 to 2 cm below the inferior border of the mandible.[30] In cadaver studies, deoxycholic acid causes myelin sheath damage when exposed to the marginal mandibular nerve.[34] Compromise of the marginal mandibular nerve leads to reduced function of the depressor muscles of the lip and can result in an asymmetric smile (▶ Fig. 8.5).

Compromise of the mentalis results in deficits of lip eversion.[30] "Pseudomarginal mandibular nerve injury" was originally reported in rhytidectomy literature to describe deficits resulting from injury to the cervical branch of the facial nerve.[35] Pseudomarginal mandibular nerve injury results in a clinically asymmetric smile, similar to a true marginal mandibular nerve injury. However, in pseudomarginal mandibular nerve injury, lip eversion remains intact.[30]

8.2.7 Complications: Skin Ulceration and Necrosis

Skin ulceration at deoxycholic acid injection sites (▶ Fig. 8.6) has occurred in clinical trials as well as case reports and the exact frequency is not reported or known.[27,31,36]

This necrosis can lead to scarring. Immediate blanching of the skin, severe pain, and bruising/erythema in a reticulate pattern are early signs of this adverse event.[31,36] Ulceration and necrosis are thought to be a result of too superficial injections. In one case, ulceration and necrosis occurred as a late sequela after inadvertent intra-arterial injection.[27,36]

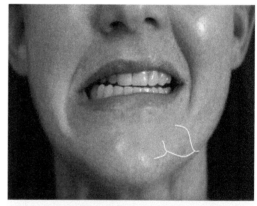

Fig. 8.5 Marginal mandibular nerve injury causes asymmetric smile. Compromise of the marginal mandibular nerve leads to reduced function of the depressor muscles of the lip, resulting in an asymmetric smile. (Used with permission from Sorenson E, Chesnut C. Marginal Mandibular Versus Pseudo-Marginal Mandibular Nerve Injury With Submandibular Deoxycholic Acid Injection. Dermatol Surg. 2018 May;44(5):733–735.)

In vitro studies of sodium deoxycholate (the salt of deoxycholic acid) have demonstrated that it acts primarily as a detergent in causing nonspecific cell lysis, which underlines the importance of proper injection technique. If skin break down after deoxycholic acid injection occurs, patients should practice diligent wound care using petrolatum- or dimethicone-based ointments or hydrocolloid dressings.[31] Three to four weeks (at the earliest) after injury, once the skin has reepithelialized, laser treatments may be considered to improve the appearance of hyperpigmentation and/or scarring in the area.[31]

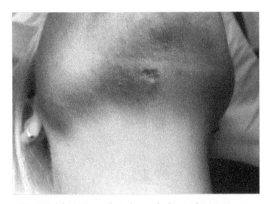

Fig. 8.6 Ulceration after deoxycholic acid injection. Skin ulceration at deoxycholic acid injection sites has been infrequently reported in clinical trials and case reports as a result of too superficial injections. (Used with permission from Lindgren AL, Welsh KM. Inadvertent intra-arterial injection of deoxycholic acid: A case report and proposed protocol for treatment. Journal of Cosmetic Dermatology. 2019.)

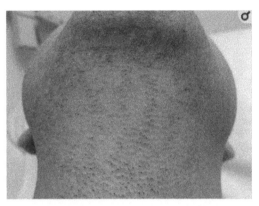

Fig. 8.7 Injection site alopecia. Submental alopecia has been reported in few male patients after deoxycholic injection. (Used with permission from Souyoul S, Gioe O, Emerson A, Hooper DO. Alopecia after injection of ATX-101 for reduction of submental fat. JAAD Case Reports. 2017.)

8.2.8 Complications: Dysphagia

In clinical trials of deoxycholic injection for SMF, dysphagia was a side effect noted in 1.6 to 2.5% of patients. Dysphagia self-resolved in all reported cases, with a median duration of 2.5 to 4 days.[9,12] Experience from clinical trials suggests that patients with current or history of dysphagia may be at increased risk of worsening condition after deoxycholic acid treatment.[27] Therefore, patients should be thoroughly screened for current or past dysphagia which may be exacerbated by submental injections.

8.2.9 Complications: Alopecia

There are multiple case reports of deoxycholic acid injection site alopecia in men. In the literature, these reported cases did note an eventual improvement in submental hair loss. It remains unknown if the injection site alopecia is temporary or if it could be permanent.[37,38] One case report which included histologic examination of the alopecic area noted increased telogen–catagen count, and proposed that local inflammation caused by deoxycholic acid led to localized telogen effluvium.[39] Male patients should be well-informed of this possible side effect. No treatment has been proposed (▶ Fig. 8.7).

8.3 Early Identification of Complications

During and immediately after deoxycholic injection, the treatment area should be inspected for early bruising or excessive bleeding. Ask the patient to smile and carefully assess for smile asymmetry. Prior to the patient's departure, education should be provided regarding normal injection site reactions (mild-to-moderate erythema, edema, anesthesia, pain). Warning signs of more serious side effects should be reviewed, including severe pain, severe swelling/edema, fever, bleeding, new or worsening dysphagia.

8.4 Managing Complications

▶ Table 8.2 summarizes key complications related to deoxycholic acid injection, avoidance techniques, and suggestions for management. One of the most critical components of managing complications is setting reasonable patient expectations prior to the procedure. For example, injection site reactions occur in a vast majority of patients, are usually mild to moderate, and resolve within 30 days. One physician with significant experience using deoxycholic acid injections for SMF treatment stated that 100% of her patients experience injection site reactions, although the procedure and side effects are well tolerated.[32] Common measures such as ibuprofen, lidocaine, and

Table 8.2 Summary of complications related to deoxycholic acid injection

Complication	Prevalence	Avoidance	Management
Injection site reactions: Pain and edema/swelling	Pain: Up to 84.6% of patients in clinical trials.[9,11,12,13] In one phase IIIb study, peak pain occurred within 1–5 min of treatment.[33] Edema/swelling: Up to 67.8% of patients in clinical trials.[9,11,12,13]	Pretreatment with ibuprofen (or similar), topical lidocaine, and injectable lidocaine are helpful.[29,32,33]	Postprocedure pain management is usually adequate with ibuprofen (or similar). Continue to apply ice after treatment.
Injection site reactions: Hematoma/bruising	Up to 72.9% of patients in clinical trials.[9,11,12,13]	After consideration of past medical history and following discussion of risks versus benefits, prescription medication and supplements with known anticoagulant activity (aspirin, etc.) may be discontinued, ideally 10 d before treatment.[29] Preinjection with lidocaine containing epinephrine is recommended to reduce bruising.[33]	If bruising occurs, the use of pulsed-dye and other lasers can assist in dissipation of bruising.[40]
Nerve injury resulting in asymmetric smile	In clinical trials, nerve injury events were temporary and resolved without sequelae in 0.9–4.3% of subjects, within a range of 4–115 d.[9,12,13]	Carefully plan treatment area to avoid "no treatment zone" described in Section 8.2.5, Common Complications. Inject only into the mid-subcutaneous space (not into platysma or deeper), avoiding injection in patients with thin, atrophic platysma or with altered anatomy from previous neck/facial procedures.[30]	All cases of nerve injury reported in clinical trials were self-limited (duration range 1–298 d, median 44 d).[9,12,13,27] Anti-inflammatory medication (ibuprofen or prednisone) could be considered, but have not been studied for this use.
Dysphagia	In clinical trials, dysphagia was noted in 1.6–2.5% of patients.[9,12]	Obtain thorough current and past health history, including any issues swallowing.	In clinical trials, dysphagia was self-resolving in all reported cases, with median duration of 2.5–4 d.[9,12]
Skin ulceration	Case reports[31,36]; exact incidence unknown.[27]	Avoid superficial injections (into the dermis).	Wound care and delay/cessation of further injections until complete resolution.
Injection site alopecia	Case reports[37,38,39]; exact incidence unknown.[27]	No prevention methods have been proposed. Male patients must be well-informed of this possible side effect.	No treatment has been proposed/studied.

ice therapy are effective in managing some injection site reactions. Other adverse events, including marginal mandibular nerve injury, dysphagia, skin ulceration, and alopecia, are usually self-limited and do not have an associated treatment recommendation.

8.5 Conclusion

In summary, in selected patients deoxycholic acid injection is a relatively safe and effective treatment for SMF. Careful consideration of submental anatomy, proper injection technique, and thorough patient screening and selection can minimize the risk of adverse events and maximize the likelihood of satisfactory aesthetic result.

References

[1] Baumann L, Shridharani SM, Humphrey S, Gallagher CJ. Personal (self) perceptions of submental fat among adults in the United States. Dermatol Surg. 2019; 45(1):124–130

[2] Raveendran SS, Anthony DJ, Ion L. An anatomic basis for volumetric evaluation of the neck. Aesthet Surg J. 2012; 32(6):685–691

[3] Thomas WW, Bloom JD. Neck contouring and treatment of submental adiposity. J Drugs Dermatol. 2017; 16(1):54–57

[4] Koehler J. Complications of neck liposuction and submentoplasty. Oral Maxillofac Surg Clin North Am. 2009; 21(1):43–52, vi

[5] Kybella (deoxycholic acid) injection [package insert]. 2018; https://www.accessdata.fda.gov/drugsatfda_docs/label/2018/206333s001lbl.pdf. Accessed November, 2019

[6] Belkyra (deoxycholic acid injection) [product monograph]. http://allerganweb-cdn-prod.azureedge. Accessed November, 2019

[7] US Food and Drug Administration. FDA approves treatment for fat below chin. 2015; https://www.fda.gov/newsevents/newroom/pressannouncements/ucm444978.htm. Accessed November, 2019

[8] Ascher B, Hoffmann K, Walker P, Lippert S, Wollina U, Havlickova B. Efficacy, patient-reported outcomes and safety profile of ATX-101 (deoxycholic acid), an injectable drug for the reduction of unwanted submental fat: results from a phase III, randomized, placebo-controlled study. J Eur Acad Dermatol Venereol. 2014; 28(12):1707–1715

[9] Jones DH, Carruthers J, Joseph JH, et al. REFINE-1, a multicenter, randomized, double-blind, placebo-controlled, phase 3 trial with ATX-101: an injectable drug for submental fat reduction. Dermatol Surg. 2016; 42(1):38–49

[10] Rzany B, Griffiths T, Walker P, Lippert S, McDiarmid J, Havlickova B. Reduction of unwanted submental fat with ATX-101 (deoxycholic acid), an adipocytolytic injectable treatment: results from a phase III, randomized, placebo-controlled study. Br J Dermatol. 2014; 170(2):445–453

[11] McDiarmid J, Ruiz JB, Lee D, Lippert S, Hartisch C, Havlickova B. Results from a pooled analysis of two European, randomized, placebo-controlled, phase 3 studies of ATX-101 for the pharmacologic reduction of excess submental fat. Aesthetic Plast Surg. 2014; 38(5):849–860

[12] Humphrey S, Sykes J, Kantor J, et al. ATX-101 for reduction of submental fat: a phase III randomized controlled trial. J Am Acad Dermatol. 2016; 75(4):788–797.e7

[13] Glogau RG, Glaser DA, Callender VD, et al. A double-blind, placebo-controlled, phase 3b study of ATX-101 for reduction of mild or extreme submental fat. Dermatol Surg. 2019; 45(12):1531–1541

[14] Humphrey SB, Ashish CB, Green LJ, et al. Improvements in submental fat achieved with the use of ATX-101 (deoxycholic acid injection) are maintained over time: three-year follow-up data from the phase 3 REFINE trials. J Am Acad Dermatol. 2019; 79(3):AB163

[15] Deeks ED. Deoxycholic acid: a review in submental fat contouring. Am J Clin Dermatol. 2016; 17(6):701–707

[16] Duncan D, Rotunda AM. Injectable therapies for localized fat loss: state of the art. Clin Plast Surg. 2011; 38(3):489–501, vii

[17] Rotunda AM, Suzuki H, Moy RL, Kolodney MS. Detergent effects of sodium deoxycholate are a major feature of an injectable phosphatidylcholine formulation used for localized fat dissolution. Dermatol Surg. 2004; 30(7):1001–1008

[18] Rotunda AM. Injectable treatments for adipose tissue: terminology, mechanism, and tissue interaction. Lasers Surg Med. 2009; 41(10):714–720

[19] Thuangtong R, Bentow JJ, Knopp K, Mahmood NA, David NE, Kolodney MS. Tissue-selective effects of injected deoxycholate. Dermatol Surg. 2010; 36(6):899–908

[20] Saedi N, Rad J. Injectable fat-reducing therapies: fat reduction. In: Orringer J, Murad A, Dover J, eds. Body Shaping: Skin Fat Cellulite. Procedures in Cosmetic Dermatology Series, vol. 91;2014

[21] Bologna J, Schaffer JV, Cerroni L. Dermatology. 4th edition. Philadelphia, PA: Elsevier; 2018: Clinical Key

[22] Jones DH, Kenkel JM, Fagien S, et al. Proper technique for administration of ATX-101 (deoxycholic acid injection): insights from an injection practicum and roundtable discussion. Dermatol Surg. 2016; 42 suppl 1:S275–S281

[23] Shamban AT. Noninvasive submental fat compartment treatment. Plast Reconstr Surg Glob Open. 2016; 4(12) Suppl Anatomy and Safety in Cosmetic Medicine: Cosmetic Bootcamp:e1155

[24] Dunican KC, Patel DK. Deoxycholic acid (ATX-101) for reduction of submental fat. Ann Pharmacother. 2016; 50(10):855–861

[25] Renaut A, Orlin W, Ammar A, Pogrel MA. Distribution of submental fat in relationship to the platysma muscle. Oral Surg Oral Med Oral Pathol. 1994; 77(5):442–445

[26] Pacifico M. Treating the submental area. Aesthet J 2019

[27] Biopharmaceuticals USFaDAK. Kybella Package Insert. Drugs@FDA: FDA-Approved Drugs. Reference ID: 4208989. FDA Drug Databases 2018

[28] Ross DS. Clinical presentation and evaluation of goiter in adults. In: Cooper DSM, Jean E, ed. UpToDate. UpToDate, Waltham, MA. Accessed December 5th, 2019

[29] Fagien S, McChesney P, Subramanian M, Jones DH. Prevention and management of injection-related adverse effects in facial aesthetics: considerations for ATX-101 (deoxycholic acid injection) treatment. Dermatol Surg. 2016; 42 Suppl 1:S300–S304

[30] Sorenson E, Chesnut C. Marginal mandibular versus pseudo-marginal mandibular nerve injury with submandibular deoxycholic acid injection. Dermatol Surg. 2018; 44(5):733–735

[31] Sachdev D, Mohammadi T, Fabi SG. Deoxycholic acid-induced skin necrosis: prevention and management. Dermatol Surg. 2018; 44(7):1037–1039

[32] Humphrey S. Management of patient experience with ATX-101 (deoxycholic acid injection) for reduction of submental fat. Dermatol Surg. 2016; 42(12):1397–1398

[33] Dover JS, Kenkel JM, Carruthers A, et al. Management of patient experience with ATX-101 (deoxycholic acid injection) for reduction of submental fat. Dermatol Surg. 2016; 42 Suppl 1: S288–S299

[34] Blandford AD, Ansari W, Young JM, et al. Deoxycholic acid and the marginal mandibular nerve: a cadaver study. Aesthetic Plast Surg. 2018; 42(5):1394–1398

[35] Ellenbogen R. Pseudo-paralysis of the mandibular branch of the facial nerve after platysmal face-lift operation. Plast Reconstr Surg. 1979; 63(3):364–368

[36] Lindgren AL, Welsh KM. Inadvertent intra-arterial injection of deoxycholic acid: a case report and proposed protocol for treatment. J Cosmet Dermatol. 2019

[37] Grady B, Porphirio F, Rokhsar C. Submental alopecia at deoxycholic acid injection site. Dermatol Surg. 2017; 43 (8):1105–1108

[38] Souyoul S, Gioe O, Emerson A, Hooper DO. Alopecia after injection of ATX-101 for reduction of submental fat. JAAD Case Rep. 2017; 3(3):250–252

[39] Sebaratnam DF, Wong XL, Kim L, Cheung K. Alopecia following deoxycholic acid treatment for submental adiposity. JAMA Facial Plast Surg. 2019; 21(6):571–572

[40] Karen JK, Hale EK, Geronemus RG. A simple solution to the common problem of ecchymosis. Arch Dermatol. 2010; 146 (1):94–95

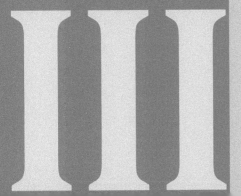

9 Laser Resurfacing

E. Victor Ross

Summary

Minimally invasive procedures on the face, although safe in general, are subject to complications and side effects. Some of these outcomes are unavoidable and are not related to operator error. However, a good understanding of local anatomy, within the context of where wounds are created with various interventions, can diminish the likelihood of short and long-term complications.

Keywords: complication, minimally invasive, face, laser, radiofrequency, safety

9.1 Introduction

Over the last 30 years many energy devices have been introduced into cosmetic medicine. One critical feature is the placement of that energy within the context of local anatomy. As one is applying the energy source, the operator should visualize where the energy is going and the immediate effect on local tissue. In energy–tissue interactions, temperature elevation is fast; however, cooling is slow, such that stacking pulses in the same area will result in a rapid local temperature increase with potentially catastrophic consequences. On the other hand, in applying a short-pulsed yellow light laser to a red area of the skin with a single pulse, only the red local targets will become hot, such that the likelihood of gross overtreatment becomes smaller.[1,2] Indeed, most good outcomes in skin are determined by finessing the cooling and heating of specific targets. The skin, especially facial skin, can withstand a thermal burden to a certain point, after which a threshold is breached and catastrophic consequences are sometimes observed.

Today not only does the practitioner need to be a savvy laser-and-light doctor, but also one needs to be aware of the nuances of radio frequency (RF) and ultrasound energy. To remain safe, the treating MD must remain vigilant in real-time assessment of the skin for superficial targets. For deeper targets, the operator must accurately predict where and when the heating will occur. In following sections, key points for energy–tissue interactions are provided to increase safety and minimize complications in facial skin.

9.2 Key Points for Maximizing Safety with Lasers and Other Energy Devices

Skin thickness varies across the face. The three components of the cutis are the epidermis, dermis, and fat. Epidermal thickness is fairly constant with exception of eyelid skin, where all three components are much thinner than their noneyelid counterparts.[3]

Most devices should be studied relative to where they heat (**see** ▶ Fig. 9.1). We can divide devices by relative depths of heating and whether they are selective or non-selective (selectivity being defined as the device preferentially targeting a small structure based on "contrast agents" such as melanin or hemoglobin)[1,4] (▶ Fig. 9.2).

Most fractional devices and other surface-heating systems are not selective; rather their targeting is based on the spatial geometry of the micro beam with respect to the general skin volume. The selectivity is based also on how long the skin is exposed to the beam, and whether a broad beam (> 1 mm) or one that is fractionated is applied.[5]

9.3 Key Points for Maximizing Safety with Shallower-Penetrating Lasers and Energy Devices

- Visualize the wound being created.
- Pay attention to the skin surface.
- Use magnification if necessary to improve feedback.
- Avoid bulk heating in this area.
- Apply surface cooling if indicated.

9.4 Fractional Laser Systems

Most fractional lasers will only penetrate up to about 1 mm even with multiple passes such that any nerve or catastrophic vascular injury is unlikely. The main danger is in overheating of the thin skin of the lower face and preauricular regions, where lower densities and depths should be applied.

One nuance of fractional lasers is that treatment is by recipe rather than endpoints. Gross blistering

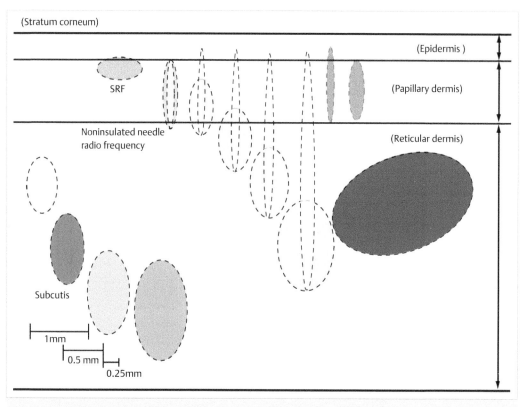

Fig. 9.1 Schematic of skin and injuries by various technologies where water is target. SRF, superficial radiofrequency.

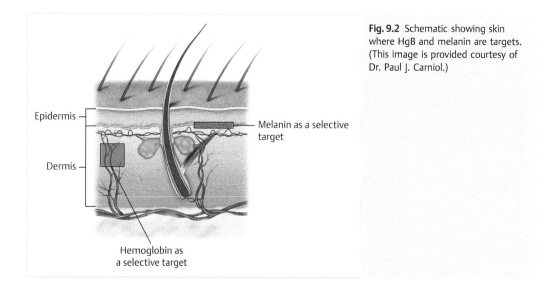

Fig. 9.2 Schematic showing skin where HgB and melanin are targets. (This image is provided courtesy of Dr. Paul J. Carniol.)

or extreme immediate tissue shrinkage should alert the operator regarding potential overtreatment; however, a key point is monitoring the system display with respect to the actual placement of scans and the number of micro beams/cm². These observations should be made within the context of surface

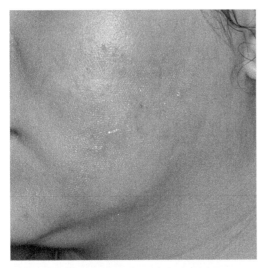

Fig. 9.3 Blister after nonablative fractional laser was carried out too quickly over too small an area such that bulk heating occurred.

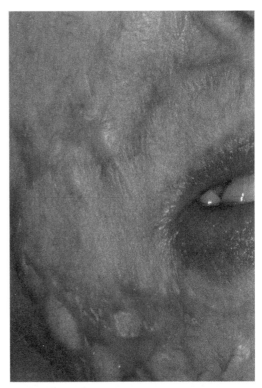

Fig. 9.4 Scarring after ablative fractional laser, settings unknown.

cooling and the size of the region that is treated. Generally speaking, applying passes over large areas will result in greater tissue cooling between passes, as there is more time between consecutive passes. For example, in providing treatment for localized scarring on the cheek, where there is only a small plaque of acne scarring, if one applies four to five passes relatively quickly, there is no opportunity for the skin to cool and overheating and blistering is possible (▶ Fig. 9.3, face blister). In general, with increasing depth and density, side effects are more likely. Also, based on surface-to-volume arguments, smaller fractional beams will cool faster than wider beams.

9.4.1 Nonablative Fractional Laser Systems

Nonablative fractional laser systems incorporate wavelengths that are poorly absorbed by water when compared to CO_2 and erbium yttrium aluminum garnet (YAG) lasers.[5] Like their ablative counterparts, the main danger is laying down the scans or pulses too close together, or not allowing for cooling between scans or between stamping motions. There are also "hybrid" lasers that include both highly absorbed and weakly absorbing wavelengths. Examples include 1,550 and 1,927 nm, and 1,470 and 2,940 nm, respectfully. In areas of preexisting melasma, any superficial heating ablative or nonablative technology, whether fractional or nonfractional, can exacerbate the condition.[6]

When using fractional lasers, the operator must know the nuances of the device to maintain safety. Most of these devices incorporate three settings: mJ/microbeam (which determines the microwound depth), pitch (space between the adjacent wounds which determines the density), and pulse interval between adjacent scans. The novice should employ all three parameters on the lower side and increase the settings as conditions allow. Many lasers include a percent coverage (cross-sectional coverage) as one of the parameters. These values should be interpreted cautiously, as manufacturers' formulas vary for the determination. For example, one fractional CO_2 laser is applied on the face with values as high as 70 mJ and 50% density on the graphical user interface (GUI), whereas another laser might show the same clinical endpoint with settings (on the GUI) as low as 30 mJ and 20% density. Scarring can result if the provider is not attuned to the nuances of a particular system (▶ Fig. 9.4).

9.4.2 Microneedling and RF Pins/Needles

A number of pin and needling systems have been applied in skin facial rejuvenation. For microneedling alone (whether using a rolling device or a sewing machine-type motorized one), most devices are well tolerated, and the procedure, with or without platelet-rich plasma (PRP), tend to be free of side effects.[7] The most serious complications are associated with infusion of nonsterile topical products into the dermis.[8] Some providers apply topical products and then use the needling systems, intending to introduce these agents in the viable skin; however, for products not designed for dermal use, risks of infection and granulomatous reactions are increased.[9] A good rule is to only infuse those compounds intended for dermal use. Track marks have also been reported with microneedling devices.[10]

RF fractional injuries are created by either deeper "needle" wounds (600–3,500 μm) or more superficial "pin" wounds (50–500 μm)(▸ Fig. 9.5). There are now over 15 systems available in the United States that deploy these pins/needles into the skin. In a typical needle configuration, 25 to 49 needles are inserted over a 1 cm² area. The needles are inserted simultaneously, reside in the skin for 50 milliseconds to 4 seconds, and depending on the setting and/or the specific device are retracted. Microwound sizes vary from very small cylinders (100 μm wide and 400 μm deep, size of "grain of sand") to larger "grain of rice-type" geometries, depending on the pulse width, needle type, and insertion depth.[11,12]

Concern has been expressed about fractional lasers interfering with previously placed fillers,

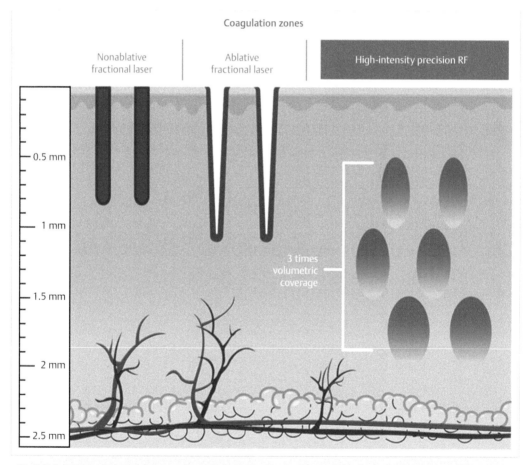

Fig. 9.5 Schematic showing relative position of injuries for fractional laser and radio frequency microneedling with insulated needles.

but most filler placement has been shown to be deeper than the deepest aspects of the vertical injuries created by these devices.[13,14] More recently, data show that some deeper needle devices might compromise fillers, but there is only one publication[15,16] that suggests a clinically impactful role for deeper devices, where Weiss et al showed that deeper RF needle devices might affect superficially placed hyaluronic acid (HA) fillers. Still, on a volumetric basis, it is unlikely that the fractional device will "dissolve" fillers to a point of changing the contour of the face.

9.5 Nonfractional Ablative Treatment

Nonfractional ablative lasers now have enjoyed over 25 years of use in skin applications (**Video 9.1**).[17,18,19,20,21] Both erbium YAG and CO_2 lasers were initially applied at total injury depths of 120 to 400 µm, depending on the application and local anatomic region. Most complications can be avoided by

playing close attention to the skin surface during treatment. The CO_2 laser, when applied such that total depths of injury (ablation + RTD) are less than 100 µm, is normally well tolerated, and barring infection or treating irradiated skin, the face should heal quickly, requiring less than 10 days to complete re-epithelialization. Avoidance of complications is primarily related to the depth of treatment. The areas where healing is most likely to be delayed are the lateral and lower cheeks, where the skin behaves much like neck skin (▶ Fig. 9.6). With the CO_2 laser, normally only one pass should be applied over the lateral face, lower face, and forehead, if one is to avoid hypopigmentation and texture changes, which are the most common long-term complications (▶ Fig. 9.7). As one proceeds toward the central face, deeper heating is tolerated. Normally more than one pass of the nonfractional CO_2 laser is applied only in the immediate perioral region, where the skin can tolerate a deeper injury. The role of wiping between successive passes has been explored in multiple studies, the most recent by Niamtu.[22,23] He found

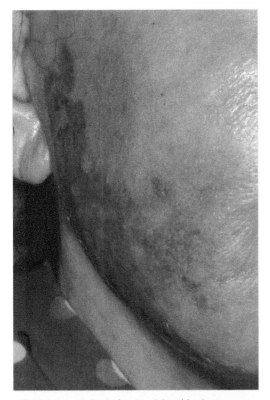

Fig. 9.6 Lateral cheek showing delayed healing versus central cheek after filly ablative laser (10 days after laser).

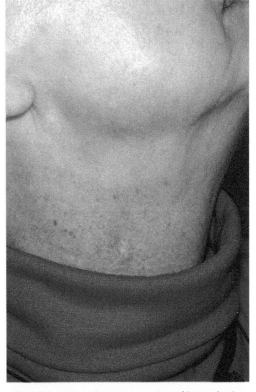

Fig. 9.7 Long-term hypopigmentation of lower cheeks and upper neck after fully ablative CO_2 laser in type II skin with actinic bronzing.

that results were similar with or without wiping, but that recovery was enhanced by not wiping between passes, presumably by allowing the denatured skin to act as a biologic dressing. Like Dr. Niamtu, we have found that perioral lines respond uniquely well to fully ablative lasers, whether CO_2 and erbium YAG.

Unfortunately, performing a series of less invasive procedures (be it fractional erbium YAG or CO_2 laser, non-ablative fractional resurfacing [NAFR], or microneedling) has not achieved satisfactory results, even after five to six treatments 6 to 8 weeks apart. If one examines the body of resurfacing literature over the last 25 years, data suggests that there is a threshold depth of injury for adequate wrinkle reduction in the perioral area, and that below this single treatment threshold, results are typically underwhelming, particularly for deeper perioral rhytides associated with severe solar elastosis. Outside of the deeper perioral lines, ablative fractional lasers work reasonably well (i.e., cheek lines).

For periorbital lines and forehead lines, neuromodulators are associated with a much more attractive benefit-to-risk ratio than energy-based interventions. Many patients will insist on lasers for all lines and rejuvenation, as they do not want to regularly come visit the clinic for a dose of fillers and neuromodulators. However, a frank discussion addressing the benefits and risks, and the complementary nature of devices, neuromodulators, and fillers, will often soften that stance. The mitigation of complications by lessening the risk of relying too much on any one intervention is a compelling argument to make for patients to decrease the overall facial complication rate.

Regarding the erbium YAG laser, the amount of material removed is typically directly proportional to the fluence per pass. Accordingly, one can calculate the total depth of injury by multiplying the pass number times the fluence, basing the amount of material removed by the fairly consistent value of 3 to 4 $\mu m/J/cm^2$.[24] Some providers rely on bleeding as a possible endpoint for erbium YAG nonfractional applications. Our experience, however, has been that bleeding is quite variable once the beam encounters the dermis. For example, a patient with telangiectasia might have brisk bleeding, and a patient with a less red face might bleed much less at the same total depth of ablation. In some patients, particularly those prone to bleeding (i.e., on aspirin), once the dermis is encountered, bleeding can be so brisk that additional passes are compromised by the blood on the surface. Using a longer pulsed

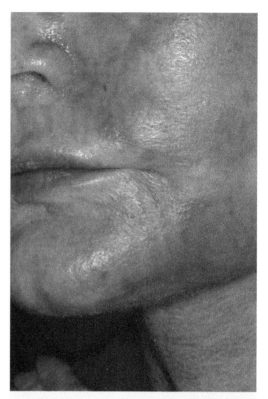

Fig. 9.8 Three months after helium plasma of cheeks showing severe erythema and mild scarring, texture changes.

erbium YAG laser can decrease bleeding by adding a bit of coagulation.[25] Also, the application of thrombin spray after several passes can reduce bleeding and allow for additional passes.

A relatively new device on the market is a helium plasma tool (J plasma), which uses RF to excite helium gas.[26] The flow rate, RF power, and operator hand speed, all determine the amount of thermal damage to the surface. Although called a cold plasma, the reaction is thermal in nature, as energy from free electrons is transferred to the skin surface. The manufacturer claims a higher degree of safety versus CO_2 lasers and other technologies, but like any thermal interaction, excessive heating has been observed (▶ Fig. 9.8).

9.6 Key Points for Maximizing Safety in the Eye Area

The periorbital areas are particularly vulnerable to injury and one must consider the distribution of

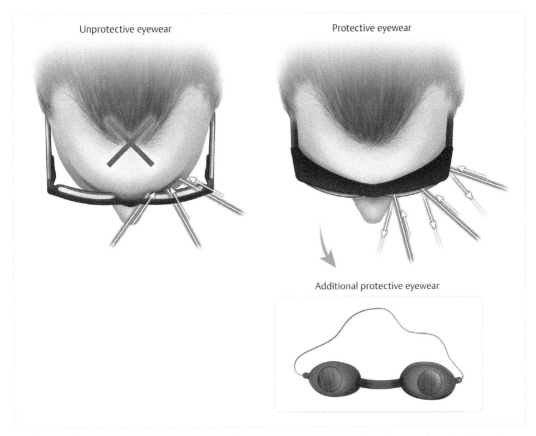

Unprotective eyewear

Protective eyewear

Additional protective eyewear

Fig. 9.9 Laser eyewear.

laser energy within the context of the microanatomic features of the globe and the surrounding tissue.

Most injuries to the eye occur when there is inadequate protection or when there is a poor understanding of the distribution of heating as a function of space and time relative to the skin surface (▶ Fig. 9.9).

The maximum permissible exposure (MPE) is the highest power density or energy density (in W/cm² or J/cm²) of a light source that is considered safe (i.e., which has a negligible probability for creating damage). These values tend to be smallest for 1,064 nm Q-switched lasers, where the short pulse creates a more violet impact on the retina than longer pulsed lasers.

The main eye concerns relate to exposure to visible light and near-infrared (NIR) visible light technologies. These wavelengths can penetrate quite deep and are likely to damage an unprotected retina. The injuries are usually irreversible (▶ Fig. 9.10). On the other hand, although corneal injuries can be severe, very superficial ones can resolve on their own, and deeper ones might be corrected by corneal surgery.

Shorter wavelengths (400–595 nm) and small spot size combinations are less likely to penetrate the thin eyelid skin. Longer wavelengths (> 755 nm) and larger spots carry a greater risk of eyelid penetration and damage to the eye's core structures (iris, cornea, and retina). For resurfacing lasers and nonablative fractional technologies, the cornea and the lens are the eye structures most vulnerable to the beam.

A conundrum is eyeliner tattoo removal. Again, the proximity of the laser beam demands insertion of an internal shield; normally an NIR laser would be applied here, but in cases where paradoxical ink darkening is a risk, ablative lasers can be applied carefully right along the lid margin. When we use resurfacing lasers in the eye area, internal eye shields are necessary when working inside the orbit.

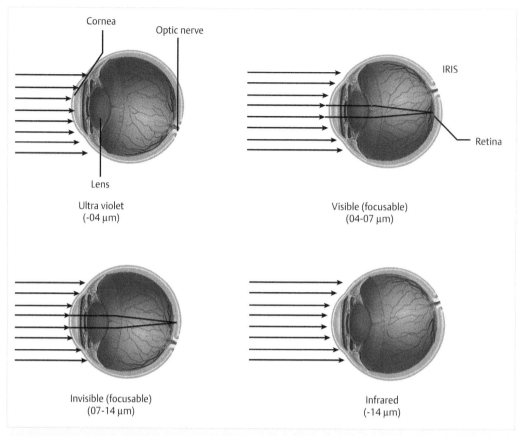

Cornea

Optic nerve

IRIS

Retina

Lens

Ultra violet
(-04 µm)

Visible (focusable)
(04-07 µm)

Invisible (focusable)
(07-14 µm)

Infrared
(-14 µm)

Fig. 9.10 Various wavelength ranges and potential injuries of eye structures.

Also, teeth should be considered a potential target for resurfacing lasers, and there have been reports of tooth injuries with erbium YAG and CO_2 lasers.[27] We normally apply wet gauze over the teeth (2 × 2 in.). A wet dental roll is an alternative.

Topical anesthetics that are more liquid in nature and are susceptible to migration across the eyelid should be avoided around the eye unless there are specifically eye safe. The pH of many of these compounds is high, and they have been implicated in corneal damage.[28] For eyelid resurfacing, particularly the upper eyelid, where it is more likely that a topical analgesic will "run" into the globe, injecting an anesthetic is preferred. We advise using 1-mL Luer lock syringe and 30-gauge needle, always maintaining the needle in a very superficial plane so that the globe is not inadvertently penetrated. The 1-mL syringe allows the operator to apply very gentle pressure so that precise placement of small volumes of anesthetic is possible. Buffered lidocaine minimizes pain greatly.

For most fractional and ablative lasers, hair is not an issue insofar as the immediate laser tissue interaction (LTI) or posttreatment sequelae, but for men, shaving on the day of treatment will minimize charring of surface hair; also a freshly shaven face enhances the absorption of topical anesthetics.

9.7 Key Points for Maximizing Safety in the Perioral/Cheek Area

Lateral cheek skin and upper neck skin is especially vulnerable to scarring after laser. The central face, thicker and endowed with more sebaceous glands,will tolerate more aggressive energy settings than the lateral and lower face. The mandibular margins and preauricular zones are particularly amenable to injury, and a feathering approach with gradually diminishing laser settings is best for the lower-third of the cheek, where the skin behaves much like the neck for wound healing. We typically apply much lower settings over the lateral cheek, both in unfacelifted and those patients who have had a facelift.

9.8 Key Points for Maximizing Safety in Different Skin Types

When laser treatments are applied to the skin, there are two mechanisms of epidermal thermal injury. One is direct damage to the epidermis based on primary melanin absorption and the other is nonselective damage to the skin where water is the chromophore (most fractional lasers). Excessive heating of the skin and delayed wound healing can result in dyspigmentation and scarring.

9.9 Ethnic Skin

Skin of color behaves for the most part like less pigmented skin with some notable exceptions. In the immediate laser tissue interaction, melanin in the epidermis can create excessive heating where visible light or NIR technologies are applied. But even when nonselective approaches are used where water is the target, although the initial reaction is identical to a light-skinned patient, the wound healing sequence can result in postinflammatory hyperpigmentation (PIH) and hypertrophic scarring.

PIH usually resolves, and for facial wounds, wound healing tends to proceed as for lighter skinned patients (▶ Fig. 9.11). One often hears of risks of hypopigmentation in darker skinned patients. While indeed this complication can occur, especially if wounds are very deep, more often

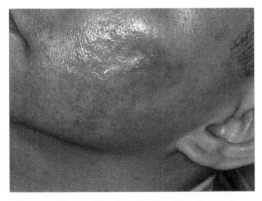

Fig. 9.11 Three weeks after ablative erbium laser in type IV patient showing early phases of hyperpigmentation.

than not, patients tend to revert to their constitutive skin color, and most cases of hypopigmentation occur when chronically bronzed Caucasian patients are treated with resurfacing lasers (▶ Fig. 9.7). Fractional lasers have been helpful in reducing the frequency of hypopigmentation in both darker and lighter patients.

To minimize postinflammatory pigmentation alterations (PIPA) and other untoward reactions after ablative procedures, a minimalist approach is favored. There are multiple proprietary ointments which promise faster healing, but with each added ingredient, there is a risk for irritation. If one is to use one of these products, we recommend applying the ointment to a small test area for a day before using over the entire treated area. Regarding skin preparation, for most laser procedures and energy-based procedures, no special preparation is necessary other than the face being free of debris. For patients at high risk of PIH, we advise a 10-day course of strong topical steroids (as soon as re-epithelialization is complete for ablative procedures and immediately after treatment in nonablative procedures) and absolute sun protection. One major conundrum in postoperative care is dermatitis and/or acne created by topical emollients. This observation is most common in the neck-and-chest area, even when these areas have not been treated. A variety of petrolatum products have been implicated, even those with no preservatives, and in some cases the rash will extend beyond the application region of treatment. Various alternative compounds have been suggested to decrease the likelihood of this phenomena, including topical silicone-based creams. In some patients, avoidance of those products with wool wax alcohol or lanolin will permit normal wound healing.

The use of preoperative hydroquinone (HQ) to prime the skin is controversial. The theory is that melanin formation will be suppressed prior to laser exposure. The only well-controlled study showed no difference in PIH based on pretreating the skin with HQ for 2 weeks versus control.[29] We normally do not pretreat the skin but rely on early intervention with steroids, HQ, and then later retinoids to suppress and treat early PIH, which tends to occur as early as 7 days after resurfacing. Our experience is that any laser procedure can create PIH; however, we have found that erbium YAG laser, so long as the depth and density of fractional wounds is small, and in cases with confluent injuries, so long as the depth of ablation is < 20 to 30 μm, that PIH is unlikely. For CO_2 laser, likewise deeper and denser injuries are more likely to result in PIH, but thresholds for PIH are smaller than for erbium laser. Most likely, the heat contributes to PIH independently from the depth of the injury.

The time to re-epithelialization and adverse effects is directly related. Every effort should be made to optimize wound healing. Short courses of PO antistaphylococcal antibiotics are advised for large surface area ablative wounds, particularly on the neck and chest.[30,31] Alternatively, one can use an ointment such as mupirocin; however with larger regions, the risk of contact dermatitis increases as it does with other older topical antibiotics such as bacitracin, polymyxin, and neomycin. For ablative procedures that involve wounds that extend beyond the epidermis, a short course of antibiotics can help to prevent bacterial infections, and vinegar soaks can be useful for decreasing gram-negative bacterial concentrations on the skin after the procedure.

9.10 Tanned/Solar-Damaged Skin

Of greater concern than a constitutively dark patient is the tanned Caucasian patient, where the skin color tends to revert to the light untanned skin after aggressive ablative treatments. The actinic bronzing observed in sunny climates requires decades to develop, such that great care must be taken not to over resurface bronzed skin.

9.11 X-Irradiated Skin

Skin that has undergone radiation therapy is especially vulnerable to laser surgery. Generally, one should reduce parameters to about 80% of normally accepted settings and test spots should be considered. We have encountered small ulcers

even with conservative settings with relatively benign interventions such as pulsed dye laser.

Remediation of injuries: Despite the best efforts of the provider, complications occur. Management should be based on a logical approach that addresses the underlying pathology. Acneiform eruptions are common after ablative and nonablative fractional lasers, and even after RF microneedling. Nonfractional lasers also can create an acne-friendly environment. Normally a 2-week course of doxycycline or topical antiacne agent is prescribed; clindamycin lotion is a preferred medication that is well-tolerated in newly laser skin. Presumably the eruption is related to disruption of the DE junction. Also for the procedures, regular application of occlusive ointments can increase the likelihood of acne. Prolonged erythema can occur, particularly in lighter skinned rosacea patients. Normally time is the best treatment, although drugs such as oxymetazoline can be applied or short courses of topical steroids used. Edema can be severe after application of aggressive resurfacing lasers, and after a time the edema descends into the neck.

Scarring and long-term hypopigmentation: These are feared side effects and typically are referred to our facility after aggressive CO_2, plasma, or erbium YAG procedures. At times, the patients present with a combination of hypertrophic scars and hypopigmentation (▶ Fig. 9.12). We normally apply conservative NAFR: four to six treatments, spaced 4 to 6 weeks apart. In these patients we also have added elidel or protopic, as well as Latisse, in the hope of cajoling the skin to produce more pigment.

Combination treatments: Combinations of resurfacing and other procedures are becoming increasingly common in dermatology. Common tandems are erbium YAG lasers and visible light technologies, or RF microneedling and NIR light applications. Also

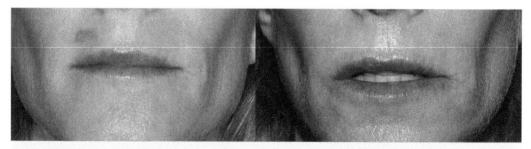

Fig. 9.12 Hypertrophic scar after erbium YAG laser, with resolution after series of sessions with pulsed dye laser and nonablative fractional lasers; pigment loss persists.

high intensity focused ultrasound (HIFU) and RF heating devices can be combined with resurfacing lasers. The array of combinations is related to strategically creating scenarios that allow for optimal outcomes and minimal risks. Some providers are combining photodynamic therapy (PDT) with not just visible light devices, but also fractional ablative lasers. To avoid complications, the provider should visualize microscopically what is occurring in the skin and proceed accordingly. For example, in performing fractional and visible light in the same session, adding bulk cooling can assist in the priming of the skin for the next installment of heat. Some lasers, such as fractional lasers, with insufficient heat extraction, can compromise the skin such that the next application overheats the surface. A layered approach to heating should be based on logic. Various manufacturers have trademark names for some of the combo approaches, such as 3D, or 360 degrees.

In the end, maximizing safety is based on commonsense and negotiating and titrating cooling and heating during the course of treatment. Patients want results with as few sessions as possible. Remember that an undertreated patient might be disappointed and require additional therapy; the overtreated patient is more likely to replace disappointment with anger. One can always "add more salt to the soup," and the prudent practitioner should abide by that rule.

References

[1] Anderson RR, Parrish JA. Selective photothermolysis: precise microsurgery by selective absorption of pulsed radiation. Science. 1983; 220(4596):524–527

[2] Altshuler GB, Anderson RR, Manstein D, Zenzie HH, Smirnov MZ. Extended theory of selective photothermolysis. Lasers Surg Med. 2001; 29(5):416–432

[3] Xu H, Fonseca M, Wolner Z, et al. Reference values for skin microanatomy: a systematic review and meta-analysis of ex vivo studies. J Am Acad Dermatol. 2017; 77(6):1133–1144.e4

[4] Anderson RR, Margolis RJ, Watenabe S, Flotte T, Hruza GJ, Dover JS. Selective photothermolysis of cutaneous pigmentation by Q-switched Nd: YAG laser pulses at 1064, 532, and 355 nm. J Invest Dermatol. 1989; 93(1):28–32

[5] Geronemus RG. Fractional photothermolysis: current and future applications. Lasers Surg Med. 2006; 38(3):169–176

[6] Cohen SR, Goodacre A, Lim S, et al. Clinical outcomes and complications associated with fractional lasers: a review of 730 patients. Aesthetic Plast Surg. 2017; 41(1):171–178

[7] Chandrashekar BS, Sriram R, Mysore R, Bhaskar S, Shetty A. Evaluation of microneedling fractional radiofrequency device for treatment of acne scars. J Cutan Aesthet Surg. 2014; 7(2): 93–97

[8] Soltani-Arabshahi R, Wong JW, Duffy KL, Powell DL. Facial allergic granulomatous reaction and systemic hypersensitivity associated with microneedle therapy for skin rejuvenation. JAMA Dermatol. 2014; 150(1):68–72

[9] Yadav S, Dogra S. A cutaneous reaction to microneedling for postacne scarring caused by nickel hypersensitivity. Aesthet Surg J. 2016; 36(4):NP168–NP170

[10] Pahwa M, Pahwa P, Zaheer A. "Tram track effect" after treatment of acne scars using a microneedling device. Dermatol Surg. 2012; 38(7 Pt 1):1107–1108

[11] Weiner SF. Radiofrequency microneedling: overview of technology, advantages, differences in devices, studies, and indications. Facial Plast Surg Clin North Am. 2019; 27(3): 291–303

[12] Hong JY, Kwon TR, Kim JH, Lee BC, Kim BJ. Prospective, preclinical comparison of the performance between radiofrequency microneedling and microneedling alone in reversing photoaged skin. J Cosmet Dermatol. 2019

[13] Farkas JP, Richardson JA, Brown S, Hoopman JE, Kenkel JM. Effects of common laser treatments on hyaluronic acid fillers in a porcine model. Aesthet Surg J. 2008; 28(5): 503–511

[14] Wu DC, Karnik J, Margarella T, Nguyen VL, Calame A, Goldman MP. Evaluation of the in vivo effects of various laser, light, or ultrasound modalities on human skin treated with a collagen and polymethylmethacrylate microsphere dermal filler product. Lasers Surg Med. 2016; 48(9):811–819

[15] Urdiales-Gálvez F, Martín-Sánchez S, Maíz-Jiménez M, Castellano-Miralla A, Lionetti-Leone L. Concomitant use of hyaluronic acid and laser in facial rejuvenation. Aesthetic Plast Surg. 2019; 43(4):1061–1070

[16] Hsu SH, Chung HJ, Weiss RA. Histologic effects of fractional laser and radiofrequency devices on hyaluronic acid filler. Dermatol Surg. 2019; 45(4):552–556

[17] Jasin ME. Regarding cutaneous resurfacing with Er:YAG lasers. Dermatol Surg. 2000; 26(8):811–812

[18] Jacobson D, Bass LS, VanderKam V, Achauer BM. Carbon dioxide and ER:YAG laser resurfacing:results. Clin Plast Surg. 2000; 27(2):241–250

[19] Grekin RC. Laser resurfacing of the face:is there just one laser? Facial Plast Surg. 2000; 8(2):153–162

[20] Fanous N, Bassas AE, Ghamdi WA. CO_2 laser resurfacing of the neck and face: 10 golden rules for predicting results and preventing complications. Facial Plast Surg Clin. 2000; 8(2): 405–413

[21] Dover JS, Hruza G. Lasers in skin resurfacing. Australas J Dermatol. 2000; 41(2):72–85

[22] Niamtu J, III. Does laser history have to repeat itself? Laser resurfacing and the risk/recovery/result ratio. Dermatol Surg. 2010; 36(11):1793–1795

[23] Niamtu J, III. To debride or not to debride? That is the question: rethinking char removal in ablative CO_2 laser skin resurfacing. Dermatol Surg. 2008; 34(9):1200–1211

[24] Ross EV, Naseef GS, McKinlay JR, et al. Comparison of carbon dioxide laser, erbium:YAG laser, dermabrasion, and dermatome: a study of thermal damage, wound contraction, and wound healing in a live pig model: implications for skin resurfacing. J Am Acad Dermatol. 2000; 42(1 Pt 1): 92–105

[25] Newman JB, Lord JL, Ash K, McDaniel DH. Variable pulse erbium:YAG laser skin resurfacing of perioral rhytides and side-by-side comparison with carbon dioxide laser. Lasers Surg Med. 2000; 26(2):208–214

[26] Gentile RD. Cool atmospheric plasma (J-Plasma) and new options for facial contouring and skin rejuvenation of the heavy face and neck. Facial Plast Surg. 2018; 34(1):66–74

[27] Israel M, Cobb CM, Rossmann JA, Spencer P. The effects of CO_2, Nd:YAG and Er: YAG lasers with and without surface

coolant on tooth root surfaces: an in vitro study. J Clin Periodontol. 1997; 24(9 Pt 1):595–602

[28] McKinlay JR, Hofmeister E, Ross EV, MacAllister W. EMLA cream-induced eye injury. Arch Dermatol. 1999; 135(7):855–856

[29] West TB, Alster TS. Effect of pretreatment on the incidence of hyperpigmentation following cutaneous CO_2 laser resurfacing. Dermatol Surg. 1999; 25(1):15–17

[30] Manuskiatti W, Fitzpatrick RE, Goldman MP, Krejci-Papa N. Prophylactic antibiotics in patients undergoing laser resurfacing of the skin. J Am Acad Dermatol. 1999; 40(1): 77–84

[31] Walia S, Alster TS. Cutaneous CO_2 laser resurfacing infection rate with and without prophylactic antibiotics. Dermatol Surg. 1999; 25(11):857–861

10 Chemical Peels

Sidney J. Starkman and Devinder S. Mangat

Summary

Patient selection is critical in enhancing the safety profile of chemical peeling. Proper intraoperative technique and tailored treatment plans to each individual patient is necessary in order to achieve desirable results. Early detection of complications can minimize the chances of scarring and long-term sequela.

Keywords: chemical peel, complications, phenol–croton oil peel, skin resurfacing, skin peel, chemoexfoliation

10.1 Background

As life expectancy and life qualities have progressed over the past century, there has been a proportionate increase in public demand for rejuvenating skin treatments. Expectedly, this has led to a surge in the options from practitioners, aestheticians, and pharmaceutical companies for skin resurfacing. The most commonly used facial resurfacing modalities currently are chemical peeling, laser resurfacing, and dermabrasion. These different variations of skin resurfacing options have been used for rhytids, actinic damage, lentigines, and dyschromias. The goal of this chapter is to describe the most commonly encountered complications of the various skin resurfacing modalities, and how to manage them. Advanced skin resurfacing, when practiced with knowledge and good technique, can yield excellent results in skin rejuvenation with a high safety profile.

10.2 Patient Selection

The first step in enhancing the safety profile of facial resurfacing is identifying both the optimal and suboptimal patient. The ideal patient must both be a physical candidate for a skin resurfacing, and also have appropriate expectations for their postoperative results. The most common complication experienced after facial resurfacing is unmet patient expectations, due to poor preprocedural discussion. Skin-specific changes, such as photodamage, lentigines, and rhytids, must be distinguished from other changes like jowling or volume loss. The ideal facial resurfacing patient will have blond hair, blue eyes, fair skin, and fine wrinkles. Of course, the vast majority of facial resurfacing patients do not fit into exact ideal criteria. Therefore, tools such as the Fitzpatrick skin type scale are used to characterize a patient's suitability (see ► Table 10.1). Additionally, patients can be rated by their skin type, complexion, texture, and photoaging, using categorizing schemes such as the one by Glogau (see ► Table 10.2).

10.3 Preoperative Guidelines

A detailed review of any patient medical conditions must be reviewed before facial resurfacing. The relative contraindications for any resurfacing procedure include diabetes, smokers, active or frequent herpes simplex virus (HSV) infections, cutaneous radiation history, hypertrophic scarring, or keloid history. Photosensitizing drugs, birth control pills, and exogenous estrogen should be avoided due to the increased risk of hyperpigmentation. With women of child-bearing age, they should also be warned not to have plans to become pregnant within 6 months after facial resurfacing, due to elevated estrogen levels of pregnancy.[1]

Isotretinoin (Accutane) is an absolute contraindication to any facial resurfacing. Skin resurfacing relies on reepithelialization from hair follicles and

Table 10.1 Fitzpatrick skin type scale

Skin type	Skin color	Characteristics
I	White; very fair; red or blond hair; blue eyes; freckles	Always burns, never tans
II	White; fair; red or blond hair; blue, hazel or green eyes	Usually burns, tans with difficulty
III	Cream white; fair with any eye or hair color; very common	Sometimes mild burn, gradually tans
IV	Brown; typical Mediterranean Caucasian skin	Rarely burns, tans with ease
V	Dark brown; mid-eastern skin types	Very rarely burns, tans very easily
VI	Black	Never burns, tans very easily

Table 10.2 Glogau skin classification scale

Group I (Mild)	Group II (Moderate)	Group III (Advanced)	Group IV (Severe)
No keratoses	Early actinic keratoses—slight yellow skin discoloration	Actinic keratoses—obvious yellow skin discoloration with telangiectasia	Actinic keratoses and skin cancers have occurred
Little wrinkling	Early wrinkling—parallel skin lines	Wrinkling present at rest	Wrinkling—much cutis laxa of actinic, gravitational, and dynamic origin
No scarring	Mild scarring	Moderate acne scarring	Severe acne scarring
Little or no makeup	Little makeup	Wears makeup always	Wears makeup that cakes on

sebaceous glands for healing, and isotretinoin prevents this from happening. It is widely recommended for all patients to stop isotretinoin for 12 to 24 months before facial resurfacing.

It is paramount to address sun exposure and smoking during the planning stages. Skin resurfacing in the faces of chronic smokers can lead to poor tissue healing, because of the microvascular damage from smoking. All current smokers should cease smoking 1 month beforehand and continue to avoid smoking for at least 6 months after the procedure. In addition, patients should be advised to avoid excessive and direct sun exposure for 6 weeks after skin resurfacing. If this is unacceptable to the patient, other options besides deep skin resurfacing should be explored.

Finally, as mentioned beforehand, the largest risk in facial resurfacing is unmet expectations by the patient. The patient and the practitioner must have agreed upon the realistic expectations of the procedure. The patient's axillary skin can represent the final result of the skin resurfacing, as long as this region has not previously received excessive sun damage.[2]

10.4 Complication Prevention

The ideal way to manage complication occurrence is to prevent them from happening in the first place, when possible. Proper preparation for facial resurfacing can greatly increase the safety profile and decrease the risks of the procedure. Patients are advised to start rigorous sunscreen usage for 3 months before the procedure in order to prevent tanning or sunburns prior to the resurfacing. Another aspect of this recommendation is to decrease the melanocyte activity before skin resurfacing.

Hydroquinone is a medication mostly used in patients with lentigines, dyschromias, or with patients with Fitzpatrick III, IV, V, and VI skin types, due to the elevated risks of postpeel postinflammatory hyperpigmentation (PIH). Hydroquinone's method of action is to block the conversion of tyrosine to L-Dopa by tyrosinase, thereby decreasing melanin production. When prescribed to those patients who meet the above criteria, hydroquinone in a concentration of 4 to 8% should be started 4 to 6 weeks before skin resurfacing. It should be restarted after the procedure once the patient's skin is ready to tolerate it.

Another beneficial drug in the preparation of facial resurfacing patients is tretinoin (Retin-A). Topical tretinoin (Retin-A) is recommended for 6 to 12 weeks before the peel. Like with hydroquinone, tretinoin should be restarted after the peel once the patient's skin is ready for its application. Tretinoin leads to increased melanin distribution, and also helps with reepithelialization.[3] Finally, another benefit of tretinoin is that it results in a uniform and thickened epidermis, which aids in the even application of the skin resurfacing modality.[4]

Tretinoin usage can begin at nighttime 6 weeks before the procedure. The dosing ranges from 0.025 to 0.1%; however, no study has shown improved results with the higher dosing. Prior to starting the medication, patients should be advised about the possible side effects of tretinoin, such as flakiness, erythema, or skin irritation. If this was to occur, the dose can be reduced, or the medication can be discontinued entirely.

10.5 Infection Prophylaxis

The first line of defense to microbial infection is the skin, and resurfacing procedures can cause breaks in the epidermis allowing microbial particles to enter. This can lead to infections by cutaneous bacterial flora, such as staphylococcal or streptococcal species. Appropriate prophylactic antibacterial coverage should begin to prevent bacterial skin infections and their resultant sequela. The senior author uses cephalexin, 250 mg four times a day, 1 day before the peel and continues it for 7 days in the postoperative period. In patients who are B-lactam sensitive, erythromycin 250 mg four times a day can be used.

Precautions should be taken to postprocedural HSV outbreaks, even if patients deny any history of herpetic vesicle breakouts. Patients should be informed that it is possible to have latent herpes infections even without any clinical history. It is recommended to start any patient with a negative history on a prophylactic dose of antivirals, acyclovir 400 mg three times a day, 3 days before and continued for at least 5 days after the peel. In patients with an observed history of herpetic vesicular breakouts, a therapeutic dose of antivirals should be used, such as valacyclovir 1 g three times day for the aforementioned time period.

10.6 Complication Management

Even with careful patient selection and strict adherence to all preparatory and intraprocedural recommendations, there is still the possibility to encounter a litany of potential complications following facial resurfacing. Early detection and management of these developing complications can be crucial to minimizing negative outcomes, and still achieving a desired result. Therefore, it is critically important for any provider offering skin resurfacing to be knowledgeable about all potential risks and also in how to quickly recognize these events. Early treatment and close postoperative care can be critical in these cases.

10.6.1 Delayed Reepithelialization

One of the more common complications following a facial skin resurfacing is prolonged skin reepithelialization times. Any area of the face that does not fully reepithelialize within 10 days should be considered prolonged. This complication is more commonly seen with deep phenol peels (Baker formula) and trichloroacetic acid (TCA) peels, versus medium-depth chemical peels or laser resurfacing.[5] It is important to rule out the presence of contact irritants or underlying infections, in cases with prolonged healing times. When these instances are encountered, it is important to bring the patients in to be checked daily and then treated accordingly, in order to minimize the risks of scarring.

10.7 Scarring

The most feared complication of facial skin resurfacing is facial scarring (see ▶ Fig. 10.1). The risk of scarring is significantly elevated in isotretinoin users, due to this medication's effects on the reepithelialization from sebaceous glands. After the patient has stopped isotretinoin for at least 12 months, the practitioner should check to confirm that the patient is clearly producing skin oils. When scar formation does occur, it will most likely begin to develop in the perioral region or over areas with prominent underlying bone structure such as the mandible or cheekbones. Scarring is most commonly caused by overly deep skin resurfacing, or from poor postoperative care. As soon as the developing scars are detected, they should be treated with silicone sheeting coverings and intralesional corticosteroids injections (Kenalog 20 mg/mL) every 2 to 3 weeks. It is recommended to exercise caution in the injections of steroids, as overinjection can lead to atrophy and skin depressions. In addition, a flash-lamp pulsed dye laser is helpful over multiple treatments to treat the erythema of the scar.

10.7.1 Infection

Bacterial infections can irritate normal wound healing and lead to scar formation. In the case of a patient presenting with signs of cellulitis or infection, an appropriate antibiotic regimen should be immediately started and continued for a 7- to 10-day course. Similarly, herpetic viral infections can be problematic for a patient's natural recovery. In the case of a herpetic outbreak despite appropriate prophylactic dosing of antivirals, a course of valacyclovir 1 g three times a day for 10 days should be used.

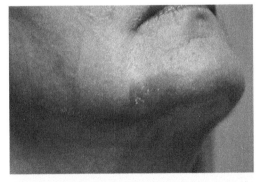

Fig. 10.1 Patient with scarring following deep chemical peel. Note that the location for scarring is often over bony surfaces, such as the mandible or zygoma.

10.7.2 Erythema and Hyperpigmentation

Postoperative erythema after skin resurfacing is common in almost all patients with deep resurfacing, and it is not unusual for it to last even longer than predicted. In patients with sensitive skin or contact dermatitis, hydrocortisone (2.5%) lotion is regularly prescribed to help with the resolution of this erythema. As this erythema eventually subsides in the weeks following the peel, something to watch out for is the development of postinflammatory hyperpigmentation. The usual scenario for this to occur is with a patient with Fitzpatrick III–VI skin types, or who exposes themselves to excessive sun exposure following resurfacing. This can be managed with a combination of 0.05% retinoic acid, 2.5% hydrocortisone cream, and 4% hydroquinone cream.

A much more severe complication than hyperpigmentation is hypopigmentation.

10.7.3 Hypopigmentation

Hypopigmentation is likely caused by phenol and its effect on the melanocyte's ability to produce melanin (see ▶ Fig. 10.2). This complication was more common in the past when deeper chemical peels such as the classic Baker–Gordon formulation were used, along with postoperative occlusive dressing applications. Hypopigmentation is unfortunately irreversible, and the potential need for makeup usage should be advised to all patients who suffer from this complication. There have been anecdotal descriptions of bimatoprost (Latisse, manufacturer:

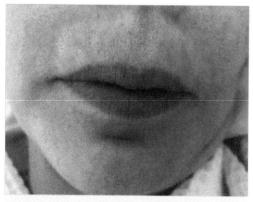

Fig. 10.2 Hypopigmentation following perioral resurfacing.

Allergan) being combined with microneedling devices for improvement of hypopigmentation.

10.7.4 Cardiac Arrhythmia

The most commonly cautioned and feared intraoperative complication of phenol–croton oil peels is cardiac arrhythmias (Video 10.1). Even in patients who have been adequately hydrated prior to the beginning of the chemical peel, a reversible cardiac arrhythmia can occur. This is especially true in any patient with an undiagnosed myocardial sensitivity. The common presentation is a supraventricular tachycardia that occurs within 20 minutes of starting the peel, and then can progress into paroxysmal ventricular contractions, paroxysmal atrial tachycardia, ventricular tachycardia, and, possibly, atrial fibrillations. The best way to manage any of these above listed progressive arrhythmias is to prevent them from occurring in the first place. As soon as a supraventricular tachycardia, or other irregular rhythm, is noted the peel should be immediately paused and adequate hydration should continue. At this point, the rhythm should eventually return to normal sinus rhythm as the phenol is cleared. Once the rhythm has returned to normal, the phenol peel may proceed carefully with attention to the rhythm monitor. In the rare instance that the rhythm does not naturally return to a normal rhythm, proper medical procedures should be undertaken for that aberrant rhythm.

10.8 Conclusion

Chemical peel, laser resurfacing, and dermabrasion all are excellent tools in the practitioner's toolkit for facial skin resurfacing. The key to consistently achieving optimal results and minimizing risks is to not dismiss skin resurfacing as trivial, and to treat it as a medical procedure, which it is. When performed knowledgeably and skillfully, skin resurfacing is predictable with excellent results. There have been many advances in the last quarter-century that now give us the ability to tailor skin resurfacing procedures to fit the characteristics of our patients on an individual level. By recognizing the correct treatment option for each patient and by exercising vigilance during the postoperative healing phase, complications can be minimized, and excellent results can be achieved.

References

[1] Brody HJ. Complications of chemical peeling. J Dermatol Surg Oncol. 1989; 15(9):1010–1019

[2] Brody HJ. Complications of chemical resurfacing. Dermatol Clin. 2001; 19(3):427–438, vii–viii

[3] Popp C, Kligman AM, Stoudemayer TJ. Pretreatment of photoaged forearm skin with topical tretinoin accelerates healing of full-thickness wounds. Br J Dermatol. 1995; 132(1):46–53

[4] Hevia O, Nemeth AJ, Taylor JR. Tretinoin accelerates healing after trichloroacetic acid chemical peel. Arch Dermatol. 1991; 127(5):678–682

[5] Szachowicz EH, Wright WK. Delayed healing after full-face chemical peels. Facial Plast Surg. 1989; 6:8–13

11 Vascular and Pigment Laser and Light Sources

Elizabeth F. Rostan

Summary

Laser treatment of vascular and pigmented lesions can be quite challenging. As with other procedures it is important to select optimal techniques and technology to optimize the outcome and minimize the risks. This chapter reviews laser and light sources for the treatment of vascular and pigmented lesions. Device and treatment parameter selection is reviewed as well as desired treatment endpoints and description of tissue effects that might indicate excessive energy and increased risk of complication. Tips on safely maximizing treatment outcomes while avoiding complications are offered as are tips on managing complications.

Keywords: laser, vascular, pigment, ideal settings, treatment endpoints, maximizing outcomes, complications

11.1 Vascular and Pigment Laser and Light Sources

Laser and light treatment of vascular and pigmented lesions has evolved to a level of safety and specificity that enables physicians to treat a variety of lesions and help numerous patients with their areas of concern.

11.1.1 Laser Treatment of Vascular Lesions

Lasers that treat vascular targets include the KTP (532 nm), pulsed dye laser (585 and 595 nm), as well as longer pulsed lasers including alexandrite (755 nm), diode (800–980 nm), and the Nd: YAG (1064 nm) lasers that emit pulses in the millisecond range. Correct choice of laser or light device as well as settings of the device are critical to achieving success in the treatment of vascular lesions.

11.1.2 Choice of Device— Wavelength and Pulse Duration

In the treatment of telangiectasia, size of the vessel is an important factor in device selection. The principle of selective photothermolysis, for these lesions, refers to site-specific, laser-induced heat injury of pigmented or vascular targets in the skin. The utilization of selective photothermolysis requires proper wavelength selection, pulse duration, and energy or fluence. An additional consideration, particularly in the treatment of vascular lesions, is spot size of the laser pulse. Larger spot sizes penetrate deeper so are better suited to deeper and larger blood vessels and small spot sizes penetrate less deeply and are best utilized in the treatment of small, superficially located vessels.

Selection of pulse duration is based on vessel size. Choosing the correct pulse duration is key to both appropriate selective heating and effective destruction of the blood vessel target as well as avoiding side effects and injury. Too short a pulse duration can lead to rupture of the blood vessel due to very rapid heating and side effect of purpura. Think of a water-filled balloon popping. This is a photoacoustic/cavitation reaction, and, in the case of linear blood vessels, repair mechanisms have been shown to lead to recovery and revascularization of the vessels; however, in the treatment of some vascular lesions, such as cherry angiomas and vascular birthmarks, this can be a desired endpoint. Too long a pulse duration can lead to spreading of heat beyond the target to surrounding tissue and can lead to nonspecific heat-induced injury in the surrounding structures—dermis and epidermis. Think of a heating coil turned on to spread heat to melt ice or snow—peripheral injury to the ice and snow. The ideal heating time is long enough to adequately heat the target without violent rupture while still slightly less than the time that allows spread of heat to adjacent tissue. This ideal heating time and confinement of laser-induced heat to the target without transfer or spread to surrounding tissues can be defined by thermal relaxation time or TRT.[1] TRT is the time required for cooling of the laser target to 50% of the temperature achieved immediately after laser impact. The TRT can be estimated by using this calculation: TRT in seconds is approximately equal to the square of the diameter of the target in millimeters—a 0.1-mm blood vessel would be expected to have a TRT of about 10 ms. Larger blood vessels require longer pulse durations and smaller blood vessels are best targeted with shorter pulse durations.

Proper selection of wavelength is also critical to safe and effective treatment of vascular lesions.

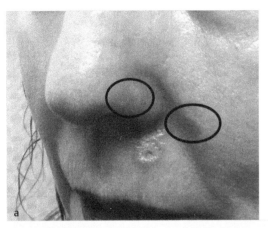 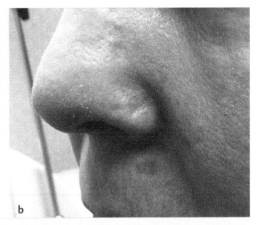

Fig. 11.1 **(a)** One week after 1,064-nm laser treatment of veins in the perinasal area with frank ulceration and signs of tissue damage (*circles*)—darkening and mild scabbing. **(b)** Scarring noted in areas 6 weeks after laser treatment.

Both patient skin color and size and depth of the vascular target must be taken into consideration. Superficial lesions are best targeted by shorter wavelengths whereas longer wavelengths penetrate deeper into the skin and are better suited for deeper blood vessels. Caution must be exercised when treating larger blood vessels. As described earlier, the heating of a large vein can act as a conduit of that heat to the surrounding tissue and damage the surrounding tissue. Blisters to frank ulceration can occur over the blood vessel with atrophic scarring—a particularly vulnerable area is the nasal ala (▶ Fig. 11.1a, b). In addition, damage to tissue can appear later as evidenced by atrophy over the treated vein with no obvious immediate injury (blistering or ulceration) at the time of the laser treatment (▶ Fig. 11.2). To avoid this complication, carefully select a pulse duration that most closely matches the vessel size and slowly increase energy while observing for vessel reaction after each laser pulse—vessel darkening or vessel shrinkage. At the same time careful cooling of the skin is critical to protect the skin overlying the blood vessels. We often employ measures above what is offered within the laser device itself (contact or cryogen cooling) by applying handheld ice packs to the area immediately before and after each laser pulse. Forced cool air can be used for additional cooling of the skin but cannot be used during firing of the laser pulse if cryogen cooling is deployed as there is potential for the air to blow the cryogen off target.

11.1.3 Enhancing Outcomes in the Treatment of Vascular Lesions

It is crucial to recognize clinical endpoint in treating vascular lesions. The goal is vascular damage without damage to surrounding structures. When treating linear vessels, the vessel may disappear immediately, or you may see spasm or coagulation of the vessel which is seen clinically as shrinkage of the vessel and darkening of the color of the vessel (Video 11.1). When treating larger blood vessels or larger blue veins, particularly on face or neck areas, careful observation for blood vessel response without too violent or rapid a response and without any skin contraction over the vessel is crucial. This slight retraction of the skin may mean there is too much heat transfer to the skin and potential for skin damage. Rupture of the vessel can be seen also as purpura but this is not always a desired endpoint.

When treating diffuse redness such as seen in rosacea, each laser pulse should generate a fleeting darkening of the treated area, or transient purpura, that does not result in persistent purpura. Typically, test pulses are done at initial treatment settings looking for this fleeting or transient purpura change with several seconds of waiting to be sure the change does not persist to true purpura (Video 11.2, and ▶ Fig. 11.3). If no transient purpura is seen, the energy can be increased in small increments until transient but not persistent purpura is observed (Video 11.2). Several methods of enhancing outcomes from laser treatment of vascular targets have been proposed and are

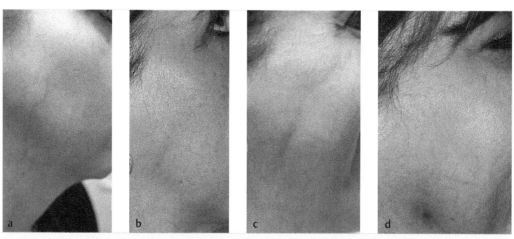

Fig. 11.2 **(a)** Blue vein before treatment. **(b)** Mild hyperpigmentation and atrophy at rest, 4 months after long-pulsed 1064 nm laser treatment. **(c)** Exaggeration of atrophy and retraction noted with animation. **(d)** Correction with filler.

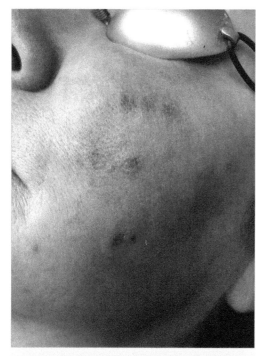

Fig. 11.3 Photo of cheek shown in Video 11.3. The areas of slight purple color persistent immediately after laser impact have developed mild purpura. The other areas that demonstrated transient or flashing purpura—a purple color that quickly disappears—show no purpura but normal postlaser treatment mild erythema and edema.

commonly utilized by many practitioners particularly when treating conditions that are typically difficult to treat with a laser. These conditions include the erythema associated with rosacea—flushing and the so called "background" erythema or redness which gives a "ground glass" red appearance to the skin that does not seem to blanch with pressure and can be seen almost as a skin color on close exam between every pore or pilosebaceous unit (▶ Fig. 11.4). Several methods can be used to enhance laser outcomes. One is to increase the target by inducing flushing or vessel dilation by heating the skin using heating pads or wraps (we use a microwaveable heating pad called Bed Buddy®) or air-activated hand warmers (Hothands®).[2] Another is to increase blood flow with measures as simple as having the patient rest with head below knees immediately prior to laser treatment. Application of topical niacin to induce vascular flushing/dilation has been shown to increase efficacy of pulsed dye laser in the treatment of vascular flushing and rosacea.[3,4] Another method using the 595-nm pulsed dye laser is called pulse stacking and refers to applying closely timed, sub-purpuric consecutive pulses to the target to increase vascular clearance[5] (Video 11.3).

Occasionally, a large vascular lesion or bleb such as a large cherry angioma, nodules within a port wine stain, venous lake, or pyogenic granuloma will require treatment. Pulse stacking with the 595-nm laser can be effective, and the excess heat

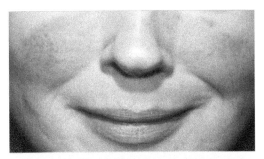

Fig. 11.4 Erythema on cheek that is characteristically more challenging to resolve with laser treatment and may require techniques to enhance outcome of laser treatment (heating, pulse stacking) as well as numerous treatments for best results.

delivered to the nodular lesion can help shrink or contract the nodule (▶ Fig. 11.5a, b). A long wavelength laser such as 755-nm or 1,064-nm laser can be utilized to treat larger vascular lesions, but caution must be exercised as it is easy to overheat these large targets and damage surrounding skin leading to ulceration, poor wound healing, and scarring. Another option is to compress the vascular bleb with a glass slide and pulse the laser over the slide. Additional cooling may be necessary as the glass slide may block the cooling associated with the laser (cryogen or contact cooling). My preferred treatment protocol is to start with the 595-nm pulsed dye laser with pulse stacking initially and then with glass slide compression if

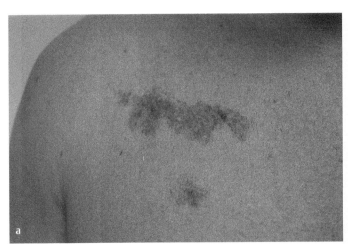

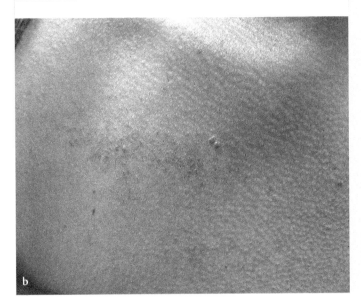

Fig. 11.5 (a) Port wine stain with nodules. **(b)** Eight weeks after pulsed dye laser treatment with pulse stacking over nodules.

needed and move to a longer wavelength laser only if the 595 nm does not produce the desired endpoint. When using a longer wavelength laser on these larger vascular lesions, always start with a moderate pulse duration (10–30 ms) and lower energy and gradually increase energy until a desired endpoint is achieved. Cool target before and in between pulses and do not rapidly stack or repeat pulses.

Summary of Steps to Success in Laser Treatment of Vascular Lesions

1. Choose correct laser/wavelength:
   a) Shorter wavelengths for smaller, superficial vessels and diffuse erythema (532 nm KTP, IPL, 585/595 PDL).
   b) Longer wavelengths for larger, deeper vessels (755-nm long-pulsed alexandrite, 800- to 980-nm diode, 1,064-nm long-pulsed Nd:YAG).
   c) Longer wavelengths (1,064 nm) are safer for darker skin types. Caution in darker skin types (Type V, VI) using wavelengths shorter than 1,064.
2. Match pulse duration to vessel size:
   a) Small veins respond best to shorter pulse durations—typically 6 to 20 ms. Be careful not to completely compress very fine telangiectasia or diffusely red areas as you will lose your target.
   b) Larger veins require longer pulse durations. Blood vessels 0.2 mm up to 1 mm have TRTs of 20 ms up to 300 ms. Caution with larger vessels—it is best to be slightly less than the TRT of the vessel to prevent heat transfer and damage to surrounding structures.
3. Utilize skin cooling:
   a) Epidermal cooling is critical, particularly when treating larger blood vessels.
   b) Pre- and postcooling can improve safety and provide complication-free outcomes when treating larger vascular targets. Caution if forced cool air is used for additional skin cooling when using cryogen cooling paired with laser pulse.
4. Recognize treatment endpoints: Key target responses indicate appropriate treatment: transient or flashing purpura, light purpura (a very light purple color), vessel spasm or contraction, immediate disappearance of vessel, evidence of intravascular thrombosis in vein/vessel, or rupture of blood vessel.
5. Don't miss warning signs: Be immediately aware of danger signs of excessive heat or transfer of heat: loud "pop" noise with laser impact, graying or whitening of skin, excessive edema or frank blistering, dark purpura (dark gray or black color), or excessive pain.
6. Exercise caution in vulnerable areas: Reduce laser energy by 10 to 20% on thin or fragile skin areas such as neck, chest, forehead, nose, and ankle areas.
7. Improve outcomes by enhancing target: Increase blood flow via heat, gravity, or niacin-induced flushing, consider pulse stacking, utilize a glass slide to compress raised lesions.

11.2 Laser Treatment of Pigmented Lesions

A variety of lasers can be utilized for the treatment of pigmented lesions. Melanin and tattoo ink are the common target chromophores when treating pigmented lesions, but the location in the skin (epidermal, dermal, mixed) varies as does the size of the chromophore. In addition, the degree of competing chromophores—skin type and tanning—can play a significant role in laser removal of pigment.

11.2.1 Nanosecond and Picosecond Lasers (1,064 nm, 755 nm, 532 nm)

Nanosecond pulse durations such as provided with Q-switched lasers can ideally treat many superficial pigmented lesions such as solar lentigines, ephilides or freckles, and café au macules. Deeper lesions—such as Nevus of Ota and Ito, and tattoos—can also be targeted with the Q-switched lasers but longer wavelengths to reach a deep target are more ideal (755 nm and 1,064 nm). The target chromophore in these lesions is the melanosome whose size appropriately matches the nanosecond pulse duration in Q-switched lasers.[6] Tattoo pigment particles are smaller than melanosomes, and the nanosecond pulse as well as ultrashort picosecond pulse produces a photomechanical or photoacoustic rupture, not selective heating via photothermolysis. When using the Q-switched laser for pigment removal, the visual endpoint of treatment is mild-to-moderate whitening of the skin overlying the target without lifting, blistering, or ablation/splatter of the skin. A mild snapping sound is typically heard on laser impact; however, a loud snap or pop-on laser impact may indicate too high an energy (Video 11.4). Excessive tissue or target reaction or excessive absorption of

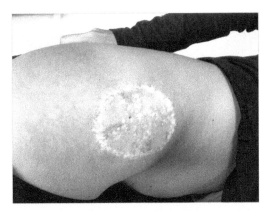

Fig. 11.6 Hypopigmentation in tattoo after laser tattoo removal.

laser energy in the upper layers of skin can lead to hypopigmentation and scarring (▶ Fig. 11.6). When treating lentigines, a shortcoming of the 532-nm laser might be mild purpura or petechiae as hemoglobin is also a target at this wavelength. In addition, when numerous lentigines are present, treatment with a small spot size, Q-switched laser can be a time-consuming task as each lesion must be treated individually. One technique that has been effective for treatment of certain pigmented lesions including melasma, postinflammatory hyperpigmentation, and café au lait macules is low fluence Q-switched 1,064-nm laser treatments directed over the entire lesion for a series of treatments spaced 2 to 4 weeks apart (Video 11.5).[7,8,9,10,11,12,13,14,15]

11.2.2 Long-Pulsed Lasers (532 nm, 595 nm, 755 nm, 800–890 nm, 1,064 nm)

Lasers with pulse durations in the milliseconds can target pigment of larger size particles such as the pigment in hair follicles and nevi. Also, these longer pulsed lasers can be utilized to treat many of the same lesions targeted by the Q-switched lasers. Although the target is the very small melanosome, in many lesions, such as café au lait macules and lentigines, this melanosome is diffusely dispersed throughout the epidermis creating a pigment layer that can be targeted with the longer pulsed lasers with an estimated TRT of 2 to 3 ms.[16] In the treatment of these pigmented lesions no cooling of the skin is used and in the case of the pulsed dye laser, compression of the skin is done to compress blood vessels in the area and disperse

the hemoglobin target in these blood vessels so that all the laser energy is targeted to the pigment. The visual treatment endpoint is slight darkening or ashy gray discoloration of the target and mild erythema in the treatment area (Video 11.6 and ▶ Fig. 11.7a–c). Blistering or skin elevation or disruption is a sign of excessive energy and excessive tissue reaction that might impair healing and lead to hypopigmentation or scarring (▶ Fig. 11.8).

Long-pulse lasers are also used for treatment of unwanted hair with the target being the pigment within the hair follicle. Light-colored hair—white, gray, blonde, and red—has minimal or no pigment, and laser hair treatments that rely on pigment in the hair are not effective.

The longer wavelength 1,064 nm is best for laser hair removal treatments in darker skin types and should be the only wavelength used in skin types V and VI. Various methods of skin cooling in devices cool the upper layer of skin so that the laser energy can penetrate deeply to reach the target of the pigment in the hair follicle.

11.2.3 Light Sources

Intense pulsed light (IPL) is broad spectrum light (typically wavelengths of 515–1,200 nm) delivered through a large crystal. Because of the numerous wavelengths, various aspects of sun damaged skin can be treated including superficial pigmented lesions. Treatment with the IPL is best suited to diffuse lentigines and generalized dyspigmentation commonly seen in sun damaged skin of lighter skin types. IPL is not an ideal device for darker skin types. An advantage of IPL can be in treating larger areas such as entire arms, chest, face very efficiently and the targeting of additional changes of sun damage such as erythema and texture changes. Treatment endpoint when using IPL for pigment lesion removal is mild erythema and/or slight darkening of the target. Deep or dark redness and/or excessive edema in the exact shape of the handpiece is a sign of too much energy. Test spots should be done, with wait time to see tissue response develop, to determine the ideal energy before proceeding with treatment of a large area. Because the IPL is delivered through a large crystal, large areas can be treated efficiently but the wrong setting will produce large areas of unwanted side effects—blistering, redness, and potential hypopigmentation (▶ Fig. 11.9a–d).

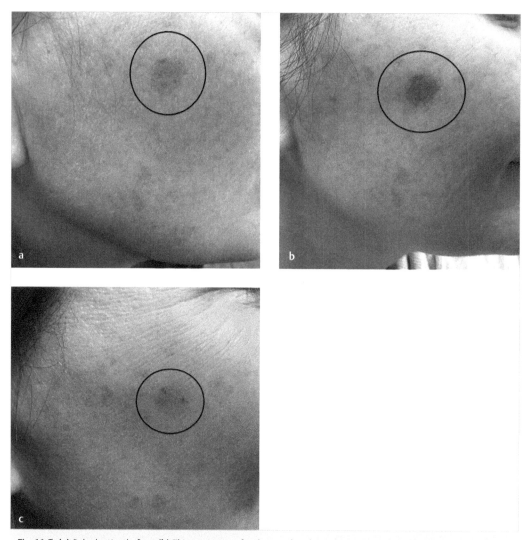

Fig. 11.7 **(a)** Solar lentigo before. **(b)** Thirty minutes after long-pulse alexandrite 755-nm laser treatment showing mild erythema and darkening of the lentigo with no blistering or skin disruption—an ideal tissue reaction. **(c)** One week after treatment with mild erythema still present.

11.2.4 Pigment Nonspecific Lasers

Fractional lasers are a very effective way to target superficial and mid-dermal pigment. The target of fractional ablative and nonablative lasers is dermal water. Impacts of the laser create what are called microthermal zones or MTZs. A treatment with a fractional laser creates thousands of these MTZs that measure 70 to 150 microns in diameter. Healing results in extrusion of these zones of thermal injury, and pigment is pushed out of the skin via this healing. Both ablative and nonablative fractional lasers have been shown to be effective for pigment removal. A 1,927-nm nonablative

fractional laser is absorbed more superficially; thus, it is very effective for superficial pigment. Fully ablative erbium and CO_2 lasers are also effective for pigment, but downtime and healing issues make their use less common. Because the erbium is so superficially absorbed, it can be used to carefully target individual pigmented lesions both on and off the face.

11.2.5 Combination of Lasers

A combination of lasers can be used to more effectively treat pigment. Pretreatment with a Q-switched, long-pulsed laser or IPL prior to fractional ablative or nonablative laser treatment yields better results in the treatment of dyspigmentation associated with sun damage.[17,18] Combinations of lasers can be used when treating other conditions as well, including CALMs, nevi and Becker's nevi, and tattoos.[19] The sequence of lasers is as follows: treatment with the pigmented laser device of choice is done first, then the fractional laser procedure is done. My preference is to do the pigmented laser first, without numbing, then topical numbing cream is applied for 45 to 60 minutes prior to fractional laser.

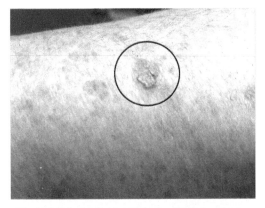

Fig. 11.8 Solar lentigo immediately after long-pulse alexandrite 755-nm laser with no cryogen cooling. Blistering and mild disruption and lifting of the skin is noted—signs of excessive tissue reaction.

Tips for Success in Treating Pigmented Lesions

1. Color of the lesion versus background skin color:
   a) Contrast is critical. Success of pigmented lesion removal depends on the contrast of the pigmented spot and the patient's skin color. The ideal situation is a very dark pigmented lesion on very light-colored skin. As the contrast narrows between color of the target and color of the background skin, the likelihood of successful treatment narrows and risk of adverse effect increases.
   b) With any laser whose target is pigment, careful exam for and questioning about tanning is essential to avoid burning of the tanned skin.
   c) Caution with tattoo removal and hair removal in darker skin types. A longer wavelength laser—1,064 nm—is ideal for skin types IV and darker and may be the only safe choice for removal of pigmented lesions in skin types V and VI.

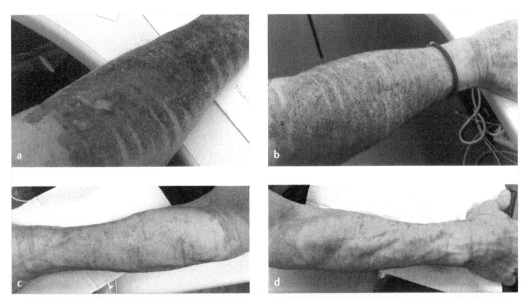

Fig. 11.9 (a, b) Patient photo of forearms 5 days after IPL treatment for sun damage showing excessive tissue reaction—pronounced erythema and bronzing, scabbing, and blistering. **(c, d)** One month after the IPL treatment showing hypopigmentation in the shape of the IPL handpiece as well as confluent hypopigmentation.

2. Select a device for pigment removal based on both color of target lesion and patient skin color:
   a) Q-switched 532-nm lasers are more effective for lighter pigmented spots but more likely to produce postinflammatory hyperpigmentation and vascular effect can cause redness or purpura.
   b) Long-pulse lasers (595 nm, 755 nm, IPL) are better to treat larger surface areas and diffuse sun damage; however, there is more risk of effect on background skin color. If there is minimal contrast between lesion and skin color, these devices should be used at very low energy or not used at all.
   c) For diffuse pigmentation, a fractional laser device can yield excellent results in pigment. These results can be enhanced by combining the fractional treatment with pretreatment with one of the above devices—Q-switched or long-pulse laser or IPL. In darker skin types, type IV skin or darker, fractional nonablative laser alone may be the only appropriate choice for pigment removal.
   d) Fully ablative devices—erbium or CO_2—can be used to remove some lightly pigmented textured lesions such as lightly colored, thin seborrheic keratoses, sharply demarcated lentigines on legs and arms, and porokeratoses. Downtime, erythema, and PIH can make treatment with these devices challenging for patient and physician.
3. Adjust laser energy for density of target color:
   a) For very dark targets—darkly pigmented lesions, dark tattoos, areas of very thick hair density—adjustment of energy to lower settings is needed to avoid delivering too much heat to area.
   b) With subsequent treatments, color, hair, or ink density should be diminished by the previous treatments and energy levels may be increased.
4. Recognize treatment endpoints:
   a) Slight whitening of target and mild snap when using Q-switched lasers for pigmented lesions including tattoos. Mild purpura may occur also.
   b) Subtle darkening or ashy gray discoloration of target and very mild redness when using long-pulse laser or IPL.
   c) Mild perifollicular edema with laser hair removal.
5. Do initial test spots to find ideal treatment setting based on the signs listed above. Settings may have to be changed based on area being treated—i.e., moving from face to neck—and

based on target—area of darker pigment (more target) versus a lighter pigmented lesion. Always be on lookout for signs of excessive energy and excessive tissue reaction:
   a) Excessive whitening of target when using Q-switched lasers and excessive darkening or graying when using long-pulse laser.
   b) Blistering, lifting, or disruption of skin overlying target.
   c) Exaggerated erythema or edema especially with IPL devices. If a footprint of the rectangular handpiece is visible on treated skin, then it is likely that the energy is too high or the patient is a poor candidate for IPL. Also, extensive edema in the treatment area of laser hair removal—edema that extends beyond perifollicular edema—can be a sign of excessive heat deposition in the area that can lead to side effects.
   d) More than moderate pain with treatment. Mild discomfort is to be expected but a lot of pain should be a red flag for the laser operator to stop treatment and evaluate skin for signs of excessive energy. Consider not using topical numbing as this can mask the sign of excessive pain.
6. Success with tattoos:
   a) Use as large a spot as possible for deep penetration.
   b) Ideal treatment interval is 8 to 12 weeks.
   c) Caution with cosmetic tattoos (red or flesh colored) and white tattoos. These may contain iron oxide which can turn dark with laser impact. Always do a test spot. White tattoo ink may be blended into other colors to create a lighter shade. These colors can also turn black with laser treatment.
   d) Colors other than black, blue, and red respond poorly to laser tattoo removal.
   e) Exercise caution with laser treatment of tattoos with evidence of allergic reaction within the tattoo. Localized, generalized, and even systemic allergic reactions have been reported with laser tattoo removal in the presence of allergic reaction using both Q-switched lasers as well as high-energy pulsed lasers (CO_2).[20,21,22,23,24,25]
   f) Application of a topical agent (glycerol or a water-soluble gel (e.g., Surgilube®) to the skin prior to laser treatment can reduce epidermal scatter of laser photons and potentially increase photon energy that reaches the tattoo pigment deeper in the skin, thus enhancing outcomes.[26,27]

11.3 Managing Complications from Laser Treatment of Vascular and Pigmented Lesions

Expected posttreatment changes after laser treatment of vascular and pigmented lesions include mild edema, purpura, vein darkening, darkening of individual pigmented spots, or diffuse pinpoint darkening that resembles a coffee ground appearance, and mild flaking and crusting of pigmented lesions with subsequent exfoliation of these areas. Postinflammatory hyperpigmentation is sometimes an expected outcome especially when treating darker skin types. In addition, when treating more dense vascular lesions or vascular lesions located on the lower extremity, hemosiderin deposition from blood vessel rupture can result in brown dyspigmentation present for weeks to months.

Complications from laser treatment of vascular and pigmented lesions can include excessive erythema and edema as well as blistering and more severe crusting to frank erosions and ulcerations. At the first signs of excessive laser energy, a change of settings can minimize complications. Early recognition and treatment of complications can minimize long-term sequelae such as hypopigmentation and hypertrophic or atrophic scarring.

Wound care to promote healing of any skin erosions is critical as well as protecting areas from friction and trauma. Once the epithelium is healed, a silicone-based scar gel may be initiated. Early intervention with low-fluence pulsed dye laser treatment on areas of erythema or induration can speed clearance of erythema and minimize subsequent scar formation. If scarring occurs, there are many interventions to treat the scarring including some of the devices that caused the scarring.

11.4 Conclusion

Successful laser treatment of vascular and pigmented lesions requires choosing the correct device and settings as well as recognition of the signs of both appropriate and concerning tissue and target reactions. Early change of settings and early intervention with complications can prevent more serious sequelae and permanent scarring. Treating vascular and pigmented lesions at ideal settings will yield satisfying results for both patient and clinician.

References

[1] Fitzpatrick R, Goldman M, eds. In Cutaneous Laser Surgery. 2nd ed. St. Louis, MO: Mosby; 1999

[2] Kashlan L, Graber EM, Arndt KA. Hair dryer use to optimize pulsed dye laser treatment in rosacea patients. J Clin Aesthet Dermatol. 2012; 5(6):41–44

[3] Cho SB, Lee SJ, Kang JM, et al. Treatment of facial flushing by topical application of nicotinic acid cream followed by treatment with 595-nm pulsed-dye laser. Clin Exp Derm. 2009; 34(7):e405–e406

[4] Kim TG, Roh HJ, Cho SB, Lee JH, Lee SJ, Oh SH. Enhancing effect of pretreatment with topical niacin in the treatment of rosacea-associated erythema by 585-nm pulsed dye laser in Koreans: a randomized, prospective, split-face trial. Br J Dermatol. 2011; 164(3):573–579

[5] Rohrer TE, Chatrath V, Iyengar V. Does pulse stacking improve the results of treatment with variable-pulse pulsed-dye lasers? Dermatol Surg. 2004; 30(2 Pt 1):163–167, discussion 167

[6] DierickxC. Laser treatment of pigmented lesions. In: Goldberg D, ed. Laser Dermatology. Berlin, Germany: Springer; 2005

[7] Yue B, Yang Q, Xu J, Lu Z. Efficacy and safety of fractional Q-switched 1064-nm neodymium-doped yttrium aluminum garnet laser in the treatment of melasma in Chinese patients. Lasers Med Sci. 2016; 31(8):1657–1663

[8] Sim JH, Park YL, Lee JS, et al. Treatment of melasma by low-fluence 1064 nm Q-switched Nd:YAG laser. J Dermatol Treat. 2014; 25(3):212–217

[9] Choi JE, Lee DW, Seo SH, Ahn HH, Kye YC. Low-fluence Q-switched Nd:YAG laser for the treatment of melasma in Asian patients. J Cosmet Dermatol. 2018; 17(6):1053–1058

[10] Choi M, Choi JW, Lee SY, et al. Low-dose 1064-nm Q-switched Nd:YAG laser for the treatment of melasma. J Dermatol Treat. 2010; 21(4):224–228

[11] Brown AS, Hussain M, Goldberg DJ. Treatment of melasma with low fluence, large spot size, 1064-nm Q-switched neodymium-doped yttrium aluminum garnet (Nd:YAG) laser for the treatment of melasma in Fitzpatrick skin types II-IV. J Cosmet Laser Ther. 2011; 13(6):280–282

[12] Ghannam S, Al Otabi FK, Frank K, Cotofana S. Efficacy of low-fluence Nd:YAG 1064 nm laser for the treatment of post-inflammatory hyperpigmentation in the axillary area. J Drugs Dermatol. 2017; 16(11):1118–1123

[13] Cho SB, Park SJ, Kim JS, Kim MJ, Bu TS. Treatment of post-inflammatory hyperpigmentation using 1064-nm Q-switched Nd:YAG laser with low fluence: report of three cases. J Eur Acad Dermatol Venereol. 2009; 23(10):1206–1207

[14] Kim S, Cho KH. Treatment of procedure-related postinflammatory hyperpigmentation using 1064-nm Q-switched Nd:YAG laser with low fluence in Asian patients: report of five cases. J Cosmet Dermatol. 2010; 9(4):302–306

[15] Kim HR, Ha JM, Park MS, et al. A low-fluence 1064-nm Q-switched neodymium-doped yttrium aluminium garnet laser for the treatment of café-au-lait macules. J Am Acad Dermatol. 2015; 73(3):477–483

[16] Kono T, Shek SY, Chan HH, Groff WF, Imagawa K, Akamatsu T. Theoretical review of the treatment of pigmented lesions in Asian skin. Laser Ther. 2016; 25(3):179–184

[17] Manuskiatti W, Fitzpatrick RE, Goldman MP. Treatment of facial skin using combinations of CO_2, Q-switched alexandrite, flashlamp-pumped pulsed dye, and Er:YAG lasers in the same treatment session. Dermatol Surg. 2000; 26(2):114–120

[18] Chan CS, Saedi N, Mickle C, Dover JS. Combined treatment for facial rejuvenation using an optimized pulsed light source followed by a fractional non-ablative laser. Lasers Surg Med. 2013; 45(7):405–409

[19] Weiss ET, Geronemus RG. Combining fractional resurfacing and Q-switched ruby laser for tattoo removal. Dermatol Surg. 2011; 37(1):97–99

[20] Bernstein EF. A widespread allergic reaction to black tattoo ink caused by laser treatment. Lasers Surg Med. 2015; 47(2): 180–182

[21] Yorulmaz A, Onan DT, Artuz F, Gunes R. A case of generalized allergic contact dermatitis after laser tattoo removal. Cutan Ocul Toxicol. 2015; 34(3):234–236

[22] Stephan F, Moutran R, Tomb R. Hypersensitivity with angioedema after treatment of a tattoo with Nd:YAG laser. Ann Dermatol Venereol. 2010; 137(6–7):480–481

[23] England RW, Vogel P, Hagan L. Immediate cutaneous hypersensitivity after treatment of tattoo with Nd:YAG laser: a case report and review of the literature. Ann Allergy Asthma Immunol. 2002; 89(2):215–217

[24] Zemtsov A, Wilson L. CO_2 laser treatment causes local tattoo allergic reaction to become generalized. Acta Derm Venereol. 1997; 77(6):497

[25] Ashinoff R, Levine VJ, Soter NA. Allergic reactions to tattoo pigment after laser treatment. Dermatol Surg. 1995; 21(4):291–294

[26] Vargas G, Chan EK, Barton JK, Rylander HG, III, Welch AJ. Use of an agent to reduce scattering in skin. Lasers Surg Med. 1999; 24(2):133–141

[27] McNichols RJ, Fox MA, Gowda A, Tuya S, Bell B, Motamedi M. Temporary dermal scatter reduction: quantitative assessment and implications for improved laser tattoo removal. Lasers Surg Med. 2005; 36(4):289–296

12 Radiofrequency and Microneedle Radiofrequency

Steven F. Weiner

Summary

Radiofrequency has been used in medicine for over 50 years and in aesthetics since the early 2000's. It's indications are for improving skin tone, laxity, and the appearance of scars, particularly acne scars. Unlike lasers, the energy delivered to the skin or deeper structures is not chromophore dependent and is reliant on the flow of energy between electrodes. While promoted as being safe for "all skin types", darker skin types are more susceptible to complications, primarily PIH. The various complications associated with RF treatments will be discussed and precautionary measures needed to prevent them. Treatments for the complications are included as well.

Keywords: radiofrequency, RF, RFM, skin tightening, neck and jawline treatment, RF safety, noninvasive cosmetic treatments, noninvasive cosmetic treatments, radiofrequency burn, radiofrequency fat loss, RFAL, post-inflammatory hyperpigmentation, PIH, scarring

12.1 Introduction

Radiofrequency (RF) use in minimally invasive facial rejuvenation dates to the first FDA-approved device for periorbital wrinkles in 2002. The indications were expanded to face and body in 2004 and 2006, respectively. Since then, there have been dozens of RF devices approved with various forms of delivery systems which have been proven to improve skin laxity/quality/tone, wrinkles, acne scars, acne, hyperhidrosis, pore size, and striae.

12.2 Science of RF

RF creates oscillating electrical current (millions of cycles per second), causing vibration and collisions between charged molecules, thus resulting in production of heat as described by Belenky et al.[1] Electrical energy is converted to thermal energy as resistance in the tissue is met.[2] Energy transfer is dictated by Ohm law: Energy $(J) = I^2 \times R \times T$ (where I = current, R = tissue impedance and T = time of application). Impendence is dependent on skin hydration, electrolyte composition, collagen content, temperature and other variables.[3] Unlike lasers which use a photothermal energy (selective photothermolysis), RF energy is independent of pigmentation/skin type, and is strictly an electrothermal effect. The RF devices used in aesthetic procedures range from 0.3 to 10 MHz. Depth of penetration is inversely proportional to frequency used.[4]

12.3 Neocollagenesis

The heat generated by RF leads to immediate collagen contraction as the heat liable bonds within the triple helical collagen strands are broken. Temperatures below 65 °C lead to various degrees of collagen denaturing which is followed by an inflammatory cascade which includes heat shock proteins and new collagen formation. If temperatures exceed 65 °C, coagulation of the dermal tissues is possible and what follows is a more robust response leading to replacement of the RF thermal zone (RTZ) with collagen, elastin, hyaluronic acid, and other extracellular matrix.

RF is not dependent on a chromophore as lasers are, so theoretically, RF is "safe for all skin types." Where lasers have difficulty when there are competing pigmentary targets in darker skin types, RF can transmit its energy to the dermal tissues based solely on the impedance (not skin type), current, and time variables as per Ohm law. However, darker skin types will be more susceptible to complications from RF such as postinflammatory hyperpigmentation (PIH).

12.4 Methods of RF Delivery

There are two methods of delivering RF energy through the skin—monopolar and bipolar.

Monopolar RF: The energy flows from an active electrode within the operator's handpiece to a grounding pad (passive electrode) placed distally on the patient's body. Early RF devices used monopolar RF, and it is still a popular technology in current devices. Its advantage is energy can be deposited rather deeply from a surface electrode—deep dermis and fibroseptal network.

Bipolar RF: The energy flows between two adjacent electrodes, all contained within the operator's handpiece. The depth of penetration (for the transepidermal devices) is postulated to approximate ½ the distance between the electrodes although this is not universally accepted. Higher energies can be delivered with bipolar than monopolar, but the depths are less (▶ Table 12.1).

Table 12.1 Complications chart

Complications	Treatment
Prolonged swelling/Erythema	Low-level laser therapy, steroids PO/topical, observation, laser for erythema
Postinflammatory hyperpigmentation	Peels, hydroquinone, tretinoin, lasers
Burn/scar	Occlusive dressings, topicals, silicon, lasers, microneedling
Fat loss	Fillers, fat grafting, subcision
Textural abnormalities	Observation, laser, retreat
Dysesthesia, neuropraxia	Observation—almost all return
Acne flare/infection	Oral and/or topical antibiotics

12.5 Safety Measures

The threshold for epidermal burn is 44 to 45 °C and it is also time dependent. The conundrum is that optimal collagen stimulation with the dermis is at temperatures of 65 to 70 °C.[5] Impendence of the epidermis and subcutaneous fat is intrinsically higher than the dermis, so the energy naturally travels to the area of least resistance. However, extraordinary measures are needed to protect the epidermis from heating. These include:

1. Cooling—most common method utilized (cryogen, cooling footplate, air chiller).
2. Motion—by moving heat source, you can create a field effect and less likely to have hot spots.
3. Temperature/Impedance feedback—limits/ controls RF delivered when critical limits are reached to give safer pulses.
4. Infrared (IR) camera—monitors skin temperature.
5. Topicals—steroids, growth factors, platelet rich plasma (PRP), antibiotics, occlusive serums can expedite healing and reduce downtime.
6. Low-level laser therapy (LLLT)—proven to improve downtime—swelling, erythema, and probably reduces burn risk.
7. Insulatedneedles (RF microneedling)—helps protect epidermis from heating.
8. Settings—giving lower energies with more passes gave similar results with less risks and discomfort. Also, in darker skin types, less energy is recommended to avoid PIH risks.

12.6 Patient Selection

Preprocedure counseling is key for patient satisfaction, particularly important when online reviews are so ubiquitous. The definition of downtime varies among patients, and it's imperative to explain that there will be swelling, and erythema (bruising in invasive RF) in almost all RF cases. In addition, optimal results can take a series of treatments and take up to 3 months to see the final result. Complete understanding of expected outcomes with the possibility of minimal or no result must be explained. The provider mustn't overly promote a particular RF technology without also mentioning alternatives such as lasers, peels, and surgery. RF skin tightening has its limitations and a surgical candidate will most likely not appreciate the changes RF has to offer. The best patients are using RF as a preventative measure ("prejuvenation") or those that aren't quite ready for surgery and desire a mild tightening.

RF outcomes are the direct result of how one's body reacts to the heat generated from the treatment. This requires an immune response for healing and production of collagen and elastin. Patients with the following conditions should be treated with caution:

1. Impaired immune function.
2. Immunosuppressive medications.
3. Extreme solar damaged skin.
4. Areas of prior radiation therapy.
5. Negative metabolic state.
6. Keloid formers.

12.7 Complications

The complications of RF are generally rare and have been reported to be 2.7% in one large study of a monopolar device.[6]

12.7.1 Prolonged Swelling, Erythema, Discomfort

Swelling, erythema, and discomfort can be considered universal to most RF procedures. Depending on the technology used, this can last from a day to up to 7 days or longer. Patients have different perceptions of downtime and tolerances to these side effects. If patients are counseled upfront, usually they will understand postprocedure. To expedite swelling resolution, sleeping upright for at least 2 days is helpful. LLLT has been shown to expedite the healing process and has no negative side effects.[7] Erythema can be improved with topicals (calming gels or steroids). If prolonged, a vascular laser can expedite resolution. It is imperative to quell any prolonged skin inflammation in a darker skin individual to minimize the PIH risk and aggressive measures including steroids, and/or Nd:YAG laser might be required. Discomfort needs to be assessed for other complications such as infection but can usually be controlled with acetaminophen. The inflammatory response is required for RF results so refrain from NSAIDs and minimize steroid use if possible.

12.7.2 Postinflammatory Hyperpigmentation (PIH)

When there is prolonged inflammation of the skin, melanocytes respond with excessive melanin production. It is more likely to occur in darker skin types III–VI. If there is epidermal redness and inflammation for a week or longer, measures must be considered to reduce this or risk PIH: LLLT, steroids, sun protection, lasers (532, 585, or 1,064 nm), and hydroquinone.[8] In fact, prevention of PIH with tretinoin (0.5%) and hydroquinone (4–8%) for 3 weeks pre- and 1 month postprocedure would considerably decrease the risk of PIH if there are concerns. In darker skin, it is advisable to use low-to-medium settings to reduce postprocedure sequelae. Since the insertion point for injection RF and radiofrequency-assisted liposuction (RFAL) is at risk for trauma, it is imperative to not make this hole too small or accumulate too much heat in this area.

12.7.3 Second-Degree Burn

A second-degree burn is the most dreaded complication of a RF rejuvenation procedure because of the potential for long-term scarring. In a study by de Felipe et al, the incidence of second-degree burn was 2.7% in a retrospective study of 290 patients (755 treatments).[9] A burn can be caused by exceeding the epidermal threshold of 44 °C for several minutes while higher temperatures require less time.[10] If there is a malfunction in the epidermal cooling mechanism or operator error such as pulse stacking, too much overlap, or improper

cooling between passes, supercritical temperatures can be obtained. Subablative RF devices that use the footplate as the return electrode have an arcing risk if the handpiece is not flush with the skin or there is blood/fluid on the skin preventing optimal contact. Similarly, there are cases of burns around the grounding electrode most likely related to arcing at the point of contact. Injection RF and RFAL can risk superficial or full-thickness burn if the electrodes are placed too superficial, even with the integrated temperature feedback. In injection RF, if the internal electrode exceeds 44 °C, it can heat the skin surface if the IR camera isn't monitored. RFAL can arc if the skin electrode isn't properly positioned. If a blister or Nikolsky sign is recognized, immediate cooling is needed. Inspection of the device for any evidence of malfunction must be performed and a decision to continue, replace the tip, or terminate the treatment should be determined. Wound care for the burn then ensues: topicals, occlusive dressing, debridement, LLLT, PRP, and extracellular matrix (amnion, porcine bladder matrix). If there is scarring, lasers, microneedling, PRP, and surgical excision might all be beneficial.

12.7.4 Fat Loss

A complication of monopolar RF devices is excessive heating of the subcutaneous fat which can lead to apoptosis. Heat will dissipate as it goes deeper into the tissues; it is possible that the energy traverses the fibroseptal network and secondarily heats the surrounding fat.[11] This complication is rare because the impedance is high in fat and apoptosis requires a prolonged temperature elevation. Volume loss from fat atrophy becomes evident several weeks after treatment. Remedies include subcision, fillers, or fat grafting.[12]

12.7.5 Textural Abnormalities

If the operator is not precise with their pulses—malalignment, skipped areas, incomplete pulses, inconsistent pressure on footplate—there will be a risk of skin irregularities, divots, grid marks/patterns, and uneven results.[13] When uncoated needles/pins are used, there is a risk of prolonged healing and subsequent scarring. To treat these problems: observation (most issues resolve), topicals (growth factors, tretinoin) lasers, or repeat treatment is recommended.

12.7.6 Acne Flair/Infection

It is not uncommon, particularly in acne-prone patients, to have an exacerbation. If this risk is recognized beforehand, pre- and posttreatment topical and oral antibiotics is useful. With the radiofrequency microneedling (RFM) devices, infection can be introduced through the microneedling channels and sterile technique must be followed. Following RFM, small pustules can mimic acne but is often a superficial infection which requires oral antibiotics. Care in selection of skin care after RFM is essential because there are cases of granuloma and infection with inappropriate topicals.[14]

12.7.7 Dysesthesia/Neuropraxia

Numbness, pain, or dysesthesia as the result of nerve injury can occur from RF. These injuries will almost always resolve in several weeks. Only with the RFAL device is marginal mandibular nerve weakness possible and this will also resolve with no therapy.

12.7.8 Seroma/Cyst

With RFAL it is possible to have a fluid collection which may need to be drained. Occasionally, a sebaceous cyst can form after RF which would require excision or drainage.

12.8 Conclusion

RF's widespread use in the face and neck for laxity, wrinkles, acne scars, and textural abnormalities is not without its complications, albeit rare. There are measures outlined above to minimize the risks and optimize the results. Education and training are essential for providers and operators to understand the etiologies of the complications.

References

[1] Belenky I, Margulis A, Elman M, Bar-Yosef U, Paun SD. Exploring channeling optimized radiofrequency energy: a review of radiofrequency history and applications in esthetic fields. AdvTher. 2012; 29(3):249–266

[2] Gold MH. The increasing use of nonablative radiofrequency in the rejuvenation of the skin. Expert Rev Dermatol. 2011; 6 (2):139–143

[3] Schepps JL, Foster KR. The UHF and microwave dielectric properties of normal and tumour tissues: variation in dielectric properties with tissue water content. Phys Med Biol. 1980; 25(6):1149–1159

[4] Beasley KL, Weiss RA. Radiofrequency in cosmetic dermatology. DermatolClin. 2014; 32(1):79–90

[5] Clementoni MT, Munavalli GS. Fractional high intensity focused radiofrequency in the treatment of mild to moderate laxity of the lower face and neck: a pilot study. Lasers Surg Med. 2016; 48(5):461–470

[6] Weiss RA, Weiss MA, Munavalli G, Beasley KL. Monopolar radiofrequency facial tightening: a retrospective analysis of efficacy and safety in over 600 treatments. J Drugs Dermatol. 2006; 5(8):707–712

[7] Calderhead RG, Kim WS, Ohshiro T, Trelles MA, Vasily DB. Adjunctive 830 nm light-emitting diode therapy can improve the results following aesthetic procedures. Laser Ther. 2015; 24(4):277–289

[8] Davis EC, Callender VD. Postinflammatory hyperpigmentation: a review of the epidemiology, clinical features, and treatment options in skin of color. J ClinAesthetDermatol. 2010; 3(7):20–31

[9] de Felipe I, Del Cueto SR, Pérez E, Redondo P. Adverse reactions after nonablative radiofrequency: follow-up of 290 patients. J CosmetDermatol. 2007; 6(3):163–166

[10] Abraham JP, Plourde B, Vallez L, Stark J, Diller KR. Estimating the time and temperature relationship for causation of deep-partial thickness skin burns. Burns. 2015; 41(8):1741–1747

[11] AlNomair N, Nazarian R, Marmur E. Complications in lasers, lights, and radiofrequency devices. Facial PlastSurg. 2012; 28 (3):340–346

[12] Dawson E, Willey A, Lee K. Adverse events associated with nonablative cutaneous laser, radiofrequency, and light-based devices. SeminCutan Med Surg. 2007; 26(1):15–21

[13] Willey A, Anderson RR, Azpiazu JL, et al. Complications of laser dermatologic surgery. Lasers Surg Med. 2006; 38(1):1–15

[14] Soltani-Arabshahi R, Wong JW, Duffy KL, Powell DL. Facial allergic granulomatous reaction and systemic hypersensitivity associated with microneedle therapy for skin rejuvenation. JAMA Dermatol. 2014; 150(1):68–72

13 Complications of Platelet-Rich Plasma and Microneedling

Amit Arunkumar, Anthony P. Sclafani, and Paul J. Carniol

Summary

Platelet-rich plasma (PRP) and microneedling are generally well-tolerated procedures with low rates of adverse events, though a limited number of severe and potentially avoidable complications have been reported.

PRP treatments employ the direct delivery of growth factors for use in facial rejuvenation, recovery after facial surgery, and wound healing, including the treatment of alopecia and facial volumization. Adverse events are generally mild, infrequent, and include transient pain during injection and shortly thereafter, injection site erythema, swelling, bruising, pruritus, postinflammatory hyperpigmentation, and skin dryness. Rare but severe reported complications include a systemic allergic reaction and irreversible blindness following periocular PRP injection.

Microneedling, also known as percutaneous collagen induction therapy, involves repeatedly puncturing the skin with fine needles in order to induce endogenous production of collagen, and is employed for treatment of acne vulgaris, scars, photodamage, dyspigmentation, skin rejuvenation, hyperhidrosis, and androgenetic alopecia. Adverse events include erythema, pain, edema, scalp pruritus, and fine superficial bleeding, resolving within hours to days. Less common side effects reported include transient lymphadenopathy, telogen effluvium, acne flare-ups, milia, bruising, scabbing, flushing, oozing, transmission of blood-borne pathogens in the absence of universal precautions, and local and systemic hypersensitivity reactions.

Complications can often be circumvented by appropriate patient and region selection, proper technique, and strict adherence to good clinical practice and universal precautions. An in-depth understanding of these issues is essential to ensure safe use and maximize outcomes.

Keywords: percutaneous collagen induction, platelet-rich plasma, platelet-rich fibrin

13.1 Platelet-Rich Plasma—An Introduction

Platelet-based treatments, commonly referred to collectively as platelet-rich plasma (PRP), employ the direct delivery of growth factors for use in facial rejuvenation, recovery after facial surgery and wound healing.[1] Autologous PRP-based aesthetic treatments allow the surgeon to deliver a functional wound healing response to a targeted area or, in the absence of a wound, to stimulate the production of viable blood vessels, fat cells, and collagen deposits that appear to persist over time.[2] In facial plastic surgery, common indications for PRP include the treatment of alopecia and facial volumization including the treatment of superficial rhytids, depressed scars, and deep nasolabial folds. PRP has also been described for wound healing in facelifts, facial implants and lateral osteotomies. The most common growth factors concentrated in these preparations include platelet-derived growth factor, transforming growth factor-beta, vascular endothelial growth factor, epidermal growth factor, and insulin-like growth factor.[1] These growth factors are chemotactic for monocytes, fibroblasts, stem cells, endothelial cells, and osteoblasts and mitogenic for fibroblasts, smooth muscle cells, osteoblasts, endothelial cells, and keratinocytes.[1]

Autologous PRP can be prepared expediently and at point-of-care by a wide range of manual or fully automated protocols which typically begin with collection of peripheral blood in a vacuum-sealed collection tube with an anticoagulant, followed by multiple centrifugation steps with or without a separator gel in order to isolate a platelet-rich fraction, which is injected using a 30-gauge needle into the dermis, subdermis, or preperiosteal plane as needed.[3]

For a given PRP preparation and protocol, the surgeon should consider the fibrin density, leukocyte content, and degree of standardization of the procedure.[4] PRP, can be subcategorized as one of four types: pure PRP, leukocyte-enriched PRP, pure platelet-rich fibrin, or leukocyte-enriched platelet-rich fibrin.[4] The inclusion of leukocytes in PRP is controversial—while leukocytes produce vascular endothelial growth factor, important for the promotion of angiogenesis, they are also associated with the production of matrix metalloproteinases, which are known to have catabolic effects on extracellular matrix proteins including collagen.[4,5,6,7] The fibrin network may protect growth factors from proteolysis, serve as a more robust scaffolding structure for

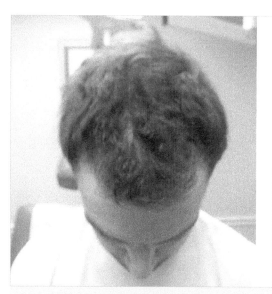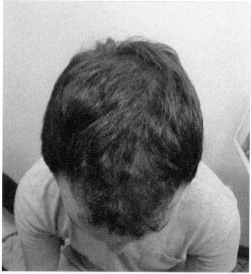

Fig. 13.1 PRP treatment for hair loss. (Source: Platelet-Rich Plasma Principles and Practices. In: Hausauer A, Jones D, ed. PRP and Microneedling in Aesthetic Medicine. 1st Edition. Thieme; 2019.)

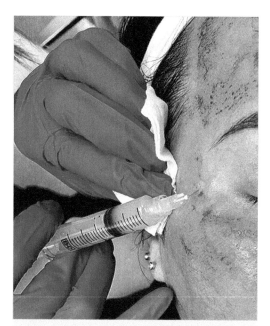

Fig. 13.2 PRP injected after microneeding. (Source: Platelet-Rich Plasma Principles and Practices. In: Hausauer A, Jones D, ed. PRP and Microneedling in Aesthetic Medicine. 1st Edition. Thieme; 2019.)

wound repair, and facilitate longer persistence and resistance to washout of platelet products at the site of injection.[2]

Applications of PRP include treatment of alopecia with subcutaneous or intradermal scalp injections (▸ Fig. 13.1).[8] Acne scars or depressed scars are treated with subcision followed immediately by subdermal injection of PRP (▸ Fig. 13.2).[3] Fine rhytids are injected intradermally. Deeper folds and volume deficient areas are injected at the dermal-subdermal border.[3] Areas requiring significant volume augmentation may be injected into deep fat (mid-face) or preperiosteally (suborbital hollows).[3] Surgical applications of PRP include augmented autologous fat transfer, in which PRP is mixed with fat (generally in a 1:2–3 ratio) just before fat injection; rhinoplasty, in which PRP is injected along the lateral osteotomy site; and rhytidectomy, in which PRP is placed in a thin layer over the flap bed before closure.[3]

PRP allows for volume restoration without substantial inconvenience to the patient, and is minimally invasive with a negligible associated recovery time. Few complications related to PRP material have been described and more often can be attributed to poor patient or region selection, injection technique, or failure to follow good clinical practice and universal precautions.[9,10] An in-depth understanding of these issues is essential to ensure safe use and maximize outcomes.

13.2 Platelet-Rich Plasma—Avoiding, Identifying, and Managing Complications

Adverse events secondary to PRP are mild, infrequent, and include transient pain during injection and shortly thereafter, injection site erythema, swelling, bruising, pruritus, postinflammatory hyperpigmentation, and skin dryness (▶ Fig. 13.3).[11,12] After treatment, intermittent application of cool compresses to the injected regions for the first few hours decreases swelling, bruising, and discomfort.[13] Massaging the region for the first several hours should be avoided as this may cause washout of the PRP.[13]

While granulomas and nodularity have been reported following injection of synthetic fillers, the only reports of granulomatous sequelae from PRP occurred in two patients with either known or

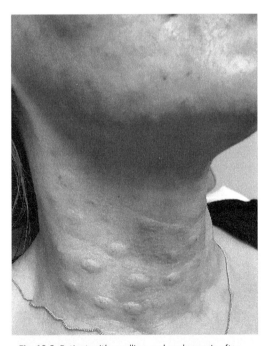

Fig. 13.3 Patient with swelling and ecchymosis after injection of PRP. (Source: Other Considerations, Combinations, and Complications. In: Hausauer A, Jones D, ed. PRP and Microneedling in Aesthetic Medicine. 1st Edition. Thieme; 2019.)

suspected subclinical sarcoidosis, a systemic granulomatous disease that can occur at sites of cutaneous injections.[14,15] As such, if sarcoidosis is suspected in patients considering PRP, further diagnostic work-up is mandatory. Though unreported for aesthetic applications, PRP injection of a tibial bone cyst has been implicated in the development of a systemic allergic reaction, thought to be predicated on a reaction to the calcium citrate anticoagulant used in preparing the injectate.[16]

Multiple systematic reviews on the use of PRP for androgenetic alopecia, the most studied aesthetic application of PRP, have shown no reports of bacterial, viral, or mycobacterial infections, folliculitis, panniculitis, allergic reactions, hematoma or seroma formation.[8,17] However, as with any invasive procedure, good clinical practice and universal precautions are imperative. Proper labeling and handling of blood samples, processing only one patient's blood at a time and following universal precautions are all important in ensuring patient safety.

Severe adverse events are uncommon and few have been reported. While visual complications from synthetic cosmetic fillers have been reported, PRP is not often used as a physical filler but rather for the growth factors it contains. Nevertheless a single case of irreversible blindness and cerebral infarct seen on magnetic resonance imaging (MRI) following periocular PRP skin rejuvenation treatment in the glabellar region performed by an unlicensed practitioner has been reported. The authors hypothesize that the technique employed in a region close to the supraorbital and supratrochlear arteries may have caused intra-arterial injection with retrograde flow of the platelet clot and resultant occlusion of the ophthalmic artery and regions of the middle cerebral artery. In this case, the patient presented to an ophthalmologist on the day after treatment with glabellar injection site skin necrosis, restricted ocular motility, and ophthalmic artery occlusion on dilated fundus exam. MRI demonstrated extraocular muscle ischemia, optic nerve infarction, and right frontal, parietal, and occipital lobe infarction. Thromboembolic and vascular evaluations were negative. Since the patient presented outside of the window for treatment with tissue plasminogen activator, treatment was limited to ocular massage, topical brimonidine 0.2%, topical timolol 0.5%, oral steroids, and empiric IV antibiotics for possible infectious etiology of periorbital swelling. Ocular motility returned to normal, but at one year, the patient's vision remained no light perception. At one year, residual scarring and hard nodules were present in the right glabellar region with scar tissue.[18]

Familiarity with facial vascular anatomy along with maintenance of the injection plane within an intradermal rather than subdermal plane when appropriate may reduce the risk of vascular compromise.[18] Awareness, early recognition, and urgent treatment of vascular complications are essential. To minimize the risk of vascular complications, it is pragmatic to inject the smallest possible volume capable of producing the desired effect in small and discrete aliquots, aspirate prior to each injection, avoid adulteration of PRP preparation with unapproved fillers, and employ smaller needles (30–32 gauge) with prudent technique and the judicious use of pressure.[19]

13.3 Microneedling—An Introduction

Microneedling, also known as percutaneous collagen induction therapy, involves repeatedly puncturing the skin with fine needles in order to induce endogenous production of collagen, and is employed for treatment of acne vulgaris, scars, photodamage, dyspigmentation, skin rejuvenation, hyperhidrosis, and androgenetic alopecia.[20,21] Microneedling typically employs a roller or stamp with multiple needles, typically ranging from 0.5 to 1.5 mm in length, which pierce the stratum corneum and papillary dermis, and can be combined with PRP therapy.[21,22,23] Focused mechanical injury triggers an inflammatory and wound healing cascade, resulting in the release of growth factors and collagen deposition.[20]

13.4 Microneedling—Avoiding, Identifying, and Managing Complications

In general, microneedling is associated with a low rate of adverse events, with transient erythema and postinflammatory hyperpigmentation most commonly reported.[21,24] Microneedling can be performed as an independent procedure or together with radiofrequency in which case it is frequently referred to as microneedling radiofrequency. Radiofrequency is also discussed in chapter 12. Radiofrequency microneedling can be performed utilizing unipolar or bipolar radiofrequency. Radiofrequency microneedling can be seen in Video 13.1. Minor complications identified by several review articles include erythema, pain, edema, scalp pruritus, and fine superficial bleeding, resolving within hours to days depending on the size of needle employed.[23,25] Less common side effects reported include transient lymphadenopathy, telogen effluvium, acne flare-ups, milia, bruising, scabbing, flushing, and oozing.[25,26] Erythema can be temporary (3–5 days) and dryness often subsides over 1 to 2 weeks.[27,28] In one series of 210 procedures of PRP with microneedling for alopecia, 14% of patients experienced scalp pruritus ($n = 30$), 1.4% transient hair shedding 4 to 6 weeks postprocedure with improvement at 6 to 8 weeks ($n = 3$), and 1.9% transient cervical lymphadenopathy ($n = 4$).[26] As with any invasive procedure, a theoretical risk of infection exists though it has not been reported, and histologic examination 24 hours posttherapy reveals an intact epidermis.[21,23]

Contraindications to microneedling include anticoagulant medications or coagulopathy that may result in excessive bleeding; active or recurrent herpes infection/herpes labial is, which may predispose to reactivation and possible scarring after minor trauma; presence of overlying skin infection, skin cancer, warts, or solar keratoses; and a history of severe keloid tendency in which each pinprick may result in a keloid (these patients can often be identified by presence of keloids on palms of hands or soles of feet).[29]

Postinflammatory hyperpigmentation (PIH), a reactive hypermelanosis of the skin that occurs when cutaneous inflammatory mediators stimulate melanocytes to increase production and transfer of melanin to surrounding keratinocytes, has infrequently been described and most often spontaneously resolves in the setting of microneedling.[30,31,32] Photoprotection after microneedling is routinely recommended to minimize the risk of PIH. A single study with inadequate postprocedure photoprotection associated with PIH observed gradual improvement in PIH in a subset of patients when subsequent strict photoprotection was subsequently implemented.[33] In general, because the natural history of PIH is to improve slowly, medical therapy is not necessary in all patients and when employed its purpose is to accelerate resolution, and may include consideration of topical hydroquinone, retinoids, azelaic acid, and/or chemical peels.[34]

Two case series report a "tram track" effect following microneedling with a dermaroller, referring to papular scars in a linear pattern in the distribution of the dermaroller.[30,33] The authors noted a 20 to 30% improvement in these scars with 0.025%

topical tretino in gel after 3 months, though no long-term follow-up is described.[33] Precautionary measures to minimize the risk of this complication include using needles sized less than 2.0 mm, adjusting the degree of pressure applied to the dermaroller when such an effect is identified, and heeding caution when microneedling over bony prominences. Although not well described in the current literature it is possible to develop scarring from radiofrequency microneedling. The scarring potentially can be due to the actual needles or the effects of the radiofrequency energy.

With current technology, it is important during a microneedling procedure to align the needles so they are perpendicular to the skin surface and not at an oblique angle. If they enter the skin on an angle this could lead to development of short track marks. These marks may be shorter but similar to the marks reported using a dermaroller.[30,33]

Local and systemic hypersensitivity reactions have been reported twice, both with the concurrent application of topical products not approved for intradermal injection with microneedling, and in a patient with known nickel-sensitive contact dermatitis who underwent microneedling with needles composed of 8% nickel bound to surgical grade stainless steel alloy.[35,36] In the first case series, biopsy-proven facial granulomatous reactions and a case of systemic hypersensitivity were thought to be predicated on the introduction of immunogenic particles into the dermis that potentiated persistent delayed-type hypersensitivity reactions.[35] In this series of three patients, initial treatment with topical and oral corticosteroids was ineffective while therapy with doxycycline hydrochloride and minocycline hydrochloride led to partial or complete resolution.[35] The ineffectiveness of corticosteroids coupled with successful treatment with tetracycline antibiotics suggests a possible biofilm infection of metal particles in this case.[19] In the second series, systemic antibiotics were ineffectual, patch testing revealed reaction to nickel sulfate, and hospitalization with oral and topical corticosteroid treatment led to gradual improvement over 2 weeks.[36] It is important to avoid the application of nonapproved topical agents with microneedling and to ensure that microneedle composition does not include known allergens in patients with a history of or suspected contact dermatitis.

Two patients contracted HIV infection during a "Vampire Facial" (a combination of microneedling and topical PRP) at an unlicensed New Mexico spa; appropriately sterilized equipment would have rendered this complication otherwise impossible given the autologous nature of PRP, and highlights the need for appropriate practitioner training, good clinical practice, and universal precautions.[9,10]

In summary, PRP, microneedling, and microneedling radiofrequency are generally minimally invasive, well-tolerated, and relatively safe procedures, with negligible associated recovery times and limited adverse event profiles. The majority of reported complications can be circumvented by appropriate patient and region selection, proper technique, and strict adherence to good clinical practice and universal precautions.

References

[1] Sclafani AP, Azzi J. Platelet preparations for use in facial rejuvenation and wound healing: a critical review of current literature. Aesthetic Plast Surg. 2015; 39(4):495–505

[2] Sclafani AP, Saman M. Platelet-rich fibrin matrix for facial plastic surgery. Facial Plast Surg Clin North Am. 2012; 20(2): 177–186, vi

[3] Sclafani AP. Safety, efficacy, and utility of platelet-rich fibrin matrix in facial plastic surgery. Arch Facial Plast Surg. 2011; 13(4):247–251

[4] DohanEhrenfest DM, Rasmusson L, Albrektsson T. Classification of platelet concentrates: from pure platelet-rich plasma (P-PRP) to leucocyte- and platelet-rich fibrin (L-PRF). Trends Biotechnol. 2009; 27(3):158–167

[5] Werther K, Christensen IJ, Nielsen HJ. Determination of vascular endothelial growth factor (VEGF) in circulating blood: significance of VEGF in various leucocytes and platelets. Scand J Clin Lab Investigation. 2002; 62(5):343–350

[6] Kobayashi Y, Saita Y, Nishio H, et al. Leukocyte concentration and composition in platelet-rich plasma (PRP) influences the growth factor and protease concentrations. J Orthop Sci. 2016; 21(5):683–689

[7] Cui N, Hu M, Khalil RA. Biochemical and biological attributes of matrix metalloproteinases. Prog Mol Biol Transl Sci. 2017; 147:1–73

[8] Badran KW, Sand JP. Platelet-rich plasma for hair loss: review of methods and results. Facial Plast Surg Clin North Am. 2018; 26(4):469–485

[9] Koenig D. Two test positive for HIV after "Vampire Facial." https://www.webmd.com/hiv-aids/news/20190430/two-test-positive-for-hiv-after-vampire-facial. Published April 30, 2019. Accessed May 1, 2020

[10] New Mexico Department of Health. Free testing for persons who received any injections.https://nmhealth.org/news/alert/2019/4/?view=762. Published April 29, 2019. Accessed May 1, 2020

[11] Gupta AK, Carviel JL. Meta-analysis of efficacy of platelet-rich plasma therapy for androgenetic alopecia. J Dermatolog Treat. 2017; 28(1):55–58

[12] Hesseler MJ, Shyam N. Platelet-rich plasma and its utility in the treatment of acne scars: a systematic review. J Am Acad Dermatol. 2019; 80(6):1730–1745

[13] Sclafani AP. Platelet-rich fibrin matrix for improvement of deep nasolabial folds. J Cosmet Dermatol. 2010; 9(1):66–71

[14] Serizawa N, Funasaka Y, Goto H, et al. Platelet-rich plasma injection and cutaneous sarcoidal granulomas. Ann Dermatol. 2017; 29(2):239–241

[15] Izhakoff N, Ojong O, Ilyas M, et al. Platelet-rich plasma injections and the development of cutaneous sarcoid lesions: a case report. JAAD Case Rep. 2020; 6(4):348–350

[16] Latalski M, Walczyk A, Fatyga M, et al. Allergic reaction to platelet-rich plasma (PRP): case report. Medicine (Baltimore). 2019; 98(10):e14702

[17] Chen JX, Justicz N, Lee LN. Platelet-rich plasma for the treatment of androgenic alopecia: a systematic review. Facial Plast Surg. 2018; 34(6):631–640

[18] Kalyam K, Kavoussi SC, Ehrlich M, et al. Irreversible blindness following periocular autologous platelet-rich plasma skin rejuvenation treatment. Ophthal Plast Reconstr Surg. 2017; 33 (3S) Suppl 1:S12–S16

[19] Sclafani AP, Fagien S. Treatment of injectable soft tissue filler complications. Dermatol Surg. 2009; 35 Suppl 2:1672–1680

[20] Badran KW, Nabili V. Lasers, microneedling, and B platelet-rich plasma for skin rejuvenation and B repair. Facial Plast Surg Clin North Am. 2018; 26(4):455–468

[21] Hou A, Cohen B, Haimovic A, Elbuluk N. Microneedling: a comprehensive review. Dermatol Surg. 2017; 43(3):321–339

[22] Doddaballapur S. Microneedling with dermaroller. J Cutan Aesthet Surg. 2009; 2(2):110–111

[23] Hartmann D, Ruzicka T, Gauglitz GG. Complications associated with cutaneous aesthetic procedures. J Dtsch Dermatol Ges. 2015; 13(8):778–786

[24] Epstein JH. Postinflammatory hyperpigmentation. Clin Dermatol. 1989; 7(2):55–65

[25] Mujahid N, Shareef F, Maymone MBC, Vashi NA. Microneedling as a treatment for acne scarring: a systematic review. Dermatol Surg. 2020; 46(1):86–92

[26] Stojadinovic O, Morrison B, Tosti A. Adverse effects of platelet-rich plasma and microneedling. J Am Acad Dermatol. 2020; 82 (2):501–502

[27] AlQarqaz F, Al-Yousef A. Skin microneedling for acne scars associated with pigmentation in patients with dark skin. J Cosmet Dermatol. 2018; 17(3):390–395

[28] Cohen BE, Elbuluk N. Microneedling in skin of color: a review of uses and efficacy. J Am Acad Dermatol. 2016; 74 (2):348–355

[29] Fabbrocini G. Complications of needling. In: Tosti A, Beer K, De Padova MP, eds. Management of complications of cosmetic procedures: handling common and more uncommon problems. Springer; 2012:119–124

[30] Pahwa M, Pahwa P, Zaheer A. "Tram track effect" after treatment of acne scars using a microneedling device. Dermatol Surg. 2012; 38(7 Pt 1) 7pt1:1107–1108

[31] Gadkari R, Nayak C. A split-face comparative study to evaluate efficacy of combined subcision and dermaroller against combined subcision and cryoroller in treatment of acne scars. J Cosmet Dermatol. 2014; 13(1):38–43

[32] Tomita Y, Maeda K, Tagami H. Mechanisms for hyperpigmentation in postinflammatory pigmentation, urticaria pigmentosa and sunburn. Dermatologica. 1989; 179 Suppl 1:49–53

[33] Dogra S, Yadav S, Sarangal R. Microneedling for acne scars in Asian skin type: an effective low cost treatment modality. J Cosmet Dermatol. 2014; 13(3):180–187

[34] Saedi N, Dover J. Postinflammatory hyperpigmentation. UptoDate. Wolters Kluwer; 2020

[35] Soltani-Arabshahi R, Wong JW, Duffy KL, Powell DL. Facial allergic granulomatous reaction and systemic hypersensitivity associated with microneedle therapy for skin rejuvenation. JAMA Dermatol. 2014; 150(1):68–72

[36] Pratsou P, Gach J. Severe systemic reaction associated with skin microneedling therapy in 2 sisters: a previously unrecognized potential for complications? J Am Acad Dermatol. 2013; 68(4):AB219

Section IV

Lipo Reduction: Avoiding and Managing Complications

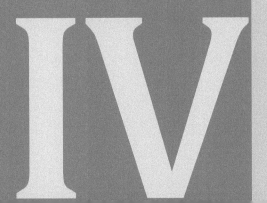

14 Liposuction

Brandon Worley and Murad Alam

Summary

The ability to provide contour to the body by adding or removing adipose tissue provides the cosmetic surgeon with a power tool to meet the needs of their patients. For the face and neck, there are special considerations that need to be observed in order to ensure optimal outcomes while minimizing risks. The following chapter will help to describe the techniques to address important areas on the face, submental area, neck and other anatomic areas as well as how to manage any complications should they arise.

Keywords: liposuction, body contouring, fat transfer, face, neck, complications

14.1 Background

Liposuction removes focal adipose accumulation improving localized body contour. Traditionally, liposuction, which entails vacuum-assisted transcutaneous cannula suction of subcutaneous fat using a crisscross or triangulation pattern and multiple port sites, was performed exclusively under general anesthesia or conscious sedation. The advent of liposuction under local anesthesia alone began in 1987 with Jeffrey Klein who pioneered tumescent technique with an extremely dilute solution of lidocaine and epinephrine. This allowed for reduced complications related to intraoperative blood loss and overall increased safety. Other recent developments in liposuction technology have increased its ease, speed, and versatility.

However, consumer data shows a decrease in the overall number of liposuction procedures in favor of noninvasive body sculpting modalities. These include radiofrequency, ultrasound, cryolipolysis, and laser fat reduction treatments. Patients appear to prefer procedures with lower recovery time and few side effects, even at the cost of achieving only mild-to-moderate results with a series of multiple noninvasive treatment sessions as compared to a dramatic benefit after a single liposuction procedure.

Consideration of patient preferences and needs through the preoperative and postoperative periods, along with planning the procedure at a point in time that is best for the patient, can help ensure postprocedure compliance that leads to an optimal result. Providers should be familiar with the changing technologies and patient choices pertaining to body contouring so that they can best address the common combination of localized skin laxity and excess adipose tissue. Prevention, minimization, and management of adverse events remain important. In this chapter we will focus on addressing contouring of the face and neck through liposuction while ensuring patient safety.

14.2 Preoperative Evaluation

As with any surgical procedure, preoperative evaluation is essential for reducing risk and ensuring good outcomes. A thorough history should be elicited that includes reasons for seeking treatment, patient expectations of treatment, past medical history, current medications and oral supplements, any potential factors contributing to poor wound healing (e.g., diabetes, chronic renal insufficiency, uncontrolled hypothyroidism, poor nutritional status, poor scar appearance), assessment of bleeding risk, and likelihood of compliance with postoperative instructions.

While diabetic patients using insulin pumps have recently been shown to develop paradoxical adipose hypertrophy of treated areas with noninvasive cryolipolysis, this has not been reported with liposuction. Diabetics are generally at greater risk of infection and poor wound healing.

Medications that should be avoided prior to liposuction include anticoagulants, nonsteroidal anti-inflammatories (NSAIDs), and supplements that have anticoagulant properties such as gingko, ginseng, garlic, saw palmetto, feverfew, and fish oil. Phytocoumarins can also interact with anticoagulants and other medications to increase the risk of major bleeding events.[1,2] Medications and supplements that can potentiate bleeding should be discontinued 2 weeks prior to liposuction. Alcohol should also be avoided.

Careful and meticulous documentation of the discussion of the risks and benefits of the procedure along with substances to avoid is an essential part of the informed consent procedure. In addition, ensuring a patient understands the likely degree of postprocedure contour improvement is critical for patient satisfaction.

Absolute contraindications to liposuction include severe obesity, a patient seeking the procedure as a weightloss solution, body dysmorphic disorder, and scarring or altered anatomy from prior surgery in the area. Consideration of earlier keloidal scarring, bleeding episodes, allergic reactions to lidocaine, incidences of poor wound healing, and unstable psychiatric condition may lead to a decision not to proceed, thereby helping prevent avoidable adverse events and patient dissatisfaction.

Appropriate patient selection greatly increases the likelihood of subsequent patient satisfaction. Patients who do not have reasonable expectations of the likely cosmetic benefits of the procedure, demand guarantees of success, or see the procedure as a way to solve a life challenge are not ideal candidates. All patients should be advised that a "touch-up" may be needed. Preoperative discussion should identify those who, regardless of the result, will not be satisfied or will be unwilling to engage in additional adjunctive treatment to achieve the desired aesthetic goal. In some cases, noninvasive modalities for fat reduction may be appropriate alternative treatment avenues.

Written preoperative and postoperative instructions are typically provided to the patient along with verbal communication of the most common and important adverse events. It is helpful to provide recommendations on nutrition and exercise to help with maintenance of results. Consultation with experts in these areas may be sought when appropriate. Lifestyle changes may need to be implemented prior to the procedure. The best results are seen in those who are at or slightly above their stable body weight. Extreme dieting prior to liposuction is highly inadvisable, as patients are likely to gain this weight back postprocedure, even if not at the anatomic site that underwent treatment. Ultimately, provision of emotional support of the patient from the time of preoperative consultation until after the postprocedure recovery leads to greater patient satisfaction.

14.2.1 Physical Examination and Laboratory Evaluation

For facial and neck liposuction, the surgeon identifies the high and low contours along with free margins and aesthetic subunits. The main areas of concern are the pretragal sulcus, nasolabial fold, malar fat pad, neck, and submental fat (▶ Fig. 14.1). It can be helpful to use a skin marker

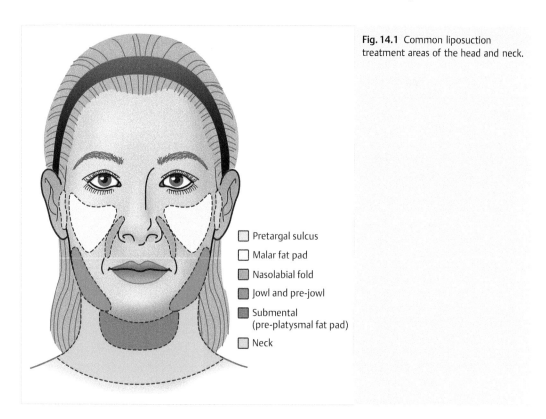

Fig. 14.1 Common liposuction treatment areas of the head and neck.

- Pretargal sulcus
- Malar fat pad
- Nasolabial fold
- Jowl and pre-jowl
- Submental (pre-platysmal fat pad)
- Neck

to identify, fully visualize, and then confirm with the patient, the primary areas of concern. Scars or traumatic wounds that may restrict postoperative skin contraction should be identified and shown to the patient. For submental fullness, assessment of skin laxity, platysmal laxity, anterior digastric hypertrophy, and adipose collection at the site allows the generation of a complete plan to treat these diverse elements. The masseter muscle and the overlying malar fat pad largely account for the cheek and jaw contour. The pretragal sulcus and nasolabial folds are less impacted by the underlying anatomy. Skin laxity can be assessed by the "snap test" where gently pulling on and then releasing the skin at the neck or area of interest shows the ability of the skin to easily return to its original position. A longer time to return to back to its original position (i.e., positive snap test) predicts an increased likelihood of persistent laxity after the liposuction procedure.

The surgeon is aware of the angles (e.g., cervicomental angle) and depressions that are considered youthful and natural for the patient's ethnic background, gender, and social group. For example, Western cultures prefer oval face shapes in women and more squared jawlines in men, while Asian cultures prefer an oval face shape with V-tapered jawline down to the point of the chin.[3] Correction outside of these norms may lead to a suboptimal result, and a dissatisfied patient.[4]

Baseline photographs are taken in profile without neck extension, oblique at 45 degrees with the nasal tip on the cheek, and portrait view to show all the relevant contours and depressions for later comparison. Software is available to simulate typical results, which can aid the preoperative discussion. Recognition of the need for platysmaplasty, partial resection of the anterior belly of the digastric muscle, or surgical neck lifting in conjunction with liposuction may also contribute to selection of an optimal treatment approach. Preoperative ultrasound of the neck can assist in distinguishing skin or fat abnormalities from problems arising from muscle dysfunction.[5] While there are no data to support anterior digastric muscle neuromodulator injections to reduce submental fullness, this may still be considered by some. Cases have been reported of such injections used to address hypertrophy from traumatic overbite. Caution should be exercised if attempting to surgically reduce anterior digastric bulk as this muscle is involved in speaking and chewing. Any attempt to manage muscle mass, as well as scar modification by laser or surgery, may need to be completed prior to correction of fat deposits. For cheeks or malar fat pads, masseter hypertrophy is typically managed with neuromodulators prior to evaluating a patient as a candidate for liposuction.

Further aspects of preoperative planning include obtaining vital signs, assessing the volume of tissue to be removed, measuring weight and BMI, testing local neuromuscular function, and checking the level of vascular perfusion. Documenting a baseline neuromuscular evaluation allows for comparison in the postoperative period if there is a question of nerve injury. Any indications of compromised, altered, or atypical vascular anatomy in the area of the procedure are documented. While surgical technique is planned in a manner to avoid vascular injury, atypical anatomy can increase such risk during the procedure. Basic laboratory blood testing, including CBC, electrolytes, creatinine, INR, PTT, hepatitis B and C, β-hCG, and HIV, is suggested. This is especially true if larger volume liposuction is planned. An electrocardiogram and other tests of the cardiovascular or pulmonary systems may be relevant in the context of particular patient comorbidities.

14.2.2 Anesthetic Planning

Selecting an anesthetic plan is a key preparatory step. Tumescent anesthesia without general anesthesia is believed to be the safest method to perform liposuction as it avoids risks and complications associated with general anesthesia. Patients are also able to assist the surgeon by indicating any feelings of pain or discomfort when the surgical plane is too superficial or there is a pending thermal injury from energy-based devices. If general anesthesia is chosen due to the need for concurrent adjunctive surgical procedures, the patient should be counseled regarding the increased risks of cardiovascular issues, venous thrombosis and vascular complications, and skin injury and delayed healing. For awake analgesia, tumescent liposuction with 55 mg/kg of patient body weight is known to be safe. This dose is recommended by the American Society for Dermatologic Surgery based on existing safety data in the literature.[6] Klein and Jeske have recommended 45 mg/kg for liposuction to increase the margin of safety.[7] However, there is no evidence that levels even greater than 55 mg/kg are unsafe, and the reluctance to use these is based more on the absence of confirmatory safety data than any reports of adverse events with higher doses. Each IV bag of tumescent solution typically contains 1 g lidocaine with 1 mg epinephrine

Table 14.1 Drug interactions with tumescent lidocaine anesthesia

	Enzyme		
	CYP3A4 inhibitor (increase toxicity)	CYP3A4 inducer (reduce effectiveness)	CYP1A2 inhibitor (increase toxicity)
Drug	HIV protease inhibitors	Anticonvulsants	Smoking
	Azole antifungals	Barbiturates	Cimetidine
	Nondihydropyridine calcium-channel blockers	Rifampicin	Ciprofloxacin
	H2 antihistamines (e.g., ranitidine, cimetidine)	Oral steroids	Erythromycin
	Amiodarone	HIV reverse transcriptase inhibitors	Ropivacaine
	Quinolone antibiotics	St. John wort	R-warfarin
	SSRI		
	Sildenafil		
	Grapefruit		

Note: The complete list of CYP3A4 inhibitors is extensive. A selection of relevant medications encountered in practice is provided.

in 100 mL, plus 10 mEq of 8.4% sodium bicarbonate in 10 mL, both added to 1,000 mL of 0.9% saline. In the context of diabetes or hypoalbuminemia, treatment with macrolides (given associated CYP3A4 or 1A2 inhibition), fluoroquinolones, or selective serotonin reuptake inhibitors, and use of lidocaine without epinephrine or general anesthesia (see ▶ Table 14.1), a larger margin of safety may be preferable. In these cases, it has been suggested that the maximum tumescent lidocaine dose be 45 mg/kg.[7] A simplified method to calculate the maximum safe volume is: [dose of lidocaine × weight (kg)/10] × [1/ concentration of lidocaine].[8] For a patient of average weight (approximately 70 kg), approximately 4 L of 0.1% lidocaine tumescent fluid is considered safe. Delivery of the solution is typically through a power-assisted infusion cannula, or 60-mL syringe for smaller areas. The syringe-based method is often useful for the face and neck.

Though volumes may vary, the cheek and neck often require 125 to 150 mL of tumescent fluid for each side. The postauricular areas and posterior neck may take 125 mL per side. Therefore, for a typical bilateral facial procedure approximately 600 mL of tumescent lidocaine may be appropriate (▶ Fig. 14.2). Smaller volumes infused with a syringe may be best for the pretragal area and nasolabial folds if one of these is the only area of concern.

Some patients may require preoperative oral analgesia, light sedation, anxiolytics, and antiemetics to tolerate the procedure. The decision to administer additional medications in the setting of tumescent liposuction should be individualized. Many patients who are nervous about the procedure can be guided through liposuction successfully with reassurance and distraction techniques.

14.2.3 Selecting the Right Tools to Optimize Aesthetic Results

Body contouring has undergone a paradigm shift in recent decades, with a renewed understanding of the distinction between fat reduction on the one hand, and tightening of adjacent skin and muscle, on the other. The evolution of technology to permit the surgeon to address all the relevant soft tissue layers has allowed for better overall outcomes. In many cases, combining various modalities may be best for achieving optimal results.

Traditional cannula and vacuum-assisted suction remains the mainstay of body contouring. Suction cannulas are hollow metal tubes with blunt patient-facing ends and holes near distal tip. Cannulas are manufactured in various bores as well as in different lengths, and also differ in the number, shape, configuration, and size of their holes. Specialty cannulas may have a circumferential array of holes for fat harvesting, or forked blades for lysis of fascial or subcutaneous adhesions. Fat reduction by cannula typically occurs via manual mechanical tunneling or power-assisted oscillation. Mechanical removal is by the physical disruption of the adipose structure into lobules, the additional benefit of hydrosection if tumescent anesthesia is used. The skill of the surgeon guides maintenance of an adequate surgical plane and sufficient force to remove the fat. To avoid oversuctioning of a small area, the suction cannula is

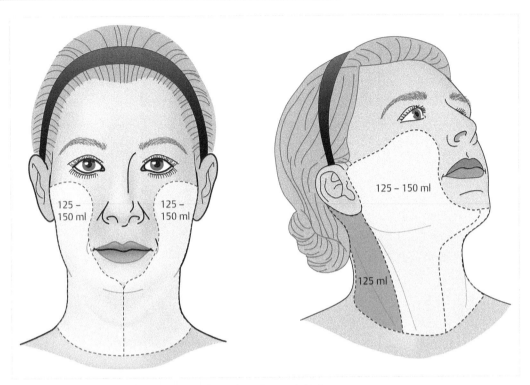

Fig. 14.2 Tumescent anesthesia pattern for the neck, jawline, and cheeks.

moved back and forth in long strokes comprising most of its length, and in a fanning motion laterally. The vibratory action of an oscillating cannula facilitates passage through subcutaneous tissue, thereby sparing some physical effort for the surgeon. Vibration also speeds adequate treatment of fibrous regions or areas of prior surgery, provides vibratory sensory stimuli to distract the patient and increase comfort, and may reduce the risk of shearing adjacent tissue.

Energy-assisted liposuction with radiofrequency, ultrasound, 1,064-nm laser, or 1,470-nm laser has been reported to increase the pace of removal, purportedly by liquefaction or destruction of the fat prior to suctioning. Further, use of energy devices may contribute to skin tissue shrinkage and sculpting of the cosmetic subunits in "high-definition" procedures that even etch the underlying muscle. Some degree of targeted skin tightening may thus be achieved in a single procedure. Energy device used in combination with liposuction delivers either heat or shock-wave-based disruption of the fat lobules. For tightening of the overlying skin, the local skin temperature needs to reach approximately 46 °C. Nonthermal ultrasound may thus not achieve as much skin tightening as radiofrequency, infrared laser, or thermal ultrasound. The disadvantage of delivering heat during liposuction is an increased risk of subcutaneous thermal injury to the skin and dermal plexus vessels. Thermocoupled devices that provide real-time temperature feedback to the operator are available to reduce the risk of injury. If fat transfer of the lipoaspirate is being considered, then traditional or nonthermal ultrasound-assisted liposuction may be considered as they may preserve a higher fraction of viable autologous fat and stem cells for grafting. In using energy devices with traditional liposuction, the operator needs to be familiar with their benefits and risks, and able to prevent thermal injury to the skin and vasculature.

Inappropriately superficial liposuction can increase the risk of skin injury. So-called "high-definition" techniques offer accentuation of the edges of aesthetic landmarks and muscle boundaries by using cannulas to etch the skin or muscle while attempting to preserve the subdermal plexus. Additional familiarity with this approach is advisable before employing it in a live patient.

The overall benefits of body contouring associated with liposuction can be increased in magnitude with the adjunctive use of noninvasive or minimally invasive modalities such as energy-device actuated skin tightening. For those patients who are poor surgical candidates or desire a shorter recovery, noninvasive or minimally invasive modalities may be used as solitary treatments, albeit with the expectation of less noticeable results or the need for an increased number of treatments. Nonsurgical reduction of adipose tissue using physical modalities (i.e., heat, cold, shock-waves) can be accomplished using cryolipolysis, external and internal radiofrequency heating, thermal and nonthermal (shock-wave) ultrasonographic adipolysis, and infrared (commonly Nd:YAG 1,064 nm) laser lipolysis. Indirect comparison of clinical studies shows a comparable reduction in adipose tissue volume of approximately 20 to 25% after a series of treatments with each of these methods. The best results are in those who have focal fat deposits and a BMI < 30.

Interestingly, despite the lack of heat delivery, cryolipolysis appears to be able to achieve an adjunctive reduction in skin laxity. It has been postulated that dermal fibroblasts may initiate collagen deposition in the skin due to the stretching and suction of the cryolipolysis device or cold stimulation. Heat-based laser, radiofrequency, and ultrasound devices use long wavelength energy to induce an adequate temperature for fat destruction while avoiding inducing thermal injury of the skin. External ultrasound or radiofrequency devices that target the deep dermis and fascia specifically are sometimes used with heat-based liposuction devices. In addition to serving as primary treatment modalities, noninvasive and minimally invasive fat reduction methods may also be useful for fine-tuning, adjusting, or touching up the results of a liposuction procedure.

Additional adjunctive techniques can improve body contour before or after liposuction. Specifically, postoperative electromagnetic stimulation (EMS) of the underlying muscle has been reported to facilitate skin tightening. EMS has shown effectiveness in reducing abdominal ptosis and narrowing the diastasis recti. Clinical studies have used treatment protocols of four treatments divided over 2 weeks, with a twice a year maintenance schedule for the abdomen. Early data suggests augmentation of liposuction results for the abdomen if EMS treatment is started within 48 hours after the procedure. Data on the face are more preliminary.

Laxity of the face and neck can be treated by other modalities as well. Definition of the jawline may be sharpened with neuromodulator application along the lower face. Since platysmal laxity or digastric hypertrophy may contribute to submental fullness and suboptimal neck contours, neck rhytides may be reduced with neuromodulator application when platysmal bands are present. The platysma may be surgically addressed by either platysmaplasty (e.g., corset platysmaplasty) or a minimallyinvasive percutaneous approach.[7,9] There are no controlled studies regarding these procedures.

14.3 Procedure

14.3.1 Cannulas

Cannulas differ in length from 3 to 14 inches and vary in bore from 10- to 18-gauge. The bore, cannula hole characteristics, and tip architecture correlate to the level of aggressiveness the cannula can provide. Medium-to-low aggressive cannulas (▶ Table 14.2) are most useful for finely sculpting an area with small fat deposits to ensure controlled, precise removal. Aggressive cannula designs like the Keel Cobra are generally used for debulking on nonfacial body sites when a large accumulation of fat is present. A helpful rule is that aggressive cannulas tend to be higher gauge, more tapered at the point, and possess larger holes near the tip. Ensuring that the cannula holes remain on the ventral side during suctioning can help to reduce the chance of skin dimpling. On the face and neck, short, fine bore cannulas, such as the 3-inch 18-gauge, are commonly used. These are sufficient because of the small volume of fat needing to be removed, and are helpful for minimizing trauma to the abundant important superficial neurovascular structures.

14.3.2 General Principles of Surgical Technique

Suction techniques for each area of the head and neck are similar; however, there are subtle site-specific differences in the selection of appropriate cannula (▶ Table 14.3). Treating multiple contiguous locations during the procedure can prevent sharp cutoffs or lines of demarcation, and blend the face or neck shape. Similarly, triangulation, or suctioning the site from two or three distinct entry points, helps minimize the risk of contour deformities and contributes to an overall even contour.

Table 14.2 Comparison of invasive and non-invasive techniques for body contouring

Modality	Mechanism of action	Advantages	Disadvantages
		Invasive	
Manual liposuction	Shearing +/– vibratory separation of lobules	• Minimal adjacent tissue injury • Lowest cost of equipment	• Prolonged procedure time compared to others • No skin tightening
Radiofrequency-assisted liposuction	Heat-based liquefaction and skin tightening	• Skin tightening • Improved atraumatic fat removal • Reduced procedure time	• Caution needed to avoid tissue injury
Laser-assisted liposuction	Heat-based liquefaction	• Skin tightening • Improved atraumatic fat removal • Reduced procedure time	• Caution needed to avoid tissue injury
Ultrasound-assisted liposuctions	Sonic disruption and lysis of the fat	• Improved atraumatic fat removal • Reduced procedure time	• Caution needed to avoid tissue injury • No skin tightening
		Noninvasive	
Cryolipolysis	Adipocyte death by water crystal formation	• Skin tightening • Minimal downtime • Noninvasive • No operator required	• Requires multiple treatments • Requires multiple cycles to address both sides • Relies on consumables
High-intensity ultrasound	Shockwave	• Minimal downtime • Noninvasive	• Requires multiple treatments • Requires operator
Nd:YAG laser lipolysis	Laser-induced liquefaction	• Minimal downtime • Noninvasive • Addresses full area in one cycle	• May not have similar efficacy to other treatments[a]
Radiofrequency	Heat-induced liquefaction	• Skin tightening • Minimal downtime • Noninvasive • Addresses full area in one cycle	• Possibility of burns
Electromagnetic stimulation	Indicated only for inducing muscle hypertrophy	• Enhances the results of liposuction for those wanting an athletic look	• No fat reduction

[a]No direct comparison studies.

After photographs are taken, treatment areas are marked and the patient is sterilely prepped and draped. For the neck and submental areas, a supine position with neck hyperextension is preferred. Some surgeons prefer elevation of the head to 45 degrees to facilitate a natural line of cannular insertion from the mentum down the neck. Port holes are made by incision or a punch biopsy tool (1-, 1.5-, or 2-mm punch) in areas that are easily hidden or along relaxed skin tension lines. For the neck, these sites are typically an inch below the pinna and slightly recessed below the point of the chin beyond the terminal lip of the jaw. Tumescent anesthesia is administered by blunt needle or spinal catheter attached to a 30- or 60-mL syringe. While warmed fluid is used to minimize the risk of hypothermia in larger cases, this is not typically necessary on the head and neck. Warming may also encourage bleeding due to vasodilation. Passive warming of the patient with blankets, or active warming with a forced warm air blanket, may be preferred. The rate of infusion of tumescent fluid is typically 100 mL/min with a 30- to 45-min delay after infusion and before suction for full anesthesia to set in. Blanching of the overlying skin will occur when anesthesia has taken full effect. The subdermal area, mid-fat, and deep fat should all be infused. Laterally, an area about 1 inch

beyond the area to be treated should be infused, and should be blanched prior to the start of suction.

The suction cannula is inserted nearly vertically at first, and then quickly leveled to an angle of 20 to 30 degrees to avoid injury to deep structures. After the cannula is safely inserted into entry port, it is advanced radially to create tunnels, like the spokes of a wheel (▶ Fig. 14.3) into the areas that were pre-marked for treatment. Pinching of the skin with the nonoperative hand to tent the subcutaneous tissue allows for maintenance of a consistent depth. The surgeon should control the cannula with their dominant hand while their guide hand folds the skin over the cannula. Pinching of the skin and guiding the cannula to pierce through the pinched tissue bulk decreases the depth of aspiration; on the other hand, pinching with the palm and then guiding the cannula below the pinched tissue increases the depth of treatment. Such maneuvers guide the depth of the cannula tip to remove fat from the different depths of adipose layer. Changing between

Table 14.3 Aspiration cannulas

Aggressiveness	Type	Size
High	Capistrano	10 or 12 G
	Keel Cobra	3 or 3.7 mm
	Mercedes	10 or 12 G
	Pinto	10 or 12 G
	Toledo	10 or 12 G
	Capistrano	14 G
	Klein	12 G
	Accelerator/Triport	3 mm
Medium	Dual Port	2.5 mm
	Fournier	2.5 mm
	Keel Cobra	2.5 mm
	Texas	2.5 mm
	Capistrano	16 G
Low	Klein	14–18 G
	Spatula	2–3 mm

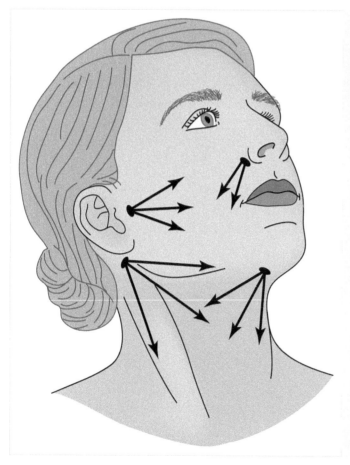

Fig. 14.3 Relevant surgical anatomy for liposuction procedures of the head and neck. The marginal mandibular and mental nerves are shown along with the course of the facial artery. These structures have variable courses between patients. Preoperative evaluation of submental fullness is required as it may be a combination of fat, hypertrophy of the anterior digastric, skin laxity, and platysma laxity.

grips is more important for areas on the trunk and extremities, but can be useful also for areas of increased fat density on the head and neck. During the tunneling process at delicate sites, suction is minimal and any energy-based assistance is kept off. Once initial tunneling is completed, the more assertive suction removal can start. As a general rule, overcorrection should be avoided as this can create contour deformities and a skeletonized look or overlying skin rippling and dimpling. When there is doubt regarding the prudence of further fat removal, it is recommended that the operator pauses and assesses the progress of the procedure. More fat can always be removed later. "Feathering," or more conservative fat removal at the margins of a cosmetic unit or subunit, helps blend the overall results without leaving demarcation lines between cosmetic units.

During the procedure, the surgeon should be mindful of the character of the aspirate being removed. A pale, straw-colored to yellow aspirate is ideal. Some serosanguinous fluid mixed within the aspirate is acceptable. Frank blood should lead to a reassessment of cannula position and active exploration to ensure no major vessels have been injured. When vigorous suction with repeated readjustment of the angle and direction of the cannula yields little to no aspiration of additional fat, treatment at that site is likely completed.

14.3.3 Malar Fat Pad and Cheek Contouring

The typical patient may complain of increased cheek fullness that causes them to appear puffy or overweight. This manifestation of cheek enlargement can occur for a variety of reasons, including normal interpersonal variation, but it may also be related to weight elevation, metabolic disease, or medications. Before liposuction is considered, it is appropriate to consider any exacerbating factors that can be modified without surgery through counseling, behavioral change, or medication management. Masseter hypertrophy, which may reduce the benefit of a liposuction procedure, may be treated with neuromodulator injections.

Entry points for facial liposuction are typically preauricular and perinasal. Alternatively, direct needle aspiration of subcutaneous fat can be performed. Keeping entry points away from the mid-cheek most effectively conceals any associated scar. The surgeon should be careful not to overcorrect the cheek, thereby engendering a sunken look and risking aging the face by removing natural structural support. A "touch-up" procedure can always be performed months later, once a steady state devoid of postprocedure edema is observable, should more fat removal be required. Typical cannula types for the head and neck are of low-to-medium aggressiveness, commonly Capistrano or Klein (i.e., spatula) tips of 1 to 2 mm diameter. Smaller cannulas are used for feathering toward the edges of the fat pad and sculpting of depressed areas like the pretragal sulcus that define the cheek. Combination treatment with rhytidectomy may be selected when significant skin laxity, sagging, and jowling is present. Concomitant rhytidectomy provides the advantage of direct visualization of the lateral aspects of the malar pad.

14.3.4 Treatment of the Nasolabial Fold and Pretragal Sulcus

The nasolabial fold and pretragal sulcus can be treated with a 1- to 2-mm cannula to create natural folds that are blunted by fat accumulation. Gradual fat removal is desired, with frequent checking of the intraoperative result to prevent overcorrection. Treatment of these areas is often combined with treatment of other nearby areas, such as the jowl of malar fat pad. Sculpting of the elevated portion of nasolabial folds to soften and smoothen excessive deepening may be accompanied by lysis of any adhesions to mimetic muscles by blunt dissection with the cannula to provide a gently undulating contour.[8,10] Correction of lateral volume loss with hyaluronic acid injections or rhytidectomy should be considered when appropriate. Care should be taken prior to suctioning adjacent to a deepened nasolabial fold to ensure that it does not make it even deeper.

14.3.5 Treatment of the Jowl

A preoperative evaluation can determine whether the jowl is a result of excess fat deposition or mid- and lateral face age-related volume loss. In general, volume loss should be corrected by soft tissue augmentation (i.e., not liposuction) at the most superior aspect first, with subsequent lesser treatment to the inferior areas. This helps to elevate mid- and lower-face structures while accentuating the "V-shape" of the face, which is an indicator of youth. The jawline can be redefined by adding hyaluronic

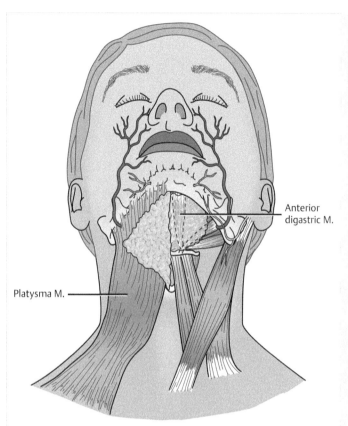

Fig. 14.4 Entry ports for access and treatment of the face and neck. Radial, spoke-wheel treatment patterns are preferred in their ability to prevent contour deformities. The use of multiple ports for one treatment area helps to further blend the overall result.

Anterior digastric M.

Platysma M.

acid filler deeply 1.5 cm anterior to the posterior border of the mandible while retracting laterally during injection. Thereafter, use of additional filler for definition along the mandible and correction of any other depressions can be considered. Some injectors use a long 25-gauge cannula for filler injections along the posterior mandibular border but the choice of bore and length of the cannula, and the decision of whether to use a cannula or a needle, varies among experts.

If, in fact, excess adiposity is present in the lateral jowl fat pads, but this excess is modest in volume, noninvasive modalities like chemical adipocytolysis with deoxycholic acid or cryolipolysis with tips specially designed for the neck may be considered instead of liposuction. There are no comparative studies of the effectiveness of liposuction versus chemical adipocytolysis or cryolipolysis for lateral jowls.[11,12] Rhytidectomy may be added as an adjunctive procedure for those with significant skin laxity.

If liposuction is the preferred procedure, being mindful of the underlying anatomy will mitigate

the risk of injury to the marginal mandibular nerve and facial artery along the mandibular border (▶ Fig. 14.4). The facial artery lies approximately 3 cm anterior to the masseteric tuberosity. The marginal mandibular nerve course is complex and can vary between right and left as well as between patients. Anatomic studies vary in terms of its most inferior location—2 cm below and 0.2 cm above the mandibular border. The most common point of its crossing of the mandibular border is 2.8 cm anterior to the border of the masseter.[13,14,15] During liposuction, care should be taken to avoid cannula motions that course perpendicular to the jawline at the point where the nerve is expected to cross. If this is not done, the nerve can be snagged by the cannula, and a nerve palsy resulting in unilateral paralysis can persist for weeks to months. After avoiding important neurovascular structures, feathering and careful extraction of the adipose tissue underneath the mandibular border along with focal removal of the descended lateral jowl fat pads will provide the most aesthetic result (▶ Fig. 14.5b). Unlike some other sites discussed in

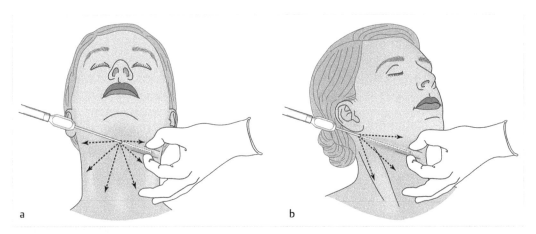

Fig. 14.5 Liposuction technique. Representation of the creation of ports and treatment pattern for the submental **(a)** and jowl and neck **(b)**.

this chapter, the jowls are amenable to superficial liposuction with a high degree of safety.[16]

14.3.6 Submental Liposuction

Submental liposuction begins with the creation of an entry point by punch biopsy tool or scalpel incision 1 mm posterior to the submental crease. The anatomic location of incision placement in this area is critical to prevent exaggeration of the submental crease after scar contracture during the healing process. Some surgeons support using a larger 2- to 3-mm cannula while others use a 1- to 2-mm cannula due to the benefit of the smaller entry site in the contest of the limited fat to be removed. The advantage of an incision is that a platysmaplasty or, in rare cases, the removal of the postplatysmal fat pads can be achieved if the incision is extended. Notably, platysmaplasty may cause elevation of the deep fat pad and make its removal unnecessary. Regardless of the method used to make it, the entry site should be slightly larger than the size of the cannula to reduce trauma to the skin edges.

Subcutaneous cannula tunneling without suction is typically commenced to include the boundaries of the chin, anterior border of the sternocleidomastoid, and the thyroid notch. An alternative to this is blunt dissection with Metzenbaum scissors. Once the tissue has been loosened, cannula suction is initiated. Throughout the procedure, the surgeon should pause to palpate the target areas to ensure progress toward a smooth, even contour. Bulges and irregularities indicate uneven liposuction and

dimpling indicates oversuctioning at a point or septal attachments that should be lysed. As the submentum lies underneath the main entry site, care should be taken to prevent overtreatment from multiple passes to treat distal sites. An excessive submental depression may simulate a "cobra" deformity, in which the oversuctioned tunnels created permit superficial tissue to contract into the new dead space. One way to avoid oversuctioning at the submentum is to turn off suction when removing and reinserting the cannula; alternatively, care can be taken to redirect the suction cannula during fanning without pulling back all the way. To assist with definition of the mandibular border, a 2-mm cannula is often used. This is rotated parallel to the mandibular border and conservative liposuction is performed. Because the marginal mandibular nerve branch and facial artery can run superficially in some patients or have atypical courses, particular caution should be exercised. The target is the fat immediately under the jawline and not over the mandibular border (▶ Fig. 14.5a). Aspirating fat over the mandibular border reduces jaw definition. Feathering with an additional pre- or postauricular entry site helps a smoother, defined contour and also reduces the risk of a "cobra" deformity. This also aids in creating secondary fibrosis along the neckline that helps the skin contract into a tighter position, hugging the underlying muscle.

Enhancements to submental liposuction include chin enhancement or reduction, and rhytidectomy. Rhytidectomy may be needed in combination with liposuction for some patients with advanced skin laxity or extensive photodamage. Noninvasive lipolysis (e.g., cryolipolysis) can correct small residual fat deposits if they persist after the procedure. A helpful rule to measure microgenia is to hold a cotton swab vertically and perpendicular to the lower vermillion border. This demonstrates the amount of chin projection that could be corrected as the point of the chin should ideally touch the cotton swab. It is important to consider prognathia, retrognathia, and micrognathia prior to determining how much chin projection to correct. Hyaluronic acid injection or surgical revision can be performed based on the clinical situation.

14.3.7 Facial and Periorbital Autologous Fat Transfer

Patients who have developed skeletonization in the periorbital area or more generalized facial lipodystrophy and who do not desire soft tissue augmentation with hyaluronic acid or poly-L-lactic acid may benefit from autologous fat transfer. The overall goal of fat transfer is to restore the youthful contours and fullness of the face. Understanding of the 3D anatomy of the fat pads of the face should guide restoration of areas that have undergone loss over time. Based on recent anatomic studies, maps of superficial and deep facial fat pads are now available. Primary areas that may benefit include the upper orbital rim and eyelid, nasojugal groove, orbitomalar groove, malar cheek, and nasolabial fold. Augmentation should also be ethnically appropriate, given different patterns of aging and fat atrophy or herniation in Caucasian, African-American, Latino, Asian, Indian-subcontinent, and racially mixed populations.

Minimally traumatic methods of fat harvesting tend to result in improved graft survival.[17] There is ongoing debate as to the ideal method that produces the most viable and functional adipocytes for injection. The principal techniques for acquisition of the fat to be transplanted are vacuum aspiration, syringe aspiration, and surgical excision. Recent experimental as well as some clinical studies support direct fat excision over aspiration.[18,19] Qin et al[19] suggests that en block grafting helps to preserve the architecture and structure of the graft to provide the most natural volume correction. Larger grafts can be made into smaller aliquots for use in areas where the latter are needed. Adipocytes in conventional lipoaspirates have been found by some investigators to be up to 90% less viable compared to fresh samples or low negative pressure-aspirated fat.[17,20] Graft

viability in lipoaspirates is further affected by cannula size. Larger cannulas induce less cellular trauma than smaller cannulas.[21,22]

The modern technique for fat harvesting described by Coleman[23] involves using a blunt, 3-mm, 2-hole cannula connected to a 10-mL syringe for lipoaspiration. Use of tumescent anesthesia increases patient comfort and minimizes bleeding. After the cannula is inserted into the harvest site, the surgeon creates gentle negative pressure by retraction of the plunger. Suitable harvest sites include the abdomen, trochanteric region, and inner thighs. Micro- and nanofat grafts harvested with small 0.7-to 1-mm-diameter cannulas may be used to treat the eyelids, lips, or other areas that may benefit from small grafts.[24,25] The mechanism of action whereby micrografts that are relatively devoid of adipose tissue provide augmentation, though not well understood, is thought to be related to the retention of a large proportion of adipose-derived stem cells (ASCs). These pluripotent stem cells are able to differentiate into adipose tissue at the site of placement, where they provide volume and skin regeneration. ASCs have also been found to improve graft survival while reducing fibrosis, calcification, and pseudocysts.[26]

Before implantation, autologous fat or ASC grafts may be rinsed with crystalloids, and further cleaned of impurities by filtration or sedimentation, with or without centrifugation. The goal is to remove collagen, blood, and cellular debris to avoid causing false increases in volume and unwanted inflammation. Centrifugation of less than 50 g has been found to be superior to other methods in terms of more favorable outcomes and lack of nodule formation after transfer.[27,28,29,30] Common practice is centrifugation at 3,000 rpm for 3 minutes. This causes fractionation into lipid, fatty tissue, and blood layers. The lipid supernatant can be poured out of the syringe or absorbed by sterile gauze. The blood fraction is ejected from the syringe prior to fat reimplantation.

For reimplantation, a small incision or entry port is created at the border of the relevant cosmetic unit or in a hidden area where the graft is to be injected. Cannulas smaller than 14-gauge are required to reduce the risk of central necrosis and graft failure.[22] Additionally, serial implantation of small aliquots over multiple sessions can avoid the problem of graft failure at the center of larger volume grafts, given that postimplantation revascularization starts at the periphery and proceeds slowly. Microinjection cannulas of 18 to 25 gauge have been used[31,32] and are likely to be most helpful for areas where smaller volumes are needed. Otherwise, the reimplantation of a fat graft is similar to placement of soft tissue filler, in that injection is performed during withdrawal of the cannula and a fanning pattern may be used for even and feathered placement. Injections are placed in multiple levels of the subcutaneous tissue to create an even contour. Anecdotal evidence suggests when larger grafts where central ischemia may occur are placed in locations such as the malar cheek, overestimating the volume required by 25 to 50% may lead to a better cosmetic result. The risks of swelling, bruising, intravascular injection (particularly, if using a needle for injection), and potential graft failure, as well as the possible need for multiple treatments, and the likelihood of progression of fat loss with aging or weight decreases should be discussed with the patient prior to the fat transfer procedure.

14.3.8 Liposuction of Other Body Sites

Though mostly outside the scope of this chapter, the described liposuction techniques and procedures can be modified to apply to the abdomen, axilla, arms, calves, breast, upper back, torso, and extremities. Medical indications for liposuction include axillary hyperhidrosis, gynecomastia, lymphedema, and upper back adipose deposition from metabolic disease.[33] The guiding principles for liposuction at these other sites are generally the same as for face-and-neck liposuction, but the underlying anatomy of other body areas may be less altered by aging-related changes. Triangulation and feathering become particularly crucial when large volumes are removed, as is often the case on the abdomen and thighs. In addition to the usual potential complications, postprocedure laxity of the skin is a greater concern off the head and neck. On the body, the volume of fat removal may be much greater and the subsequent tendency of the skin to retract may be insufficient to compensate. During liposuction on the abdomen, where there are multiple fascial layers and fat compartments, it is important to adjust for depth and treat the deep, mid, and superficial fat. The surgeon should remember that the first 0.5 to 1.0 cm of the torso may be skin rather than fat or subcutis. Communicating this to patients can create appropriate expectations, given that abdominal liposuction cannot achieve the type of extremely tight contour possible with abdominoplasty, when muscle is plicated and skin is resected. Arms and thighs benefit from conservative treatment with careful intraoperative rechecking of the result. Too much fat removal from the arms can make hanging skin more noticeable and result in a skeletonized appearance that is actually less aesthetically pleasing than the preliposuction contour.

14.4 Postoperative Considerations

Whether to close entry sites with suture or leave them to heal by secondary intention is an individual decision. Very small entry sites, such as those created by 1.5- or 2-mm punch may not be amenable to subcutaneous closure with absorbable sutures. If entry sites are allowed to heal spontaneously, depending on patient characteristics, topical antibiotic ointment may be beneficial.

Swelling begins within 2 days of the procedure and peaks at approximately 2 weeks. Woody lymphedema can then develop that softens by 2 months. Complete tissue healing and return to baseline pliability are expected by 3 months. Persistence of significant pain and swelling beyond 6 weeks may be a sign of overly aggressive liposuction that may signal an increased risk for exaggerated deep scarring and contour irregularities.[34] There are no prospective studies that have definitively evaluated the length of compression required after liposuction. For the trunk, legs, and arms, many surgeons recommend daily compression for 4 to 6 weeks and reducing activity to prevent fluid accumulation and to allow the skin to contract and form new adhesions. In submental liposuction, typically, a chin strap is worn while at home and asleep for a minimum of 2 weeks. Longer term use for 6 to 8 weeks may potentially be better as this corresponds to when all edema from procedure should naturally subside. Protracted use of compressive garments may also facilitate the readhesion of the dermis to the underlying deep fat and fascia. For this reason, for patients who are able to tolerate compressive devices and are motivated to work toward optimal outcomes, surgeons may recommend that garments be worn for longer.

14.5 Minimizing Risks

Tumescent liposuction is safe. Most complications are transient and mild. Some adverse events are specific to the face and neck, while can occur after any liposuction procedure. Common, unwanted adverse effects include erythema at the entry site, diffuse erythema, bruising, edema, mild tenderness, and drainage from the insertion sites. Patients should be informed that bruising and swelling can persist for weeks. Pinpoint, hypo- or hyperpigmented scars eventually develop at the cannula entry sites. Scar pigmentation is least predictable in Fitzpatrick skin types IV to VI, who may be relatively more susceptible to develop hypertrophic or keloidal scarring. In such patients, and even in others, assessing prior scars preoperatively can help estimate the risk of poor scarring after liposuction. In rare cases, very superficial, very aggressive liposuction can lead to the creation of thin skin flaps that are poorly perfused and may necrose and slough. Other complications that may be associated with suboptimal surgical technique, such as patient hypothermia and infection close to the time of surgery due to nonsterile technique or inadequate cleaning of instruments.

Not all adverse events can be prevented. However, an understanding of the location of the adipose tissue to be treated, its changes with age, and the relevant surrounding anatomy can help to ensure good outcomes while minimizing the risk of adverse events. Sterile technique should be used during liposuction, and the patient should be assessed intraoperatively to ensure stable function and vital signs. Common as well as rare but serious side effects should be discussed before surgery with the patient and listed on the informed consent form. Answering questions about the risks can also set reasonable expectations regarding the postoperative course.

Even an outstanding outcome after liposuction may not be perfectly symmetrical since few patients are symmetrical before surgery. Patients should know to expect a good result that is not perfect. A touch-up liposuction treatment may be considered to soften fat deposits or feather areas of depression that were not visible immediately after the procedure but become apparent weeks or months later. Ideally, this possibility will have been discussed with the patient beforehand.

14.6 Management of Complications

14.6.1 Pain and Edema

Pain and edema are the two most commonly managed side effects of liposuction. These occur almost without exception, although pain is usually mild and self-remitting in a day or two. When pain is significant, in addition to the pain relief associated with the use of compression garments or devices,

pain management with 70% alcohol wiped–sterilized ice packs, acetaminophen, and ibuprofen can be very effective when used concurrently in a multimodal approach. Opioids can be considered on an individual basis as relevant to the particular clinical setting and procedure. When used, in accordance with opioid reduction strategies, the minimum number of tablets should be prescribed to balance effectiveness with the risk of diversion and accidental overdose. Metaanalysis of randomized control trials has shown that the use of a combination of pain reduction agents acting at different receptors or through more than one route can significantly mitigate opioid consumption.[35,36] Despite previous concerns, an increased risk of major bleeding events has not been observed in patients treated with NSAIDS such as ibuprofen. Specifically, metaanalysis of the available trials in plastic surgery demonstrated no significant bleeding risk with postoperative use of ibuprofen.[37] If possible, a pain management plan tailored to the patient should be implemented in the preoperative period. This allows the surgeon to consider patient preferences, prior adverse reactions, and any safety concerns that may modify pain management strategies.

Chin straps and other compression garments after liposuction reduce the risk of excess postoperative edema. Reducing activity, aspirating excess fluid, and providing lymphatic drainage massage in the early postoperative period have also been suggested. For the abdomen, allowing port sites to heal by secondary intention can help to reduce the chance of fluid accumulation by keeping open an avenue for drainage. Putting in place strategies to decrease postoperative edema enables hastened healing, increased patient comfort, and prompt formation of new attachments between the residual deep fat and the overlying skin. The use of bromelain for 5 days after surgery to reduce swelling in some surgical and aesthetic procedures is supported by weak-to-moderate evidence.[38,39] There are no specific studies regarding the use of this agent for liposuction, plastic surgery procedures, or invasive dermatologic surgery. Counseling patients regarding the likelihood of slowly resolving postoperative swelling may minimize their anxiety.

14.6.2 Vascular Complications

Patients being medicated with anticoagulants and antithrombotics are at risk for intraoperative bleeding, and should be cleared by their internist or cardiologist prior to liposuction. If possible, nonessential blood thinners, as well as all herbal and alternative medications predisposing to blood loss, should be discontinued well in advance of the procedure.

During liposuction, preservation of the subdermal plexus and nearby vessels during liposuction minimizes the risk of extensive bruising, livedo reticularis–like reactions, retiform purpura, and skin necrosis. Some bruising is virtually inevitable. However, more serious vascular complications can be prevented by maintaining a thin 3- to 4-mm band of fat below the dermis to avoid dermal injury. Liposuction that is too superficial or aggressive is most likely to result in vascular damage. The highest-risk anatomic areas are watershed areas where the small, fragile capillaries of two large or named arteries anastomose. The abdominal flanks, where the anterior and posterior circulations meet, are one example. Energy-assisted liposuction creates additional risks, as the heat imparted by ultrasound, laser, and radiofrequency devices can cause thermal coagulation of small vessels. This problem is magnified when the energy device is used superficially proximal to the dermis and when the same area of skin is treated repeatedly or for a prolonged period. Thermocoupled tips in newer devices are designed to help overcome this pitfall by providing the operator real-time feedback regarding the temperature of the overlying skin. Other strategies to reduce the risk of injury include ensuring constant motion of the cannula, allowing for sufficient recovery time between invasive procedures, and performing tumescent liposuction with the patient awake so that perceived pain can be communicated. Intraoperative pain is a sensitive indicator that can presage vascular occlusion or dermal injury associated with superficial cannula use.

Superficial bruising is common. Without intervention, bruising peaks by 1 week and resolves 2 to 4 weeks after surgery. Offering the patient treatment with pulsed-dye laser may shorten the time to resolution. Standard settings are 7.5 J/cm^2, 10-mm spot, 6-ms pulse duration, and cryogen 30 ms with a 20-ms delay for a single pass 24 to 48 hours after the onset of the bruise. For dense bruising, some advocate an additional pass with a 10-ms pulse duration or a strategy that uses lower fluences with a longer pulse duration in multiple passes.[40] Bruises that are violaceous and between 24 and 48 hours old respond more favorably. Resolution can begin within 6 hours.[41,42] Topical *arnica montana* has also been tried to reduce bruising after procedures. A small randomized control trial has shown a modest effect with topical applications at concentrations of 20%, which are higher than those in most topical products.[43] The effect of oral arnica at homeopathic doses in a randomized setting has been mixed after surgery.[44,45] More standardization of dosing and study methodology is needed before recommending this as a routine treatment for bruising.

Venous thromboembolism (VTE) after liposuction is the most common cause of mortality (23%). However, the risk is much less than 1%. All reported cases have occurred after procedures performed under general anesthesia. Early ambulation is the most important intervention to prevent venous clotting. Standard prophylaxis measures for VTE can be employed for large volume or general anesthesia cases in which the patient requires admission and will not be walking after the procedure. Prophylaxis is rarely necessary after patient-awake tumescent liposuction.

Hemorrhage and severe bleeding are unlikely for liposuction procedures on the head and neck. Body weight, supernatant volume over 1,500 mL, and prolonged operative time, medication with anticoagulants, and injury to major arteries are correlated with the extent of blood loss. Reported cases of mortality have fit within these parameters and been restricted to the abdomen. Estimates of blood loss during abdominal liposuction suggest a mean of 10 mL per liter of aspirate (± 5 mL).[46] Maximum allowable blood loss calculations predict that a 1 g/dL (10 g/L) decrease in hemoglobin or 3% drop in hematocrit correlates to a minimum of 250 mL of blood loss. However, third spacing can cause a false elevation of hemoglobin due to hemoconcentration, and this may lead to underestimation of blood loss during larger procedures. Hemoglobin levels that are safe and do not require transfusion in asymptomatic patients or those who do not appear anemic are typically 8 g/dL (80 g/L).[47]

Tumescent fluid contains epinephrine, which causes local vasoconstriction and thus minimizes the risk of bleeding. Mechanical and energy-assisted liposuctions are equivalent regarding bleeding risk, which is generally low.[48] Some intraoperative findings can suggest that abnormal bleeding is occurring. Perioperative orthostasis should initiate investigation to rule out hypovolemia or anemia. Brisk abdominal or other compartment distension with or without overlying spreading purpura may indicate hemorrhage. Developing rigidity rather than compressible fluctuance as routine with tumescent fluid may also be a cause for concern.

When hemorrhage is detected, management may require advanced cardiac life support procedures coupled with volume repletion. Randomized control trials have shown no difference between saline over colloids for volume correction in the acute setting.[49] Immediate notification of emergency services is followed by prompt transfer to an acute care facility. Fortunately, liposuction-associated hemorrhage is a rare event.

Another rare but serious adverse event is fat embolism syndrome. There are at least 17 cases reported in the literature. Typical onset is within 24 to 72 hours after surgery. Symptoms generally include rapid onset tachypnea, dyspnea, and hypoxemia. Small fat droplets may bypass the lung to reach the central nervous system. The mechanism of action whereby fat emboli develop is not fully characterized, but it is thought to be a combination of lipid entering traumatized veins[50] and C-reactive protein in a proinflammatory state after surgery inducing calcium-dependent lipid aggregation to form an embolus.[51] In general, C-reactive protein is thought to be more responsible for later-onset fat embolism. Overall mortality following a fat embolic event is approximately 10 to 15%, and related to the severity of respiratory compromise. Treatment is supportive care, and survival relies on rapid recognition and referral to specialized hospital-based services.

14.6.3 Suboptimal Aesthetic Outcomes

Pre- and postoperative photographs are critical for tracking aesthetic outcomes and managing patient expectations. Serial photographs also provide the ability to document complications in a visual medium, and then demonstrate any improvement in these over time. This ability to follow the course of complications is particularly helpful for scarring and other contour irregularities.

Scarring is a natural part of the healing process. Some development of subcutaneous adhesions is desirable to re-drape lax skin tautly and smoothly over the underlying deep fat and fascia. Cannula entry sites are also expected to close with a small scar. In some cases, especially in patients with ethnic skin, healing may be with hyperpigmentation, or hypertrophic or keloidal scarring. The probability of such suboptimal outcomes is most correlated with how previous wounds have healed. Dermal injury from overly aggressive suctioning at insufficient depth may culminate in visible tractlike scarring in line with where the cannula was advanced. Management of scarring may include intralesional triamcinolone, paring of thicker scars, microneedling, pulsed dye laser, and resurfacing. Persistent hyperpigmentation in a mature scar may benefit from topical bleaching with hydroquinones, superficial chemical peels, or low-fluence Q-switched Nd:YAG laser. Of note, topical therapies that inhibit tyrosinase like kojic acid, hydroquinone, or vitamin C cannot usually target the deeper pigment. Since hyperpigmentation also frequently resolves without treatment, patients can be reassured that improvement will also occur spontaneously, without any specific intervention, although possibly over months to years. Hypopigmentation is more difficult to treat, with excimer laser and laser-delivered prostaglandins tried with variable success.[52] Suboptimal scarring or pigmentary change in patients with phototypes IV to VI may best be managed by an expert in the care of skin of color.

Irregular contours after liposuction may result from localized or generalized oversuctioning in areas at high risk for contour deformities. On the head and neck, such risky areas include the first centimeter posterior to the chin and submental area where overtreatment can lead to a residual "cobra-deformity" or S-shaped indentation. Similar high-risk areas on the body are the trochanteric and medial regions of the thigh. In general, over-removal of fat produces a skeletonized appearance, with a rippled or crepey skin contour overlying the partially visible form and boundaries of connective tissue, veins, and muscle. During autologous fat transfer, fat graft necrosis may similarly lead to irregular contour or a return to a patient's preoperative appearance. Volume loss that occurs when tissue augmentation with fat fails can be corrected by injection with poly-L-lactic acid, calcium hydroxyapatite, hyaluronic acid augmentation, or repeat fat grafting. Adherence to proper technique and conservative treatment approaches, whether during liposuction or fat transfer, may help avoid the creation of irregular contour.

Unresolving skin laxity after liposuction is another factor that may contribute to a poor aesthetic outcome. So-called "soft skin," which is more lax and less likely to contract after fat extraction, should be identified before treatment so that the patient can be appropriately warned and counseled. When baseline skin laxity is accentuated after liposuction, treatment can be with energy-based devices such as ultrasound or radiofrequency, barbed sutures for lifting the skin, or rhytidectomy of the excess skin.

14.6.4 Perforation Injury

Death from bowel perforation is the second most common cause of death in liposuction procedures. Injuries to the bowel, gallbladder, pancreas, and spleen have also been reported. Needless to say, these are not relevant risks during liposuction of the head and neck. However, fat or muscle herniation, solid or hollow viscus injury, or large artery injury are possible. All these events are exceedingly rare. In the head and neck, the risk to critical neck structures is theoretically possible and can occur if the relatively thin platysma muscle is punctured. Ensuring that cannula insertion is in the proper plane and the cannula tip is angled properly avoids possible perforation of the muscles or tendinous insertions. When proper technique is used there is a very low chance of harm to underlying structures. Immediate pain, atypical changes in blood pressure, altered mentation, air under the muscle (as in pneumoperitoneum), or rapid bruising in dependent areas can indicate that an injury has happened. In such cases, emergent referral to general or head-and-neck surgery with hospital admission is required for further work-up.

14.6.5 Intravascular Volume Redistribution

In order to compensate for the fat removed during liposuction, the body shifts fluid to occupy the space left by the procedure. This ultimately results in third spacing into the cavity being suctioned and depletion of intravascular volume. Large-volume liposuction of 4 L of fat or greater can cause sufficient third-spacing to lead to significant hypotension, and hypotensive shock in extreme cases.[53] A large retrospective study of 4,534 patients found that removal of greater than 100 mL of fat per unit of BMI independently correlated with an increased rate of complications (OR 4.58).[54] Even with lower volumes, light headedness can result from fluid shifts combined with dehydration. Initial signs may be subtle or be detectable only when moving to an upright position. Patients should be monitored over the course of the liposuction procedure and provided oral fluids as needed.[53] Hydration prior to surgery has not been studied, but it is a reasonable precaution prior to larger cases. Ideally, the surgeon would be able to monitor heart rate and blood pressure during large-volume procedures to identify those that may need further intervention such as intravenous hydration. Practitioners may also wish to be familiar with advanced cardiac life support

procedures in the rare event of a cardiovascular collapse. Stabilization and transfer to an acute care facility is critical should this occur. Large-volume (i.e., > 4 L of fat aspirated) liposuction procedures, if attempted, should be performed in a controlled operating room setting with an anesthesiologist and adequate monitoring to assess any significant hemodynamic changes.

14.6.6 Nerve Injury

Hypoesthesia is common after liposuction due to direct mechanical or stretch injury to small cutaneous nerves. Sensation generally returns to near normal by the end of 1 year. Fascial or muscle injury can lead to muscular adhesions that may require release. Neuromas or hyperesthesia may also rarely occur. Both can be treated by oral gabapentin, tricyclic antidepressants, or local anesthetics. Neuromas are amenable to surgery. Chronic pain can be a sign of the formation of unwanted adhesions or nerve injury.

14.6.7 Infection

Soft tissue infections are rare. The reported incidence is less than 1%. Uncontrolled diabetes and immunosuppression are significant risk factors, and patients with these conditions are not ideal subjects for liposuction. Adequacy of glycemic control or glucose testing should be part of the preoperative evaluation. Some surgeons opt to premedicate with antibiotics prior to the surgery. Seven days of prophylactic oral antibiotics directed against gram-positive organisms are suggested for all larger liposuction cases, and some surgeons use prophylactic antibiotics in all cases. Coverage for methicillin-resistant staphylococcus aureus, as well as gram-negative and anaerobic organisms, may be selected, with the precise choice dependent on the practice setting, patient characteristics, and local resistance patterns. Proper surgical technique, including hand washing, maintenance of a sterile field, and proper cleaning of instruments, is crucial for ensuring the safety of the procedure.

Erythema, tenderness, blisters, or increased warmth should initiate concern, with empiric antibiotics started and therapy possibly changed once cultures and sensitivities are available. Active opening of cannula entry sites may allow drainage of collections, but additional incision and drainage may be needed for any focal collections or loculations. Ultrasound or other imaging may be needed to localize abscesses. Negative pressure wound therapy or wound packing can be employed should any cavities or ulcerations persist after significant debridement or drainage.

Risk factors for severe and necrotizing infections include age > 50, diabetes mellitus, intravenous drug use, immunosuppression, malnutrition, and peripheral vascular disease. Visceral perforation is not required for such infections to advance. Rapidly progressing erythema, severe pain, and edema may lead to cyanosis and necrosis. Emergent debridement, possible ICU admission, antibiotics, and support care are required. Toxic shock syndrome due to exotoxins of *Group A Streptococcus* or *Staphylococcus aureus* has also been described. This requires hospital admission and antibiotics (i.e., empiric: vancomycin and clindamycin). Intravenous immunoglobulin has been tried for severe cases. Atypical mycobacterium or fungal infections should also be considered if there is no response to antibiotic therapy, or if ulcers, pustular plaques, or nodules form at the treatment site.

14.6.8 Seroma

Seromas may form due to lymphatic damage resulting from excessive tissue trauma. Routine cases of moderate-to-large volume liposuction are also at elevated risk of developing seromas due to the increased associated third-spacing. Since fat removal volumes on the head and neck tend to be much smaller, seromas are uncommon on the head and neck. To minimize the risk of seromas, a compression garment should be worn consistently for at least the first postoperative week after liposuction on the trunk or extremities, and for as long as feasible after neck liposuction. An older study based on a national survey found the overall incidence of seroma after liposuction to be 1.2%. This was mostly with larger procedures that involved the abdomen.[55] Indeed, the lower abdomen and posterolateral thighs are most at risk. When seromas do occur, placement of a bulky dressing over the seroma site under the compression bandage may facilitate its resolution. Some surgeons advocate for placing a primrose or Jackson–Pratt drains after larger procedures to pre-empt any seromas. In many cases, and particularly in lower volume cases such as on the head and neck, this may be unnecessary as the immediate use of compression garments or straps can prevent accumulation of excess fluid.[56] Using just in excess of the minimum amount of tumescent fluid required may help avoid overtumescence and minimize the risk of persistent fluid accumulation.

Despite the importance of preventing seromas, and reducing the likelihood of their reaccumulation through conservative means like extra compression, an acute seroma usually cannot be managed conservatively and much be actively evacuated. Evacuation of a seroma reduces the likelihood of a poor aesthetic outcome, which will commonly occur if the seroma is allowed to persist, fibrose, and gradually become a solid nodule. Options for evacuation include needle aspiration or placement of a drain, either of which can yield copious quantities of straw-colored aqueous liquid. After evacuation, prophylactic antibiotics are prudent. Seromas may reaccumulate after being drained, and drainage procedures may need to be repeated every few days until the cavity seals. Seromas lasting more than 4 weeks are considered chronic. These may require not only aspiration but also subsequent injection of sclerosant or irritant into the cavity to promote its closure.[57] Locally injected triamcinolone acetonide 40 mg/mL has been used with seromas developing from large flap reconstructions as well as liposuction.[58] Use of tetracycline 250 mg/mL in saline has been described in case reports.[58] Recalcitrant cases may need to undergo surgical excision of the resulting pseudocyst.

14.6.9 Delayed Improvement

Though not traditionally considered an adverse event, delayed-onset aesthetic results can be frustrating for patients and surgeons. Patients should be counseled before surgery that postliposuction improvement in skin laxity as well as formation of the new skin attachments necessary for their desired contour may not be fully evident for 6 mont'hs or longer. Residual swelling may subside particularly slowly when energydevices are used in combination with traditional fat suction. Serial photography and office visits may reassure the patient. Supporting the patient through their postoperative care with frequent contacts and communications may also reduce anxiety and possibly reveal ongoing subtle improvements that they can enjoy.

14.6.10 Lidocaine Toxicity

As long as recommended volumes and doses of tumescent liposuction are used, there is little danger of lidocaine toxicity. This has been proven in multiple studies.[6,7] Still, medications and supplements may interfere with lidocaine metabolism (▶ Table 14.4), and whether any

Table 14.4 Overview of the procedural steps for tumescent liposuction

- Obtain consent:
  - Review consent form and ensure all questions are answered
  - Ensure informed consent and explanation of common and rare side effects
  - Mark excess adiposity and key contours. Review with the patient in a mirror
  - Provide preoperative analgesia, sedation or anxiolytics as indicated
- Prepare the surgical field and drape in a sterile fashion
- Infuse tumescent anesthetic:
  - Anesthetize and create port sites (e.g., punch tool) appropriate for the treatment area
  - Infuse anesthesia amount appropriate to site and 1–2 cm beyond the treatment area
  - Reposition and repeat process for any additional port sites
- Aspirate:
  - Insert the cannula with or without pretunneling depending on the body site. While beyond the opening of the port site turn on the suction and any energy assistance
  - Remove fat in a radial pattern and use a crisscross pattern using multiple port sites. Treat both sides
  - Ensure feathering at the edges of the treatment areas to smooth any contours
  - Observe and avoid danger zones
- Discharge:
  - Gently aspirate any excess fluid if present. Turn off suction and energy assistance when exiting a port site
  - Clean and apply absorbent dressings over the port sites. If on the submentum, close the port linearly
  - Apply compression garment or chin strap
  - Review postoperative instructions and provide a written summary. Provide any necessary prescriptions for analgesia or antibiotics
  - Schedule follow-up to review their progress. Suggested to call the patient postoperatively

such medications are being taken by a prospective patient should be elicited during the preoperative visit. After consultation with the patient's internist or other relevant physician, these contraindicated medications may either be held prior to surgery, or some other noninvasive method of fat reduction may be deemed more appropriate for the patient.

If lidocaine toxicity is suspected, one of the earliest symptoms in circumoral numbness,it progresses to facial numbness, tinnitus, restlessness, slurred speech, tonic–clonic seizures, hemodynamic collapse, coma, and death. Immediate cessation of the procedure and active monitoring of the patient should occur if any of these symptoms or signs manifest. Also, immediate referral to the emergency department is essential in such cases. Personnel in offices performing liposuction should also be trained in, and have the relevant equipment for, advanced cardiac life support. In larger liposuction procedures, it is also advantageous to be able to continuously or episodically monitor a patient's heart rate and blood pressure during a liposuction procedure as an additional precaution. Treatment of lidocaine toxicity consists of supportive care, with consideration of intravenous fat emulsion for those who have signs of moderate-to-severe toxicity.

14.7 Conclusions

Overall, liposuction is a safe, effective, and well-tolerated procedure. Liposuction on the head and neck is safer than body liposuction, in that smaller volumes are mobilized and the risks of larger volume liposuction are generally absent. However, special care must be taken at head-and-neck sites to avoid injury to neurovascular structures, and to minimize scarring, which can be highly aesthetically relevant on the face. Liposuction can be used in combination with other rejuvenation procedures, including fat transfer of the aspirated fat to areas of depression and volume loss, as well as neuromodulators, prepackaged injectable fillers, and lasers and energy devices.

References

[1] Di Minno A, Frigerio B, Spadarella G, et al. Old and new oral anticoagulants: food, herbal medicines and drug interactions. Blood Rev. 2017; 31(4):193–203

[2] Wang CZ, Moss J, Yuan CS. Commonly used dietary supplements on coagulation function during surgery. Medicines (Basel). 2015; 2(3):157–185

[3] Samizadeh S, Wu W. Ideals of facial beauty amongst the Chinese population: results from a large national survey. Aesthetic Plast Surg. 2018; 42(6):1540–1550

[4] Rhodes G. The evolutionary psychology of facial beauty. Annu Rev Psychol. 2006; 57:199–226

[5] Mashkevich G, Wang J, Rawnsley J, Keller GS. The utility of ultrasound in the evaluation of submental fullness in aging necks. Arch Facial Plast Surg. 2009; 11(4):240–245

[6] Svedman KJ, Coldiron B, Coleman WP, III, et al. ASDS guidelines of care for tumescent liposuction. Dermatol Surg. 2006; 32(5):709–716

[7] Klein JA, Jeske DR. Estimated maximal safe dosages of tumescent lidocaine. Anesth Analg. 2016; 122(5):1350–1359

[8] Walsh K, Arya R. A simple formula for quick and accurate calculation of maximum allowable volume of local anaesthetic agents. Br J Dermatol. 2015; 172(3):825–826

[9] Tiryaki KT, Aksungur E, Grotting JC. Micro-shuttle lifting of the neck: a percutaneous loop suspension method using a novel double-ended needle. Aesthet Surg J. 2016; 36(6): 629–638

[10] Wang J, Huang J. Surgical softening of the nasolabial folds by liposuction and severing of the cutaneous insertions of the mimetic muscles. Aesthetic Plast Surg. 2011; 35(4):553–557

[11] Montes JR, Santos E, Chillar A. Jowl Reduction With Deoxycholic Acid. Dermatol Surg. 2020; 46(1):78–85

[12] Carruthers J, Humphrey S. Sodium deoxycholate for contouring of the jowl: our preliminary experience. Dermatol Surg. 2019; 45(1):165–167

[13] Hazani R, Chowdhry S, Mowlavi A, Wilhelmi BJ. Bony anatomic landmarks to avoid injury to the marginal mandibular nerve. Aesthet Surg J. 2011; 31(3):286–289

[14] Anthony DJ, Oshan Deshanjana Basnayake BM, Mathangasinghe Y, Malalasekera AP. Preserving the marginal mandibular branch of the facial nerve during submandibular region surgery: a cadaveric safety study. Patient Saf Surg. 2018; 12:23

[15] Al-Qahtani K, Mlynarek A, Adamis J, Harris J, Seikaly H, Islam T. Intraoperative localization of the marginal mandibular nerve: a landmark study. BMC Res Notes. 2015; 8:382

[16] Matarasso A. Superficial suction lipectomy: something old, something new, something borrowed.... Ann Plast Surg. 1995; 34(3):268–272, discussion 272–273

[17] Pu LL, Coleman SR, Cui X, Ferguson RE, Jr, Vasconez HC. Autologous fat grafts harvested and refined by the Coleman technique: a comparative study. Plast Reconstr Surg. 2008; 122 (3):932–937

[18] Fagrell D, Eneström S, Berggren A, Kniola B. Fat cylinder transplantation: an experimental comparative study of three different kinds of fat transplants. Plast Reconstr Surg. 1996; 98(1):90–96, discussion 97–98

[19] Qin W, Xu Y, Liu X, Xu S. Experimental and primary clinical research of core fat graft. Zhongguo Xiu Fu Chong Jian Wai Ke Za Zhi. 2012; 26(5):576–582

[20] Pu LL, Cui X, Fink BF, Cibull ML, Gao D. The viability of fatty tissues within adipose aspirates after conventional liposuction: a comprehensive study. Ann Plast Surg. 2005; 54(3): 288–292, discussion 292

[21] Ozsoy Z, Kul Z, Bilir A. The role of cannula diameter in improved adipocyte viability: a quantitative analysis. Aesthet Surg J. 2006; 26(3):287–289

[22] James IB, Bourne DA, DiBernardo G, et al. The architecture of fat grafting II: impact of cannula diameter. Plast Reconstr Surg. 2018; 142(5):1219–1225

[23] Coleman SR. Structural fat grafting: more than a permanent filler. Plast Reconstr Surg. 2006; 118(3) Suppl:108S–120S

[24] Dasiou-Plakida D. Fat injections for facial rejuvenation: 17 years experience in 1720 patients. J Cosmet Dermatol. 2003; 2(3–4):119–125

[25] Mazzola RF. Fat injection: from filling to regeneration. St. Louis, MO: Quality Medical Publishing; 2009:373–422

[26] Matsumoto D, Sato K, Gonda K, et al. Cell-assisted lipotransfer: supportive use of human adipose-derived cells for soft tissue augmentation with lipoinjection. Tissue Eng. 2006; 12 (12):3375–3382

[27] Strong AL, Cederna PS, Rubin JP, Coleman SR, Levi B. The current state of fat grafting: a review of harvesting, processing, and injection techniques. Plast Reconstr Surg. 2015; 136(4): 897–912

[28] Botti G, Pascali M, Botti C, Bodog F, Cervelli V. A clinical trial in facial fat grafting: filtered and washed versus centrifuged fat. Plast Reconstr Surg. 2011; 127(6):2464–2473

[29] Pfaff M, Wu W, Zellner E, Steinbacher DM. Processing technique for lipofilling influences adipose-derived stem cell concentration and cell viability in lipoaspirate. Aesthetic Plast Surg. 2014; 38(1):224–229

[30] Ferraro GA, De Francesco F, Tirino V, et al. Effects of a new centrifugation method on adipose cell viability for autologous fat grafting. Aesthetic Plast Surg. 2011; 35(3):341–348

[31] Mojallal A, Foyatier JL. The effect of different factors on the survival of transplanted adipocytes. Ann Chir Plast Esthet. 2004; 49(5):426–436

[32] Nguyen PS, Desouches C, Gay AM, Hautier A, Magalon G. Development of micro-injection as an innovative autologous fat graft technique: the use of adipose tissue as dermal filler. J Plast Reconstr Aesthet Surg. 2012; 65(12):1692–1699

[33] Coleman WP III, Flynn TC, Coleman KM. Liposuction. In: Bolognia J, Schaffer JV, Cerroni L, eds. Dermatology. 4th ed. China: Elsevier; 2018: 2628–29

[34] Shiffman MA. Prevention and treatment of liposuction complications. In: Shiffman MA, Di Giuseppe A, eds. Liposuction: Principles and Practice. 1st ed. New York: Springer; 2006:333–41

[35] Elia N, Lysakowski C, Tramèr MR. Does multimodal analgesia with acetaminophen, nonsteroidal antiinflammatory drugs, or selective cyclooxygenase-2 inhibitors and patient-controlled analgesia morphine offer advantages over morphine alone? Meta-analyses of randomized trials. Anesthesiology. 2005; 103(6):1296–1304

[36] Chou R, Gordon DB, de Leon-Casasola OA, et al. Management of postoperative pain: a clinical practice guideline from the American Pain Society, the American Society of Regional Anesthesia and Pain Medicine, and the American Society of Anesthesiologists' Committee on Regional Anesthesia, Executive Committee, and Administrative Council. J Pain. 2016; 17(4):508–10

[37] Kelley BP, Bennett KG, Chung KC, Kozlow JH. Ibuprofen may not increase bleeding risk in plastic surgery: a systematic review and meta-analysis. Plast Reconstr Surg. 2016; 137(4): 1309–1316

[38] Singh T, More V, Fatima U, Karpe T, Aleem MA, Prameela J. Effect of proteolytic enzyme bromelain on pain and swelling after removal of third molars. J Int Soc Prev Community Dent. 2016; 6 Suppl 3:S197–S204

[39] Urdiales-Gálvez F, Delgado NE, Figueiredo V, et al. Treatment of soft tissue filler complications: expert consensus recommendations. Aesthetic Plast Surg. 2018; 42(2):498–510

[40] DeFatta RJ, Krishna S, Williams EF, III. Pulsed-dye laser for treating ecchymoses after facial cosmetic procedures. Arch Facial Plast Surg. 2009; 11(2):99–103

[41] Karen JK, Hale EK, Geronemus RG. A simple solution to the common problem of ecchymosis. Arch Dermatol. 2010; 146 (1):94–95

[42] Mayo TT, Khan F, Hunt C, Fleming K, Markus R. Comparative study on bruise reduction treatments after bruise induction using the pulsed dye laser. Dermatol Surg. 2013; 39(10): 1459–1464

[43] Leu S, Havey J, White LE, et al. Accelerated resolution of laser-induced bruising with topical 20% arnica: a rater-blinded randomized controlled trial. Br J Dermatol. 2010; 163(3):557–563

[44] Stevinson C, Devaraj VS, Fountain-Barber A, Hawkins S, Ernst E. Homeopathic arnica for prevention of pain and bruising: randomized placebo-controlled trial in hand surgery. J R Soc Med. 2003; 96(2):60–65

[45] Seeley BM, Denton AB, Ahn MS, Maas CS. Effect of homeopathic Arnica montana on bruising in face-lifts: results of a randomized, double-blind, placebo-controlled clinical trial. Arch Facial Plast Surg. 2006; 8(1):54–59

[46] Mangubat EA, Harbke C. Blood loss in liposuction surgery. In: Shiffman MA, Di Giuseppe A, eds. Liposuction: Principles and Practice. 1st ed. New York: Springer; 2006:347–52

[47] Carson JL, Guyatt G, Heddle NM, et al. Clinical practice guidelines from the AABB: red blood cell transfusion thresholds and storage. JAMA. 2016; 316(19):2025–2035

[48] Karmo FR, Milan MF, Silbergleit A. Blood loss in major liposuction procedures: a comparison study using suction-assisted versus ultrasonically assisted lipoplasty. Plast Reconstr Surg. 2001; 108(1):241–247, discussion 248–249

[49] Lewis SR, Pritchard MW, Evans DJW, et al. Colloids versus crystalloids for fluid resuscitation in critically ill people. Cochrane Database Syst Rev. 2018; 8(8):CD000567

[50] Wang HD, Zheng JH, Deng CL, Liu QY, Yang SL. Fat embolism syndromes following liposuction. Aesthetic Plast Surg. 2008; 32(5):731–736

[51] Hulman G. Pathogenesis of non-traumatic fat embolism. Lancet. 1988; 1(8599):1366–1367

[52] Massaki AB, Fabi SG, Fitzpatrick R. Repigmentation of hypopigmented scars using an erbium-doped 1,550-nm fractionated laser and topical bimatoprost. Dermatol Surg. 2012; 38 (7 Pt 1):995–1001

[53] Iverson RE, Lynch DJ, American Society of Plastic Surgeons Committee on Patient Safety. Practice advisory on liposuction. Plast Reconstr Surg. 2004; 113(5):1478–1490, discussion 1491–1495

[54] Chow I, Alghoul MS, Khavanin N, et al. Is there a safe lipoaspirate volume? A risk assessment model of liposuction volume as a function of body mass index. Plast Reconstr Surg. 2015; 136(3):474–483

[55] Teimourian B, Rogers WB, III. A national survey of complications associated with suction lipectomy: a comparative study. Plast Reconstr Surg. 1989; 84(4):628–631

[56] Bhave MA. Can drains be avoided in lipo-abdominoplasty? Indian J Plast Surg. 2018; 51(1):15–23

[57] ood A, Kotamarti VS, Therattil PJ, Lee ES. Sclerotherapy for the management of seromas: a systematic review. Eplasty. 2017; 17:e25

[58] Taghizadeh R, Shoaib T, Hart AM, Weiler-Mithoff EM. Triamcinolone reduces seroma re-accumulation in the extended latissimus dorsi donor site. J Plast Reconstr Aesthet Surg. 2008; 61(6):636–642

Further Readings

Chou R, Gordon DB, de Leon-Casasola OA, et al. Management of postoperative pain: a clinical practice guideline from the American Pain Society, the American Society of Regional Anesthesia and Pain Medicine, and the American Society of Anesthesiologists' Committee on Regional Anesthesia, Executive Committee, and Administrative Council. J Pain. 2016; 17 (2):131–157

Hanke CW, Sattler G, Sommer B. Textbook of liposuction. Arbingdon: Informa Healthcare;2007

Massry GG, Azizzadeh B. Periorbital fat grafting. Facial Plast Surg. 2013; 29(1):46–57

Nairns R. Safe liposuction and fat transfer. New York: Marcel Dekker; 2003

Shiffman MA, Di Giuseppe A. Liposuction: principles and practice. 1st ed. New York: Springer; 2006

15 Cryolipolysis

Aria Vazirnia and Mathew M. Avram

Summary

Cryolipolysis and deoxycholic acid injections are effective and generally safe and well-tolerated non-invasive fat removal modalities. Cryolipolysis involves the use of controlled cooling to noninvasively target and destroy subcutaneous fat. ATX-101 refers to synthetic deoxycholic acid (a bile acid), which is used to disrupt adipocyte cell membranes. Common postprocedural side effects from both may include temporary erythema, bruising, swelling, numbness, and/or tenderness/pain. However, it is important for health practitioners to be aware of rare concerning complications associated with both procedures.

Keywords: adverse events, ATX-101, complications, contouring, coolsculpt, cryolipolysis, deoxycholic acid, fat, noninvasive, panniculitis, side effects

15.1 Introduction

Body contouring and noninvasive fat removal procedures have grown strongly in popularity within the past decade. The American Society for Dermatologic Surgery (ASDS) 2019 consumer survey on dermatologic procedures shows that 58% of consumers are interested in body sculpting procedures.[1] More and more patients seek noninvasive body contouring and fat removal procedures that lack the risks associated with surgery and liposuction, which include infection, anesthesia complications, and death.[2,3] Two effective noninvasive techniques for the removal of unwanted subcutaneous fat are cryolipolysis and deoxycholic acid injections. While these are generally considered safe and effective treatment modalities,[4,5] it is important for health practitioners to be aware of associated adverse events and potential complications.

15.2 Cryolipolysis Mechanism of Action

Cryolipolysis refers to the localized application of controlled cooling to noninvasively target and destroy subcutaneous adipose tissue. The controlled cooling promotes crystallization of lipids within adipocytes, which triggers a localized panniculitis. This inflammatory response leads to

selective loss of adipocytes through apoptosis without injuring surrounding tissue. The apoptotic cells are eliminated by macrophages, a process that peaks at about 2 weeks and resolves at about 3 months.[6,7] More than 7 million procedures have been performed globally on different body sites as of 2019,[8] and cryolipolysis (CoolSculpting; Allergan, Inc. Irvine, CA) has been cleared by the US Food and Drug Administration (FDA) for reduction of fat in the flank area (2010), abdomen (2012), thighs (2014), submental area (2015), and arms/back/bra fat/area beneath buttocks (2016).[7,9] The treatment cycle involves positioning a negative pressure applicator on a region of skin overlying excess adiposity; the negative pressure helps bring the treatment area into complete contact with two cooling plates. The original treatment cycles were 60 minutes, but newer applicators such as the CoolAdvantage family of applicators have helped reduce treatment times to as low as 35 minutes.[9]

15.3 Safety Profile of Cryolipolysis

Cryolipolysis is generally considered a safe and well-tolerated body contouring procedure with minimal treatment-associated discomfort.[10,11] Studies have demonstrated no significant changes in serum total cholesterol, low-density lipoprotein (LDL), high-density lipoprotein (HDL), and triglycerides after treatment.[11] Postprocedural side effects include temporary numbness, dysesthesia, erythema, edema, induration, bruising, and/or tenderness that typically self-resolve within 14 days.[10,11,12,13] About two-thirds of patients may experience numbness in the treatment area for about 2 months after the procedure.[14,15]

A 2013 review by Stevens et al of 528 patients who underwent 2,729 cryolipolysis treatment cycles at 1,785 anatomic sites resulted in no serious adverse events; there were only three cases of mild or moderate pain.[15,16] A 2015 systematic review by Ingargiola et al highlighted the following complications after cryolipolysis—temporary erythema, bruising, swelling, dysesthesia/numbness, and pain, which resolved within a few weeks. No cases of scarring, ulceration, blistering, bleeding, infection, or dyspigmentation were noted. However, the authors noted a case of paradoxical adipose hyperplasia

(PAH), a rare but significant adverse event that will be discussed in detail later in this chapter.[3]

A 2015 review of the FDA Manufacturer and User Facility Device Experience (MAUDE) database lists 62 adverse events from cryolipolysis reported from 2011 to 2013. The MAUDE database is a record of all adverse events that patients voluntarily report after using various medical devices. Adverse events within the MAUDE database included fat hypertrophy, firmness, pain/dysesthesia, hernia, indentation, laxity of the skin, laxity of the fascia, hyperpigmentation, and edema.[17] It is unclear if the reported hernias were present before or after cryolipolysis treatment.[15,17] One limitation of the MAUDE database is that it is based upon the voluntary anecdotal reporting of physicians, other health care providers and patients. Thus, the actual incidence of adverse side effects is not elucidated within the MAUDE database. By contrast, industry reports are mandated.

Side effects from submental cryolipolysis are mild and generally self-limited. Side effects, although uncommon, include swelling, bruising, tenderness, and paresthesias.[18] Kilmer et al highlight two cases of prolonged erythema lasting 2 to 3 weeks, one incident of hyperpigmentation resolving at 4 weeks, and one patient with the sensation of fullness at the back of the throat lasting 1 to 2 months from swelling after submental cryolipolysis.[5] Lee et al discuss a rare case of marginal mandibular nerve (MMN) palsy resolving 2 months after submental cryolipolysis using CoolMini applicators (Cool Sculpting; Allergan, Inc., Irvine, CA).[18] Gregory et al highlight two rare cases of submental neuropathic pain associated with mandibular nerve injury due to submental cryolipolysis.[19] One case demonstrated sudden severe posttreatment pain of the left submental region extending toward the left ear. The second case highlighted a subacute onset of significant discomfort extending from the treatment area into the oral cavity and manifesting as dental pain.

15.4 Paradoxical Adipose Hyperplasia in Cryolipolysis

While most side effects associated with cryolipolysis are mild, well-tolerated, and occur within hours to days of the procedure, there are several rare and more notable delayed-onset symptoms. PAH is the most common, significant complication of cryolipolysis. PAH refers to large well-demarcated, painless, firm masses that develop in areas treated with cryolipolysis 2 to 6 months after treatment.[20,21] Reported cases have been noted on the abdomen, chest, back, flanks, and thighs.[9] Initially described in two patients by Jalian et al in 2014, the estimated incidence of PAH was previously thought to be 1 in 20,000 treatment cycles;[20,22] however, with more recent data, the incidence rate is estimated as 0.029% or 1 in 3,500 treatment cycles.[23] Some still believe that this incidence rate may even be underrepresented, and a study by Singh et al showed that the incidence of PAH may be as high as 2%.[24]

Histological studies on PAH are inconsistent, showing either tissue hypovascularity and adipocyte hypocellularity, or hypervascularity and adipocyte hypercellularity.[20] Jalian et al reported biopsied tissue specimens showing septal fat thickening, decreased adipocyte organization, and hypervascularity.[10,22] However, Seaman et al reported adipose tissue demonstrating hypocellularity and hypovascularity compared to controls.[10] Septal thickening and hypervascularity may represent a reactive fibrosis and angiogenesis resulting from hypoxic injury to adipocytes that have been cooled.[9]

The pathophysiology of PAH is poorly understood but appears to involve both genetic and hormonal factors.[25] A systematic review by Ho and Jagdeo showed that PAH was more common in men and in patients with Hispanic and Latino backgrounds, especially when large applicators were utilized.[9] In addition, there are several cases of PAH developing in men after pseudogynecomastia treatments, suggesting that caution must be taken when treating the male chest.[20] The negative suction from the cryolipolysis applicator has been implicated in adipocyte stimulation and proliferation.[26] Specifically, inadequate suction may lead to suboptimal cooling of the targeted tissue, thereby preventing a cold panniculitis from developing. Therefore, poor suction without the necessary panniculitis may stimulate the adipose tissue to grow larger. This idea has been demonstrated by a breast augmentation device (BRAVA, Biomecanica, Inc, Miami, FL) that uses low suction to increase fibroglandular tissue and adipose tissue within breasts.[20,27]

The treatment of choice for PAH is liposuction. No evidence of spontaneous resolution of PAH has been described to date, and therefore treatment with liposuction should be considered.[25] Liposuction is recommended between 6 and 9 months after cryolipolysis treatment to allow the newly expanded tissue to soften after a firm inflammatory phase.[25] Additional treatment with cryolipolysis is not recommended, as it may exacerbate the PAH.[9] In a case series of 11 patients, Kelley et al describe one patient with recurrence of PAH at 2 months following ultrasound-assisted liposuction, but no recurrence was noted with power-assisted liposuction.[25] Ward et al describe the use of ATX-101 (deoxycholic acid), another noninvasive fat removal modality, in the treatment of PAH.[28]

15.5 Delayed Post-treatment Pain in Cryolipolysis

While PAH is more common in men, women are at increased risk of delayed posttreatment pain with cryolipolysis. Delayed posttreatment pain refers to neuropathic symptoms, increased pain disrupting sleep at night, and/or discomfort unalleviated by analgesic medications.[11] The pathophysiology is unknown, but it is thought that there may be sensory nerve variation in women versus men, and that sensory nerves may be affected by the strong inflammation within the treated area.[11] Keaney et al conducted a retrospective study on 125 patients (27 men and 98 women) who received a total of 554 cryolipolysis treatment cycles (CoolSculpting; Allergan, Inc., Irvine, CA) for the lower and upper abdomen, flanks, back, thighs, and/or chest using one of four small applicators, a large applicator, or flat applicator.[11] A total of 19 patients (15.2%) developed delayed posttreatment pain, and all these patients were female. The pain developed on average 3 days after cryolipolysis and resolved with an average duration of 11 days. Pain was most commonly localized to the abdomen, which was also the most commonly treated area. The delayed posttreatment pain was managed with compression garments, lidocaine transdermal patches, low-dose gabapentin, and/or acetaminophen with codeine.

15.6 Miscellaneous Complications in Cryolipolysis

There are additional isolated complications associated with cryolipolysis. The device being used appears to be a major factor in these cases. Skin necrosis has been reported with the improper use of cryolipolysis. Nseir et al illustrate a case of skin necrosis on the left thigh following cryolipolysis performed without the required interface gel pad.[13] Motor nerve palsy has been reported with cryolipolysis of the arms. Lee et al reports a case of a young woman who underwent cryolipolysis to the distal upper arms with the MiCool cryolipolysis device (MiCool, Hironic Co., Seongnam,

Korea).[12] Days later, the patient developed radial nerve injury characterized by left hand extensor weakness and difficulty in lifting heavy objects. Electromyography was consistent with axonal damage to the distal branch of the radial nerve, which bifurcates at the elbow. The left hand motor neuropathy fully recovered 6 months later. Khan reports a case of cryolipolysis to the lower anterior thighs resulting in unsatisfactory contour irregularities and mild hyperpigmentation, which was later corrected with fat grafting and nonablative fractional laser, respectively.[8]

15.7 Introduction to ATX-101

In addition to cryolipolysis, the injectable compound known as ATX-101 is an effective treatment for the noninvasive removal of unwanted fat. ATX-101 (Kybella; Allergan, Inc., Irvine, CA) was approved by the FDA in 2015 for the treatment of moderate-to-severe submental fat.[15,29] However, it has been used off-label for the jowls, brassiere line fat, and lipomas.[30] The compound contains synthetic deoxycholic acid (a bile acid), which causes lipolysis by disrupting adipocyte cell membranes.[7,15,31] Submental injections are performed in recommended dosages of 0.1-mL to 0.2-mL aliquots spaced 1-cm apart from one another, using a 30-gauge 0.5-inch needle.[31] In clinical practice, other dosages are often used.

15.8 Safety Profile of ATX-101

The most common side effects from ATX-101 are erythema, edema, induration, bruising, pain, and numbness.[31,32,33] Symptoms typically resolve within 1 to 2 weeks,[31] but have been reported to take as long as 3 to 4 weeks, or more.[15] The pain and bruising are considered mild-to-moderate, but patients typically have significant swelling.[5] The injection discomfort has been attributed to the basic pH of the medication.[15] The degree of swelling is dependent on the volume of drug injected.[29] The frequency of injection-related side effects tends to decrease over subsequent treatment courses.[32,33] As with cryolipolysis, there are no significant changes in serum lipid profiles after a treatment session.[32,33] Rarer side effects include dysphagia from swelling, MMN injury, hyperhidrosis, paresthesias, and nodule formation.[34] Temporary injection site alopecia has also been reported.[32,33]

15.9 Marginal Mandibular Nerve Injury with ATX-101

MMN injury is a concerning adverse event associated with ATX-101 injections. Injury may occur from direct needle trauma to the nerve or from the edema and inflammation surrounding or compressing the nerve.[15] Branches of the MMN can be found 1 to 2 cm below the inferior border of the mandible, and the facial artery and vein cross the mandibular border anterior to the masseter at the antegonial notch. Therefore, it is recommended to avoid injecting within 1.5 cm below the inferior mandibular border.[35] In the FDA clinical trials, temporary MMN paresis was noted in 4.3% of subjects treated with ATX-101 versus 0.4% of patients treated with placebo.[32,33] All cases of MMN paresis resolved after a median of 42 days and 85 days in the ATX-101 and placebo groups, respectively.[32,33]

15.10 Vascular Complications in ATX-101

There are a few reports of intra-arterial injection with ATX-101. Sachdev et al report a case of ATX-101 injection into the facial artery causing skin necrosis despite injecting the facial artery and surrounding tissue with normal saline and starting the patient on daily aspirin.[35] Lindgren and Welsh report a case of ATX-101 injected into the submental artery, which is a branch of the facial artery.[36] The injection resulted in a mottled appearance of the skin, in addition to significant lower tooth and gum pain, jaw pain, and headache. The patient was treated with hyaluronidase injections, oral prednisone, aspirin, warm compresses, and transferred to a hyperbaric oxygen center. The pain and mottled appearance improved, but the patient developed an eschar at the injection site.[36]

15.11 Conclusion

With careful application and awareness of potential complications, noninvasive fat removal treatments with deoxycholic acid injections and cryolipolysis can be performed safely and effectively. As body contouring and noninvasive fat removal procedures continue to grow in popularity, it is important for both patients and providers to be aware of common and rare procedure-related side effects.

References

[1] American Society for Dermatologic Surgery (ASDS). 2019 Consumer Survey on Cosmetic Dermatologic Procedures. Data were collected from 3645 consumers through a blind online survey in 2019. https://www.asds.net/skin-experts/news-room/press-releases/asds-survey-dermatologists-and-digital-resources-influence-cosmetic-procedures-and-skin-care-decisions. Accessed August, 2020.

[2] Rao RB, Ely SF, Hoffman RS. Deaths related to liposuction. N Engl J Med. 1999; 340(19):1471–1475

[3] Ingargiola MJ, Motakef S, Chung MT, Vasconez HC, Sasaki GH. Cryolipolysis for fat reduction and body contouring: safety and efficacy of current treatment paradigms. Plast Reconstr Surg. 2015; 135(6):1581–1590

[4] Liu M, Chesnut C, Lask G. Overview of Kybella (deoxycholic acid injection) as a fat resorption product for submental fat. Facial Plast Surg. 2019; 35(3):274–277

[5] Kilmer SL, Burns AJ, Zelickson BD. Safety and efficacy of cryolipolysis for non-invasive reduction of submental fat. Lasers Surg Med. 2016; 48(1):3–13

[6] Avram MM, Harry RS. Cryolipolysis for subcutaneous fat layer reduction. Lasers Surg Med. 2009; 41(10):703–708. Review. Erratum in: Lasers Surg Med. 2012 Jul;44(5):436

[7] Klein KB, Bachelor EP, Becker EV, Bowes LE. Multiple same day cryolipolysis treatments for the reduction of subcutaneous fat are safe and do not affect serum lipid levels or liver function tests. Lasers Surg Med. 2017; 49(7):640–644

[8] Khan M. Complications of cryolipolysis: paradoxical adipose hyperplasia (PAH) and beyond. Aesthet Surg J. 2019; 39(8): NP334–NP342

[9] Ho D, Jagdeo J. A systematic review of paradoxical adipose hyperplasia (PAH) post-cryolipolysis. J Drugs Dermatol. 2017; 16(1):62–67

[10] Seaman SA, Tannan SC, Cao Y, Peirce SM, Gampper TJ. Paradoxical adipose hyperplasia and cellular effects after cryolipolysis: a case report. Aesthet Surg J. 2016; 36(1): NP6–NP13

[11] Keaney TC, Gudas AT, Alster TS. Delayed onset pain associated with cryolipolysis treatment: a retrospective study with treatment recommendations. Dermatol Surg. 2015; 41(11):1296–1299

[12] Lee SJ, Kim YJ, Park JB, Suh DH, Kwon DY, Ryu HJ. A case of motor neuropathy after cryolipolysis of the arm. J Cosmet Laser Ther. 2016; 18(7):403–404

[13] Nseir I, Lievain L, Benazech D, Carricaburu A, Rossi B, Auquit-Aukbur I. Skin necrosis of the thigh after a cryolipolysis session: a case report. Aesthet Surg J. 2018; 38(4): NP73–NP75

[14] Coleman SR, Sachdeva K, Egbert BM, Preciado J, Allison J. Clinical efficacy of noninvasive cryolipolysis and its effects on peripheral nerves. Aesthetic Plast Surg. 2009; 33(4):482–488

[15] Vanaman M, Fabi SG, Carruthers J. Complications in the cosmetic dermatology patient: a review and our experience (Part 2). Dermatol Surg. 2016; 42(1):12–20

[16] Stevens WG, Pietrzak LK, Spring MA. Broad overview of a clinical and commercial experience with CoolSculpting. Aesthet Surg J. 2013; 33(6):835–846

[17] Tremaine AM, Avram MM. FDA MAUDE data on complications with lasers, light sources, and energy-based devices. Lasers Surg Med. 2015; 47(2):133–140

[18] Lee NY, Ibrahim O, Arndt KA, Dover JS. Marginal mandibular injury after treatment with cryolipolysis. Dermatol Surg. 2018; 44(10):1353–1355

[19] Gregory A, Humphrey S, Varas G, Zachary C, Carruthers J. Atypical pain developing subsequent to cryolipolysis for noninvasive reduction of submental fat. Dermatol Surg. 2019; 45(3):487–489

[20] Keaney TC, Naga LI. Men at risk for paradoxical adipose hyperplasia after cryolipolysis. J Cosmet Dermatol. 2016; 15 (4):575–577

[21] Karcher C, Katz B, Sadick N. Paradoxical hyperplasia post cryolipolysis and management. Dermatol Surg. 2017; 43(3): 467–470

[22] Jalian HR, Avram MM, Garibyan L, Mihm MC, Anderson RR. Paradoxical adipose hyperplasia after cryolipolysis. JAMA Dermatol. 2014; 150(3):317–319

[23] Coolsculpting corporate website: "Coolsculpting business update." http://pro.coolsculpting.com/l/70932/2017-11-20/5nnm1p

[24] Singh SM, Geddes ER, Boutrous SG, Galiano RD, Friedman PM. Paradoxical adipose hyperplasia secondary to cryolipolysis: an underreported entity? Lasers Surg Med. 2015; 47(6):476–478

[25] Kelly ME, Rodríguez-Feliz J, Torres C, Kelly E. Treatment of paradoxical adipose hyperplasia following cryolipolysis: a single-center experience. Plast Reconstr Surg. 2018; 142 (1):17e–22e

[26] Stefani WA. Adipose hypertrophy following cryolipolysis. Aesthet Surg J. 2015; 35(7):NP218–NP220

[27] Khouri RK, Schlenz I, Murphy BJ, Baker TJ. Nonsurgical breast enlargement using an external soft-tissue expansion system. Plast Reconstr Surg. 2000; 105(7):2500–2512, discussion 2513–2514

[28] Ward CE, Li JY, Friedman PM. ATX-101 (deoxycholic acid injection) for paradoxical adipose hyperplasia secondary to cryolipolysis. Dermatol Surg. 2018; 44(5):752–754

[29] Behr K, Kavali CM, Munavalli G, et al. ATX-101 (deoxycholic acid injection) leads to clinically meaningful improvement in submental fat: final data from Contour. Dermatol Surg. 2019

[30] Sung CT, Lee A, Choi F, Juhasz M, Mesinkovska NA. Non-submental applications of injectable deoxycholic acid: a systematic review. J Drugs Dermatol. 2019; 18(7): 675–680

[31] Thomas WW, Bloom JD. Neck contouring and treatment of submental adiposity. J Drugs Dermatol. 2017; 16(1):54–57

[32] Dayan SH, Humphrey S, Jones DH, et al. Overview of ATX-101 (deoxycholic acid injection): a nonsurgical approach for reduction of submental fat. Dermatol Surg. 2016; 42 Suppl 1: S263–S270

[33] Dayan SH, Schlessinger J, Beer K, et al. Efficacy and safety of ATX-101 by treatment session: pooled analysis of data from the Phase 3 REFINE trials. Aesthet Surg J. 2018; 38(9): 998–1010

[34] Souyoul S, Gioe O, Emerson A, Hooper DO. Alopecia after injection of ATX-101 for reduction of submental fat. JAAD Case Rep. 2017; 3(3):250–252

[35] Sachdev D, Mohammadi T, Fabi SG. Deoxycholic acid-induced skin necrosis: prevention and management. Dermatol Surg. 2018; 44(7):1037–1039

[36] Lindgren AL, Welsh KM. Inadvertent intra-arterial injection of deoxycholic acid: a case report and proposed protocol for treatment. J Cosmet Dermatol. 2019

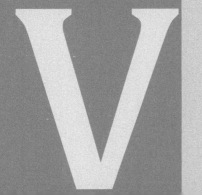

16 Thread Lift

Kian Karimi

Summary

Thread lifts have been available since 2002. Some of the complications related to these procedures were due to the use of nonabsorbable sutures for these procedures. More recently absorbable sutures have been used. This has been associated with a lower complication rate. The more frequent complications include bruising and puckering. Mild to moderate puckering is usually self-limited. Severe puckering is usually technique dependent. This may need to be treated with partial or complete removal of the thread. Although uncommon, infections have occurred requiring antibiotic therapy.

Keywords: threadlift, polydioxanone, absorbable sutures, minimal foreign body reaction, complications

16.1 Introduction

Threadlifting, or suture suspension, has emerged as a minimally invasive option for facial rejuvenation in patients who are looking for affordable options without downtime.[1,2] Although other such modalities such as neurotoxins, injectable fillers, lasers, and energy devices remain popular, they may not lift or reposition the underlying ptotic tissues.[1,3,4] Thread lifts can be used to reposition ptotic tissues. With threadlifts, recovery time is usually short, large incisions are avoided,[5] and general anesthesia is not needed[4]

Traditionally, threadlifting involves passing threads underneath the skin surface to lift the tissue. Threads are placed along a planned trajectory, pulled to lift the skin, secured and trimmed at the entry point.[6,7] Threadlifting for facial rejuvenation was introduced by Sulamanidze and colleagues in 2002.[8] These authors used bidirectional, nonabsorbable barbed suture thread (APTOS) to lift ptotic facial tissues. APTOS threads were manufactured with nonabsorbable polypropylene and designed for use in freely mobile tissue. The threads also had barbs cut at an angle and organized so they faced the midline in a bidirectional manner (▶ Fig. 16.1).[9]

Modifications of these original sutures have since been introduced,[10] each with specific features and techniques for insertion.[11] Longer than APTOS threads, bidirectional threads were made of

nonresorbable polypropylene with dents to create slant edges and sharp ends to hold tissue firmly.[9,12] Contour threads (Surgical Specialties, Corp., Reading, PA) were nonabsorbable polypropylene unidirectional threads with barbs in a helical design like DNA. The Contour thread could be fixed at the proximal end to the deep temporal fascia or other nonmobile structure. These threads received FDA clearance for midface suspension in 2005.[9]

Silhouette Soft threads (Sinclair Pharma, London, United Kingdom) consist of poly-L-lactic acid (PLLA), a biocompatible and biodegradable polymer used in biomedical and pharmaceutical applications.[10] This absorbable suture has bidirectional cones designed to lift the eyebrows and reposition the cheek, lower jaw, and neck. The cones are made of absorbable poly lactide/glycolidecopolymer (PLGA).[13] The Silhouette InstaLift is an absorbable suspension suture with cones oriented bidirectionally along the suture.[14] Sutures and cones are made with PLGA and PLLA. The Happy Lift™ (Promoitalia International S.r.l, Naples, Italy) is an absorbable, monofilament suspension thread made of caprolactone and polylactic acid.[15]

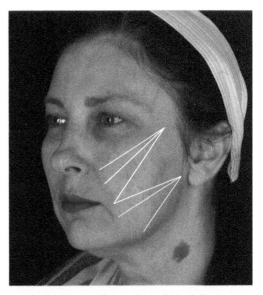

Fig. 16.1 Insertion of 18-gauge Barb 4 polydioxanone (PDO) thread cannula. Threads are placed along a planned trajectory, pulled to lift the skin, and secured and trimmed at the entry point.

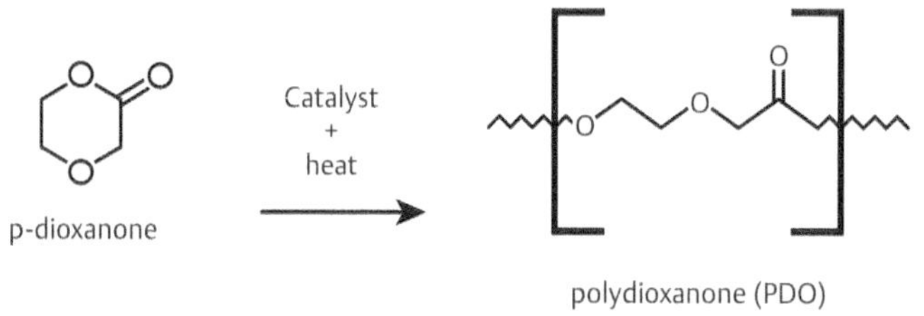

Fig. 16.2 Chemical structure of polydioxanone (PDO). PDO is a synthetic monofilament polymer, used as a biostimulator for skin and collagen rejuvenation.

The major paradigm shift in threads occurred with the introduction of dissolvable materials expected to completely dissolve within 6 to 24 months. The materials used for these threads worldwide include polydioxanone (PDO), polycaprolactone (PCL), and poly-L-lactic acid/polyglycolic acid (PLLA/PLGA). Currently in the United States, the only two approved types of dissolvable threads are PDO and PLLA/PLGA, although it is anticipated that PCL will enter the market in the near future.

The most popular type of threads used in the United States and worldwide is PDO, and thus the rest of this discussion will focus on this type. PDO is a synthetic monofilament polymer and can be used as a lifting suture to suspend ptotic tissues of the face or body, or both (▶ Fig. 16.2). PDO sutures are more pliable than their polypropylene counterparts and have more strength than other absorbable sutures.[16] Knotless PDO threads lift tissue with barbs, cogs, or molds, which adhere to tissues when the thread is inserted. This creates tension in the thread that lifts the skin tissues. The effect increases over time as collagen forms around the threads, cogs, and barbs.[2,12]

PDO threads (NovaThreads Inc., Miami, FL) are the subject of a case report of a patient presenting with sagging jowls after injection of fillers into her perioral area.[17] Fillers were used simultaneously in areas of volume and bony deficiency to enhance the result achieved by the threads because the lifting procedure may reveal volume deficits that can be corrected with dermal fillers. The procedure was well tolerated with only transient mild swelling at the insertion points (▶ Fig. 16.3).

PDO threads have been used extensively for aesthetic applications in Korea. The thread resembles a V-shape, with half of the thread residing outside the needle and the rest inside the caliber. The needle or caliber is inserted, and then removed, causing the thread to be fixed inside the skin without anchorage or knots.[18]

PDO threads are completely absorbed within 8 months after insertion with minimal foreign-body reaction.[11]

Reported novel uses of PDO threads include hair stimulation and treatment of hyperdynamic muscle movements with subsequent improvement of rhytids.[19,20]

16.2 Complications

When discussing complications of threads it is important to discern between dissolvable threads and nondissolvable threads. In general, the complications associated with nondissolvable threads are far more frequent and problematic than their dissolvable counterparts. It is important to understand and recognize the complications of permanent threads as the predecessors of today's modern and higher tech dissolvable threads.

Threadlifting with permanent threads may be accompanied by a variety of complications which include:

- Infection, rippling and puckering, asymmetry, granuloma formation, thread loss, and thread breakage.[7]
- Nerve damage and hematoma formation.[2]
- Chronic pain, hypersensitivity, palpability, and sensory impairment.[21]
- Erythema, ecchymosis, facial asymmetry, thread migration, skin dimpling, and scar formation.[1,18,22,23]

Wu and colleagues[12] treated cheeks and jowls with APTOS threads and reported thread migration (7.8%), infections and granuloma (4.9%), palpable thread ends with pain (10.8%), and dimpling with irregular wavy skin (4.9%) caused by superficial placement of threads. Threads had to be removed in all these patients. Wu and colleagues also performed WOFFLES thread lifts of the midface and jowls with results similar to those of a traditional face lift. Reported complications include knot palpability or knot exposure in the scalp, small granuloma and dimpling at the insertion point. Exposed knots were removed and the thread was cut even with the skin; dimpling was resolved by secondary skin release.

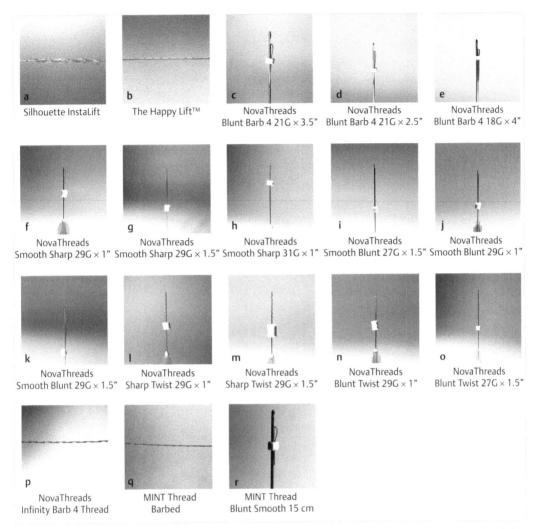

Fig. 16.3 (a–r) Chart of polydioxanone (PDO) threads. Knotless PDO threads lift tissue with barbs, cogs, or molds, which adhere to tissues when the thread is inserted.

Contour threads have been evaluated as the primary procedure in four studies,[1,6,24,25] as well as in combination with other procedures. Efficacy was variable and unpredictable,[9] while reported complications included:

- Bruising, swelling, and pinching.[24]
- Skin dimpling and visible knots.[6]
- Swelling, ecchymosis, infection, thread extrusion, palpable threads, contour irregularity, and recurrent laxity.[25]
- Intractable pain, dimpling, visible and palpable thread, thread extrusion, paresthesia, and foreign body reaction.[1]

- Contour threads lost FDA approval due to numerous postoperative complications.[7]

De Benito and colleagues studied Silhouette Soft threads over a mean follow-up time of 18 months.[26] Results were reported as "good, with high patient satisfaction." Complications reported were moderate pain in the temporal area, visible dermal pinching, temporal hematoma, asymmetry, and palpable sutures.

Lorenc and colleagues[14] described how to prevent and treat complications associated with the Silhouette InstaLift in detail. Swelling due to lidocaine injection is common and resolves within several days. Prior to the procedure, patients are advised to discontinue medically unnecessary supplements that may increase bruising (e.g., vitamin E, garlic, ginger, ginkgo). Hypersensitivity, though rare, may be treated with steroids. Irregularity and cellulitis after placement of Silhouette InstaLift sutures is possible and was recently observed and treated by the author.

This chapter describes in detail the complications associated with PDO thread lifting and how to prevent and treat them.

16.3 PDO Threads

Complications of PDO threads have been reported[1,3,11,17,18,19,22,23,27,28,29,30,31,32,33] and are summarized in ▶ Table 16.1.

An early study[1] (▶ Table 16.1) using barbed suture lifting in 29 patients showed that adverse events occurred in 69%, and early recurrence of skin laxity was noted in 45% of patients. Suh and colleagues[18] in their 31-patient study reported that 27 patients (87%) were satisfied with their PDO results while 4 patients (13%) were not satisfied. Complications included bruising (93.5%), mild postprocedure swelling (90.3%), and mild asymmetry (6.5%). These adverse events resolved within 2 weeks without treatment.

A case of mycobacterium infection after PDO thread-lift insertion has been reported by Shin and coworkers.[27] The thread-lift procedure was performed in a nonmedical cosmetic beauty salon 6 weeks before the patient presented to a hospital with itchy erythematous plaques on both cheeks. The patient had received 1 week of antibiotic therapy without improvement. Numerous cultures and stains to identify the infecting organism were negative until nontuberculous mycobacterium infection became apparent using reverse transcriptase-polymerase chain reaction, and the use of an *erm* gene polymerase chain reaction restriction fragment length polymorphism kit revealed the presence of *Mycobacterium massiliense*. The cutaneous lesion was significantly improved after 2 months of treatment with clarithromycin and amikacin. Triamcinolone intralesional injections at each visit helped to decrease the lesion size.

Kang and colleagues,[22] in treating glabellar and forehead wrinkles in Korean patients, reported skin ulceration in two patients and thread extrusion in one patient, both events attributed to inserting the threads too superficially. Resolution was achieved by removing the threads.

Karimi and Reivitis[17] reported mild swelling in the lower face which resolved without intervention 7 days later.

Yeo and coworkers[28] reported early complications from absorbable anchoring sutures after PDO thread lifts for facial rejuvenation in 144 patients. The average follow-up time was 11.1 weeks (range 0–52 wk). Complications developed in 11.1% of patients. These events were thread exposure, dimples, alopecia, undercorrection, asymmetry, and parotid gland injury. Thread exposure was noted in five patients. In two cases the thread was removed because it was palpable 1 month after thread lifting. In the other three patients the thread was removed at 2 months. Thread exposure was attributed to migration of the thread to a superficial layer followed by an inflammation reaction. Dimpling developed in three cases. One appeared after 5 days and was resolved by lightly retouching the entire area. In another case dimpling appeared at 3 weeks and disappeared 3 months after cannula dissection of the dimple.

Alopecia was noted in three patients and resolved after 5 months. This complication did not occur after widening the anchor gap. Alopecia was attributed to ischemia due to tension in the anchoring process. Undercorrection developed in two cases at 1 month and in one case at 6 months. Asymmetry was noted in one patient at 4 months. The authors suggest that an additional thread lift should be performed only after swelling from the initial lift has subsided.

Parotid gland injury occurred in one patient. When antibiotic therapy relieved symptoms only temporarily, ultrasonography at 3 months showed that the thread had passed through the parotid gland. The condition resolved 5 months later after observation and conservative treatment (i.e., retouching or widening the anchoring gap). Lawson and colleagues[34] recommend that to avoid this dangerous complication, thread lifting should be performed "carefully at the inferior side of the parotid gland and from the posterior side of the masseter to the mandible angle because they are tightly attached to superficial facial fascia and parotidomasseteric fascia."

Kim and coworkers,[29] in their 22-patient, 7-month study, reported transient edema and erythema. Yarak and colleagues[30] treated mild-to-moderate sagging of the middle and lower face in six patients. All patients experienced pain of moderate intensity

Table 16.1 Documented complications with polydioxanone (PDO) thread lifting

Reference	No. of patients	Treated area	Complication	% of patients	Treatment	Comment
Suh et al[18]	31	Face	Bruising	93.5	–	Resolved in 2 wk
			Swelling	90.3	–	Resolved in 2 wk
			Asymmetry	6.5	–	Resolved in 2 wk
Shin et al[27]	1	Cheeks	Mycobacterium infection, erythematous plaques	–	Antibiotic, steroid	–
Kang et al[22]	33	Glabella, forehead	Skin ulceration	6.1	Remove thread	Attributed to too superficial insertion of threads
			Thread extrusion	3.0	Remove thread	Attributed to too superficial insertion of threads
Karimi and Reivitis[17]	1	Lower face	Mild swelling at insertion area	–	–	Resolved within 7 days
Yeo et al[28]	144	Face (cheek)	Thread exposure	3.5	Thread removed in all patients	Due to thread migration and inflammation
			Dimples	2.1	Light retouching, cannula dissection	–
			Alopecia	2.1	–	Attributed to ischemia due to tension in anchoring process
			Undercorrection	2.1	Additional thread lift	Developed in 1 mo, 6 mo
			Asymmetry	0.7	–	4 mo
			Parotid gland injury	0.7	Observation, conservative treatment	Resolved by retouching or widening anchor gap
Kim et al[29] (Euro)	22	Nasolabial folds, cheeks	Edema, erythema	–	–	Transient
Yarakand Ribeiro de Carvalho[30]	6	Face, middle and lower third	Pain (moderate) at insertion point	100	Cold compresses	–
			Ecchymosis	33	–	–
Lee et al[31]	35	Face	Mild swelling	45.7	–	–
			Bruising	31.4	–	–
			Skin dimpling	8.5	–	Persisted for 1 mo
			Asymmetry	Repeat procedure	–	–

(continued)

Table 16.1 (continued) Documented complications with polydioxanone (PDO) thread lifting

Reference	No. of patients	Treated area	Complication	% of patients	Treatment	Comment
Ali[32]	21	Face	Thread breakage	4.8	Remove thread, repeat correctly	Injection error
Unal et al[23]	38	Face	Infection	5.2	Antibiotic	Presented at 1 mo
			Granuloma	5.2	Corticosteroid	Same
Ahnand Choi[33]	1	Cheeks	Inflamed palpable masses, cellulitis	–	Excisional biopsy, removal of thread	–
Bertossi et al[11]	160	Malar, nasolabial, mandibular	Superficial displacement of sutures into dermis	11.2	Massage followed by suture removal at 1 mo	–
			transient erythema	9.4	–	Resolved in 1 mo
			infection	6.2	Suture removal	–
			skin dimpling	6.2	Light massage by patient, resolved	–
			temporary facial stiffness	1.2	None, resolved in 7–15 wk	Resolved in 7–15 wk
Kang et al[19]	39	Malar, submalar areas	Dimpling	5.1	–	–
			Bruise	2.6	–	–
			Asymmetry	2.6	–	–
			Thread extrusion	2.6	–	–
			Malar eminence accentuation	2.6	–	–

at the insertion point immediately after the procedure and two patients reported ecchymosis.

Lee and colleagues,[31] in their 35-patient study reported mild swelling, bruising, and skin dimpling after PDO thread lift, all of which resolved without surgical intervention. One patient experienced asymmetry which was corrected with a repeat procedure.

Ali[32] reported outcomes of patients treated with PDO threads for facial rejuvenation over a 2-year period. Among 21 patients treated with PDO alone, one patient experienced thread breakage, which the author attributed to technique during the procedure. Specifically, the subcutaneous plane was missed during thread insertion and penetrated the superficial dermis, and then attempted to redirect into the subcutaneous plane. As a result, the thread was broken and had to be withdrawn.

Unal and colleagues[23] studied 38 patients treated with bidirectional barbed PDO cog threads (DongWon Medical Co. Ltd, Bucheon, Korea) for facial rejuvenation. After insertion of the threads, they prevented migration by tying threads in the same entry point to each other and burying the remaining threads into subcutaneous tissue using an 18-gauge needle. This technique did not allow the threads to float freely in the subcutaneous tissue.[35] Patients were given topical and oral antibiotics for 5 days. Although reported outcomes were good to excellent in all patients, infection developed in two patients and a granuloma appeared in two other patients, all within 1 month after the procedure. The infections were treated with additional ciprofloxacin. For granulomas, intralesional triamcinolone acetonide 10 mg/mL was injected.

Ahn and colleagues[33] reported a case of cellulitis in a woman presenting with a 3-month history of persistent, multiple inflamed palpable masses in both cheeks. The patient had undergone three courses of acupoint embedding therapy with use of PDO threads during the last 2 years. After combination antibiotic therapy failed to reduce the inflammation, excisional biopsy revealed the presence of threads which were removed. Tenderness and swelling in both cheeks resolved in 2 weeks.

In their 160-patient study, Bertossi and colleagues[11] treated deep nasolabial folds with or without midface ptosis and jowls in patients whose soft tissue thickness was sufficient to conceal the inserted threads. Reported complications included superficial displacement of the barbed threads into the dermis, erythema, skin dimpling, infection, and temporary facial stiffness for an overall complication rate of 34%. Superficial displacement of barbed

threads into the dermis occurred 1 month postoperatively and required suture removal. The patient was instructed to massage the treated area three times daily for 6 days before the threads were surgically extracted in a direction opposite that of placement. The authors suggested that this complication may have been due to their insertion technique. Erythema resolved without treatment and was absent 1 month postoperatively. Patients resolved skin dimpling by lightly massaging the treated area daily for several days or weeks. Infection required removal of the sutures by the same procedure used to remove displaced sutures. Facial stiffness resolved spontaneously in both patients within 7 to 15 weeks.

Kang and coworkers[19] reported the use of wedge-shaped PDO threads for the treatment of deep static glabellar and forehead wrinkles in 33 Korean patients. Three patients (9.1%) experienced procedure-induced complications resulting from too superficial insertion of the PDO threads. Two patients experienced skin ulcerations and thread extrusion was noted in another patient, both complications attributed to excessively superficial insertion of the PDO threads. Complications were resolved in all cases by removing the thread.

16.4 Prevention of Complications Utilizing PDO Threads

The author (KK) has utilized PDO threads (Nova Threads, Miami, FL) for nearly 5 years and has performed over 2,000 such procedures in this period of time. Prevention of complications can be achieved by considering the following:

- Patient selection.
- Proper informed consent.
- Treatment protocols.
- Posttreatment instructions and protocols.

16.4.1 Patient Selection

Patient selection is vital for positive outcomes in thread lifting. The "ideal" patient has sufficient skin thickness and subcutaneous fat to minimize the possibility of palpability of the thread, strong bony projections, and skin of sufficient pliability and mobility to permit repositioning.[17] Patients may be young, without many wrinkles or much redundant skin, or who seek slight-to-moderate improvement after rhytidoplasty (▸ Fig. 16.4).[36]

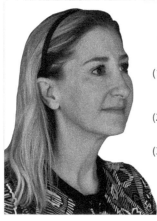

Ideal candidate

(1) Sufficient skin thickness and subcutaneous fat

(2) Strong bony projections

(3) Skin of sufficient pliability and mobility

Fig. 16.4 Ideal patient selection for polydioxanone (PDO) thread lift procedure.

Table 16.2 Potential adverse effects of polydioxanone (PDO) threads

Infection

Bruising

Thread migration

Thread extrusion

Hematoma

Cellulitis

Granuloma

Need for thread removal

Injury to deeper structures

Injury to nerves

Alopecia[a] (if placed within hair-bearing skin)

Pain (static and dynamic)

Suboptimal or worsened aesthetic result (irregularity, dimpling, puckering)

[a]If threads are placed in hair-bearing skin.

Table 16.3 Contraindications to polydioxanone (PDO) thread lifting

Immune system diseases

Pregnancy

Cutaneous neurofibromatosis

Acute illness

Psychiatric disorders (picking)

Inflammation of skin area to be treated

Nonabsorbable implant (e.g., silicone) in zone of thread insertion

Oncologic treatment (e.g., chemotherapy)

Tendency toward keloid scarring

Blood, bleeding disorders

Unrealistic expectations

The author has found that subcutaneous fat is the single most important factor to consider when utilizing lifting sutures. When utilizing the thinner sutures for mainly biostimulatory effects, this becomes less important as these types of threads are very fine (6–0 and 7–0 suture) and are placed in the immediate subdermis.

16.4.2 Patient Informed Consent

It is important to have a frank conversation with patients considering PDO threads for facial rejuvenation and/or lifting. Risks of adverse effects discussed explicitly with patients in the informed consent process are included in ▶ Table 16.2.

Fortunately there is no risk of vascular compromise, ischemia, blindness, or cerebrovascular accident when performing PDO threads. In the author's practice, a conversation is had with patients discussing "most likely" risks which include bruising, mild pain and discomfort for up to 5 days, and more rarely temporary dimpling, puckering, or irregularity which self-resolves in 95% of cases within 1 to 2 weeks.

16.4.3 Treatment Protocols

After consent has been obtained, the following treatment protocols are followed for (a) biostimulatory thread placement or (b) lifting thread placement. ▶ Table 16.3 shows contraindications to the procedure.

Biostimulatory Thread Placement

Patient's skin is prepped with either chlorhexidine only on the lower portions of the face, alcohol, or hypochlorous acid (0.01–0.03%) solution. Betadine can be used as well and is advised if entering through hair-bearing skin. Although topical anesthesia is not absolutely necessary, it is helpful in decreasing the pain associated with the procedure and can be applied for 10 to 30 minutes prior to administration of the threads. The topical is then completely removed and the skin is again prepped and allowed to dry. The author prefers the use of 29 gauge 1½ inch "smooth" NovaThreads (Nova Threads, Inc. Miami, FL) placed either next to each other, in a crisscross pattern, or in a wheel pattern, depending on the area being treated. The threads are inserted by puncturing the skin at a 30-degree angle and then immediately dropping the hub of the thread and advancing the tip of the needle in the immediate subdermis. The needle, loaded with the thread, is left in as the rest of the threads are placed in the area that skin rejuvenation is desired. Once the threads have all been placed, the needle and hub is removed by simply pulling it out and pressure is applied on any area that demonstrates bleeding. Pressure is held for 2 to 3 minutes and cool compresses are immediately applied. Following placement of the threads, topical application of platelet-rich plasma, platelet-rich fibrin, and/or arnica gel can be applied (Video 16.1, Video 16.2). The placement of PDO threads has shown to produce a robust collagen response that peaks at 1 month then slowly diminishes over the course of at least 7 months.[37] This treatment can be repeated in 6 to 8 weeks for further improvement of the skin area being treated.

Lifting Thread Placement

For placement of lifting threads the following protocol is performed in the author's practice. The face is prepped with either chlorhexidine, alcohol, or hypochlorous acid. Care is taken not to use chlorhexidine around the eyes. Oral antibiotics neither are routinely given nor are necessary prior to the procedure. The author prefers a fixationless system for a majority of his patients. Vectors are drawn depending on the patient's desires and the agreed plan and desired effect to lift any of the following areas: the brows, midface, lower third, and the submental neck (▶ Fig. 16.5). The author prefers to use preloaded threads on blunt cannulas to minimize many of the complications discussed.

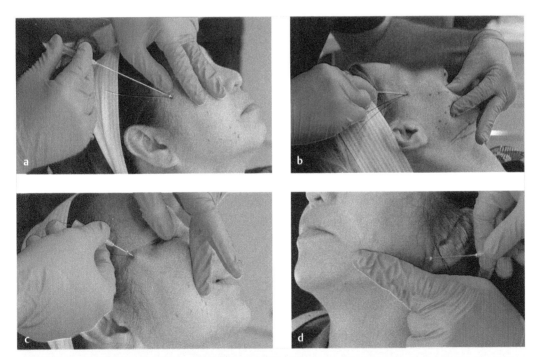

Fig. 16.5 (a–d) Thread vectors. Planning the placement of threads.

The author typically uses Nova Threads 21-gauge "Barb4" threads for the brows and submental neck, and 18-gauge "Barb4" threads or "Infinity" molded threads for the midface, lower third, and jowls and jawline (NovaThreads Inc., Miami, FL). The planned insertion points are injected with a small intradermal wheal of 1 or 2% lidocaine with 1:100,000 epinephrine. Seven to ten minutes are allowed to elapse for maximum vasoconstriction of the injected areas. Following this, the skin and surrounding areas are re-prepped and puncture of the skin is performed with a 20-gauge hypodermic needle if using 21-gauge Barb4 sutures or with a 18-gauge hypodermic needle if using 18-gauge or Infinity sutures. The needle is then removed and additional anesthesia is performed by injecting 0.3 mL of 1% plain lidocaine buffered with sodium bicarbonate (2.5 mL of 1 or 2% plain with 0.5 mL sodium bicarbonate) along each planned vector utilizing a DermaSculpt 22-gauge 2 and ¾ inch microcannula. The microcannula is then removed and the cannula that contains the preloaded thread is placed through the skin puncture and advanced subcutaneously along the drawn vector(s). While advancing the cannula, extreme care is taken to maintain a proper subcutaneous plane, avoiding superficial placement or touching the dermis. In addition, it is equally important to avoid deep placement which could put deeper structures at risk or cause prolonged pain and discomfort. As the thread is advanced, the author typically will have the tip of the cannula come slightly more superficially at the distalmost aspect of the vector to enhance the effect of the repositioning of the superficial fat compartments. The cannula is then removed and the patient is asked to animate to ensure the thread is not visible or palpable. It is also important to gently palpate the track where the thread was placed to ensure the thread is not palpable (Video 16.3, Video 16.4). If there is a significant pucker, loop, or palpable suture, this can be corrected immediately by pulling back on the untrimmed thread that comes out through the insertion point and the tissues can be re-draped (Video 16.5). If this measure does not correct the problem, the thread should be completely removed, discarded, and a new one placed. Trimming of the threads is important to perform correctly by pressing the scissors against the thread and causing a pucker at the insertion point—only after this has been achieved should the thread be trimmed to avoid the end of the thread being too close to the skin (Video 16.6,

Video 16.7). Once all of the threads are placed, the puncture points are covered either with bacitracin ointment or a small piece of cut Steri-strip, which is left on until the following day at which point the patient can remove.

16.4.4 Posttreatment Instructions and Protocols

Posttreatment instructions are provided to patient and include the following:
1. No makeup applied for 24 hours.
2. Wash gently in the direction of the lift for 1 week.
3. No exercise or excessive facial movements for 72 hours.
4. No facial massages or manipulation of the soft tissues for 1 month.
5. No energy-based devices or treatments for at least 6 weeks.
6. Cool compresses (neitherice nor ice packs) for 10 minutes of each hour for 24 hours.

16.5 Management of Complications

The most common complications (▶ Table 16.4) encountered in the author's practice are bruising and irregularity/puckering. The author serves as a medical consultant for NovaThreads, Inc. and will share his experience in managing complications and adverse events that have been reported by practitioners around the country.

16.5.1 Bruising

Arnica can be used preprocedure to help minimize bruising. Blood thinners should be avoided for 1 week prior to the procedure. If bruising is encountered, arnica gel and warm compresses can be utilized.

16.5.2 Mild-to-Moderate Puckering/Irregularity

Mild-to-moderate puckering and irregularity are the most common complications to occur after placement of heavier lifting PDO threads. These typically self-resolve; however, if a patient is extremely concerned they are typically invited back

Table 16.4 Management of complications

Complication	Treatment	Comments
Bruising	Arnica gel (pre- and postprocedure), warm compresses	Avoid blood thinners 1 wk before procedure
Puckering, mild-to-moderate/irregularity	Massage, opposite lifting vector; heat-based therapy	Usually resolve without intervention
Severe puckering/irregularity of superficial placement of threads	Remove thread only if palpable; technique requires care and patience	May require needle to widen puncture and remove thread
Infection	Oral antibiotics	If severe, IV antibiotics that cover gram-positive organisms

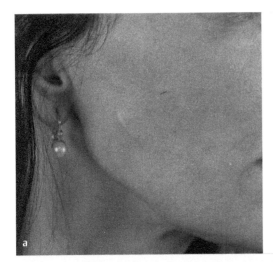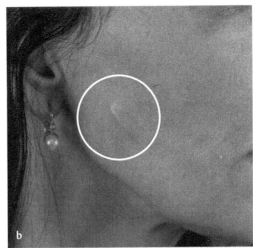

Fig. 16.6 (a, b) Thread pucker "Loop." Irregularity of superficially placed thread appearing as a "loop" under the skin.

into the practice for further assessment. If the pucker is from overcorrection or superficial placement of part of the thread, the tissues can be massaged in the direction opposite of the desired lifting vector and at times can be "unzipped" from the area of the thread causing the complication. Puckers and irregularities always resolve but can take several months to disappear if no interventions are performed. Theoretically using heat-based therapies such as topical radiofrequency may speed up the metabolism of the threads faster, although this has never been scientifically proven.

16.5.3 Severe Puckering/Irregularity of Superficial Placement of Threads

Severe puckering, irregularity, dimpling are uniformly caused by superficial placement of part of

the thread and can generally be avoided with proper technique and prevention as discussed earlier in this chapter. If a loop of thread is palpable, this may need to be removed. Removal should never be attempted if the thread is not definitively felt by touching the skin. The thread can appear as a "loop" or as a protruding "mole" (▶ Fig. 16.6, ▶ Fig. 16.7). Thread removal is performed with the following technique. The area where the thread is too superficial and palpable is marked. 1% lidocaine with 1:100,000 epinephrine is injected at this location and 7 to 10 minutes are allowed to elapse. Puncture is performed with a 20- or 18-gauge hypodermic needle. One tine of a non-toothed fine or ultrafine pickup forceps is placed through the puncture, and sweeping motions are performed until the thread is expressed, at which point it can be removed in its entirety or simply trimmed as long as no further thread is visible or

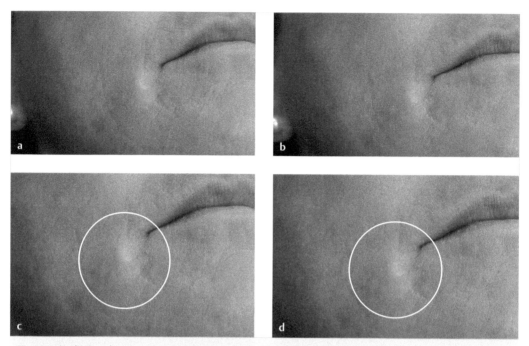

Fig. 16.7 (a–d) Thread pucker "Mole." Irregularity of superficially placed thread appearing as a "mole" under the skin.

palpable (**Video 16.8**). The author has found that patience is required to successfully perform this—one tip is that when the forceps is touching the thread, a very distinctive gritty sound and feel is appreciated when encountering the thread. In rare circumstances, the author has had to use the 18-gauge needle to widen the puncture to successfully remove the thread.

16.5.4 Infection

Infection is extremely uncommon and is estimated to occur in less than 0.1% of the time a PDO thread is placed. If an infection is encountered typically oral antibiotics are administered (doxycycline 100 mg po BID × 10–14 d or amoxicillin/clavulanate 850 mg po BID for 10–14 d). If a severe infection is encountered then the patient should be admitted for intravenous antibiotics covering gram-positive organisms. The author did manage an infection in a patient who was treated at a different facility that had a thread inadvertently penetrate the oral cavity. The practitioner simply "trimmed" the

thread instead of removing the thread from the mouth and the patient suffered a severe cellulitis reaction and was admitted to the hospital for imaging and intravenous antibiotics (▶ Fig. 16.8). The patient's infection resolved without further intervention necessary and no further sequelae now 1 year after the incident.

16.6 Conclusion

Dissolvable sutures have entered the aesthetic market and are a new tool in the aesthetic armamentarium to reposition and lift tissues. They appear to be most effective when combined with other modalities such as neuromodulators, injectable fillers, and/or blood plasma. Complications of dissolvable threads are common and frequent. Fortunately, most of these complications are mild, manageable, and temporary. Dissolvable threads appear to be a safe-and-effective new tool in the aesthetic practitioner's options for skin rejuvenation and soft tissue ptosis.

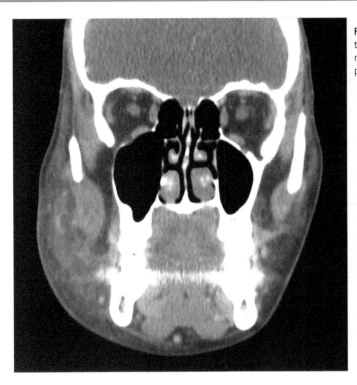

Fig. 16.8 CT scan of thread complication. Patient suffering severe cellulitis reaction from complication of thread placement.

References

[1] Rachel JD, Lack EB, Larson B. Incidence of complications and early recurrence in 29 patients after facial rejuvenation with barbed suture lifting. Dermatol Surg. 2010; 36(3):348–354

[2] Kalra R. Use of barbed threads in facial rejuvenation. Indian J Plast Surg. 2008; 41 Suppl:S93–S100

[3] Sulamanidze MA, Paikidze TG, Sulamanidze GM, Neigel JM. Facial lifting with "APTOS" threads: featherlift. Otolaryngol-Clin North Am. 2005; 38(5):1109–1117

[4] Tong LX, Rieder EA. Thread-lifts: a double-edged suture? A comprehensive review of the literature. DermatolSurg. 2019; 45(7):931–940

[5] Tavares JP, Oliveira CACP, Torres RP, Bahmad F, Jr. Facial thread lifting with suture suspension. Rev Bras Otorrinolaringol (Engl Ed). 2017; 83(6):712–719

[6] Abraham RF, DeFatta RJ, Williams EF, III. Thread-lift for facial rejuvenation: assessment of long-term results. Arch Facial Plast Surg. 2009; 11(3):178–183

[7] Tonks S. Understanding thread lifting. https://aestheticsjournal.com/feature/understanding-thread-lifting. Accessed 1 October, 2019

[8] Sulamanidze MA, Fournier PF, Paikidze TG, Sulamanidze GM. Removal of facial soft tissue ptosis with special threads. Dermatol Surg. 2002; 28(5):367–371

[9] Paul MD. Barbed sutures in aesthetic plastic surgery: evolution of thought and process. AesthetSurg J. 2013; 33(3) Suppl:17S–31S

[10] Gülbitti HA, Colebunders B, Pirayesh A, Bertossi D, van der Lei B. Thread-lift sutures: still in the lift? A systematic review of the literature. Plast Reconstr Surg. 2018; 141(3):341e–347e

[11] Bertossi D, Botti G, Gualdi A, et al. Effectiveness, longevity, and complications of facelift by barbed suture insertion. Aesthet Surg J. 2019; 39(3):241–247

[12] Wu WT. Barbed sutures in facial rejuvenation. AesthetSurg J. 2004; 24(6):582–587

[13] SarigulGuduk S, Karaca N. Safety and complications of absorbable threads made of poly-L-lactic acid and poly lactide/glycolide: experience with 148 consecutive patients. J CosmetDermatol. 2018; 17(6):1189–1193

[14] Lorenc ZP, Ablon G, Few J, et al. Expert consensus on achieving optimal outcomes with absorbable suspension suture technology for tissue repositioning and facial recontouring. J Drugs Dermatol. 2018; 17(6):647–655

[15] De Masi EC, De Masi FD, De Masi RD. Suspension threads. Facial PlastSurg. 2016; 32(6):662–663

[16] Ray JA, Doddi N, Regula D, Williams JA, Melveger A. Polydioxanone (PDS): a novel monofilament synthetic absorbable suture. SurgGynecolObstet. 1981; 153(4):497–507

[17] Karimi K, Reivitis A. Lifting the lower face with an absorbable polydioxanone (PDO) thread. J Drugs Dermatol. 2017; 16(9): 932–934

[18] Suh DH, Jang HW, Lee SJ, Lee WS, Ryu HJ. Outcomes of polydioxanone knotless thread lifting for facial rejuvenation. Dermatol Surg. 2015; 41(6):720–725

[19] Kang SH, Moon SH, Rho BI, Youn SJ, Kim HS. Wedge-shaped polydioxanone threads in a folded configuration ("solid fillers"): a treatment option for deep static wrinkles on the upper face. J Cosmet Dermatol. 2019; 18(1):65–70

[20] Bharti J, Patil P. Polydioxanone threads in androgenetic alopecia: a novel innovation. 12th International Conference and Exhibition on Cosmetic Dermatology and Hair Care,

Nov. 28–30, 2016, San Antonia,TX, USA. J Cosmo Trichol. 2016; 2:(3 Suppl):44

[21] Della Torre F, Della Torre E, Di Berardino F. Side effects from polydioxanone. Eur Ann Allergy ClinImmunol. 2005; 37(2): 47–48

[22] Kang SH, Byun EJ, Kim HS. Vertical lifting: a new optimal thread lifting technique for Asians. DermatolSurg. 2017; 43 (10):1263–1270

[23] Unal M, İslamoğlu GK, ÜrünUnal G, Köylü N. Experiences of barbed polydioxanone (PDO) cog thread for facial rejuvenation and our technique to prevent thread migration. J Dermatol Treat. 2019; 15:1–4

[24] Kaminer MS, Bogart M, Choi C, Wee SA. Long-term efficacy of anchored barbed sutures in the face and neck. Dermatol Surg. 2008; 34(8):1041–1047

[25] Garvey PB, Ricciardelli EJ, Gampper T. Outcomes in threadlift for facial rejuvenation. Ann PlastSurg. 2009; 62(5):482–485

[26] de Benito J, Pizzamiglio R, Theodorou D, Arvas L. Facial rejuvenation and improvement of malar projection using sutures with absorbable cones: surgical technique and case series. Aesthetic PlastSurg. 2011; 35(2):248–253

[27] Shin JJ, Park JH, Lee JM, Ryu HJ. Mycobacterium massiliense infection after thread-lift insertion. DermatolSurg. 2016; 42 (10):1219–1222

[28] Yeo SH, Lee YB, Han DG. Early complications from absorbable anchoring suture following thread-lift for facial rejuvenation. Arch Aesthetic Plast Surg. 2017; 23:11–16

[29] Kim J, Kim HS, Seo JM, Nam KA, Chung KY. Evaluation of a novel thread-lift for the improvement of nasolabial folds and cheek laxity. J EurAcadDermatolVenereol. 2017; 31(3):e136–e179

[30] Yarak S, Ribeiro de Carvalho JA. Facial rejuvenation with absorbable and barbed thread lift: case series with Mint Lift™. J Clin Exp Dermatol Res. 2017; 8:415–417

[31] Lee H, Yoon K, Lee M. Outcome of facial rejuvenation with polydioxanone thread for Asians. J Cosmet Laser Ther. 2018; 20(3):189–192

[32] Ali YH. Two years' outcome of thread lifting with absorbable barbed PDO threads: innovative score for objective and subjective assessment. J Cosmet Laser Ther. 2018; 20(1):41–49

[33] Ahn SK, Choi HJ. Complication after PDO threads lift. J Craniofac Surg. 2019; 30(5):e467–e469

[34] Lawson GA, III, Kreymerman P, Nahai F. An unusual complication following rhytidectomy: iatrogenic parotid injury resulting in parotid fistula/sialocele. Aesthet Surg J. 2012; 32(7):814–821

[35] Han HH, Kim JM, Kim NH, et al. Combined, minimally invasive, thread-based facelift. Arch Aesthetic Plast Surg. 2014; 20:160–164

[36] Lycka B, Bazan C, Poletti E, Treen B. The emerging technique of the antiptosis subdermal suspension thread. DermatolSurg. 2004; 30(1):41–44, discussion 44

[37] Kim J, Zheng Z, Kim H, Nam KA, Chung KY. Investigation on the cutaneous change induced by face-lifting monodirectional barbed polydioxanone thread. Dermatol Surg. 2017; 43(1): 74–80

17 SMAS Lift

Phillip R. Langsdon and Ronald J. Schroeder II

Summary

The concept of SMAS facelift involves a spectrum of SMAS manipulation ranging from imbrication or plication to undermining in a deep plane. We define a "SMAS facelift" as a facelift where the SMAS is advanced without extensive undermining of the SMAS (deep plane), followed by resuspension via plication or imbrication. This procedure is ideal for patients who have mild or moderate sagging of facial skin and soft tissue or for patients who may be predisposed to poor wound healing that necessitate a more limited dissection. This chapter covers the procedure in detail, as well as how to optimize outcomes and minimize complications.

Keywords: facelift, rhytidectomy, SMAS, rhytids, aesthetics, complications

17.1 Introduction

The facelift procedure has undergone several modifications over the past century since first explained by Hollander in 1901.[1] The various techniques differ in length and placement of the incision, the extent of undermining and dissection, and the handling of the superficial musculoaponeurotic system (SMAS). Methods include simple skin dissection, SMAS plication or imbrication, deep plane, composite, high-SMAS, extended SMAS, subperiosteal, SMASectomy, and other variations.[2,3,4,5,6,7,8,9]

For the purposes of this chapter, it is important to define a "SMAS facelift." Technically a SMAS facelift involves a spectrum of SMAS manipulation that ranges from imbrication or plication to a deep plane dissection (▶ Fig. 17.1). We define a "SMAS facelift" as a procedure without any significant undermining (> 3 cm) of the SMAS followed by resuspension of the SMAS via plication or imbrication.

17.2 Indications and Patient Selection

Although there are many variations of the facelift procedure, the goals remain the same. These include removing excess fat and repositioning tissue to achieve a more youthful, yet natural lift. The author's technique involves the removal of any excess cervical fat, repositioning the SMAS and platysma, and removing excess cervical and facial skin. Ideal candidates are those in good health with good vascularity who exhibit a loss of skin elasticity, sagging of cheek tissues and cervical platysma, and who may also have excess neck fat. Patients who enjoy average weight, an aesthetic facial bony contour, and high posteriorly positioned hyoid bone are usually better candidates than those who have thin tissues, are overweight, or who have a low-anteriorly placed hyoid.

Patients should be psychologically stable, possess realistic expectations, and demonstrate comprehension of the limitations of the facelift procedure. In the author's practice, the details are usually discussed on three occasions prior to surgery: initial consultation, preoperative instructional visit 2 to 3 weeks prior, and the day of surgery. Patients must also understand that no surgical rejuvenation procedure can remove facial asymmetries, improve the general facial deflation that occurs with aging, halt aging, remove wrinkles, or facial expression lines, or restore the deteriorated condition of skin. Other techniques, not included with the facelift procedure, might be considered or needed to address facial atrophy, wrinkles, skin deterioration, asymmetries, and/or future aging.

In the author's practice, the average facelift candidate typically undergoes a deep plane facelift. Our SMAS facelift is selected for those patients needing minimal tissue repositioning or those with a potentially compromised vascular supply. Certainly, patients with minimal-to-moderate tissue sagging do not need extensive skin undermining or extensive sub-SMAS undermining. Patients with a history of excessive smoking or medical conditions such as lupus, rheumatoid arthritis, or scleroderma are not generally good candidates for facelift procedures due to a compromised vascular supply. However, in select patients with a remote past history of smoking (minimal current social smoking of 3–4 cigarettes/d) or those with very mild cases of collagen vascular disease may be candidates for minimal skin undermining facelift-type procedures. The SMAS facelift can be done with minimal skin undermining and excellent tissue movement via SMAS repositioning.

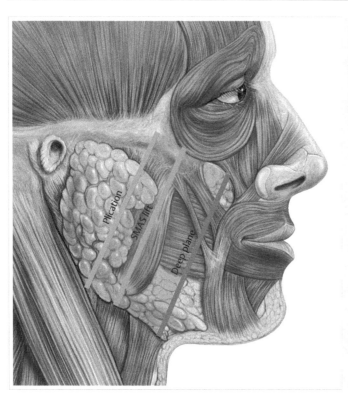

Fig. 17.1 Facelift spectrum of superficial musculoaponeurotic system (SMAS) undermining. (Adapted and used with permission from Patrick J. Lynch; illustrator; C. Carl Jaffe; MD; cardiologist Yale University Center for Advanced Instructional Media; Medical Illustrations by Patrick Lynch.)

17.3 Surgical Technique

17.3.1 Procedure Details

We have found that intravenous sedation provides excellent and safe anesthesia with a quicker gentler emergence for facelift patients. Although general anesthesia is commonly used throughout the United States, we have found it to be unnecessary. Our sedation is carried out in a state-licensed facility that must comply with safety guidelines. All emergency equipment, proper personnel, and appropriate emergency medications are available. In our facility, the patient is administered diazepam 20 mg orally, dimenhydrinate 200 mg orally, and prednisone 40 mg orally 1 hour prior to surgery. The patient is also administered an oral antibiotic. It may take an hour or slightly longer for the diazepam to have full effect. During this time, the patient is marked for incisions and injection of local anesthetic (▶ Fig. 17.2, ▶ Fig. 17.3).

The senior author believes in preserving the temporal sideburn at the level of the superior portion of the ear. Therefore, a horizontal mark is usually placed in this location to prevent the repositioning of hair to a point superior to the cephalic portion of

the ear. The resulting incision may then be reused in future facial rejuvenation procedures without the elevation of the sideburn area and loss of temporal hair. Instead of shaving the patient's hair, parted segments of temporal hair on either side of the incision are twisted and wrapped with paper tape. The mark is continued in the preauricular groove found just in front of the curvature of the auricle. In female patients, a posttragal mark (1–2 mm behind the tragus) is incorporated to hide the scar. In male patients, the incisional mark is usually carried in front of the tragus in a preauricular crease. The author usually leaves an area of non-hair-bearing skin between the tragus and sideburn in male patients. The mark then curves around the earlobe. Postauricularly, the incisional mark is carried slightly up on the posterior surface of the ear parallel to the postauricular sulcus. Some surgeons stop the incision low in the postauricular sulcus. However, the resulting bunching (even if only temporary) can be somewhat disconcerting to patients in the early postoperative period. The continuation of the postauricular incision along the posterior hairline allows for removal of excess skin and the lessening of bunching. The extent of skin undermining is marked approximately 5 cm from the incision site, circumferentially around the ear.

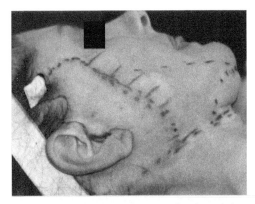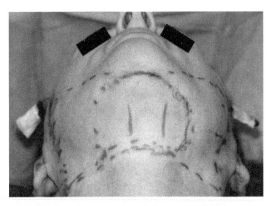

Fig. 17.2 Preoperative markings in a female, including posttragal mark and preservation of the temporal sideburn. Incisional mark is carried into the postauricular sulcus extending onto the posterior hairline forming a short gentle curve along the hairline.

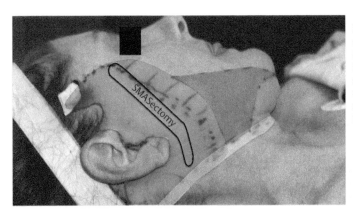

Fig. 17.3 Red area shows subcutaneous dissection extending about 2 cm beyond where SMASectomy is performed. Blue area shows submental subcutaneous dissection. Yellow area is where drain is placed. Purple area is optional for subcutaneous dissection in patients with severe skin laxity.

Local anesthesia is carried out with 1% xylocaine and 0.25% bupivacaine with 1:150,000 epinephrine along the incision lines and the borders of the areas to be undermined. A tumescent mixture of 0.3% xylocaine with 1:600,000 epinephrine is injected in the areas to be undermined. Intravenous sedation can be very helpful during the injection of local anesthesia. It is usually delayed until the oral diazepam has been fully absorbed. Intravenous sedation by the anesthetist or anesthesiologist usually makes the patient totally unaware of the application of local anesthetic.

After local anesthesia has been administered, about 10 minutes are allowed to pass in order to allow the epinephrine to take full effect for hemostasis. The skin should be noticeably blanched, which allows you to determine if additional local anesthetic is needed in certain areas. However, patients with thick skin may not have as much noticeable blanching.

The submental area is addressed first with cervicofacial liposuction and platysmaplasty as indicated.[10,11] Patients with a significantly obtuse cervicomental angle may benefit from a SMMS (submental muscular medialization and suspension) procedure for more dramatic results. SMMS is performed by excising the fat overlying the mylohyoid fascia, then suturing the anterior digastric muscles to the mylohyoid fascia in the midline to prevent a cobra deformity. The platysma muscle is then sutured to the digastric muscles in the midline (▶ Fig. 17.4).[12,13,14]

Attention is then turned to performing the SMAS facelift. A #15 blade is used to make the incisions in the preoperative periauricular markings. The incision is carried through the dermis and is beveled across the direction of the hair follicles in the hair-bearing horizontal temporal incision and the posterior hairline skin. This maneuver allows the hair to grow through the incision line.

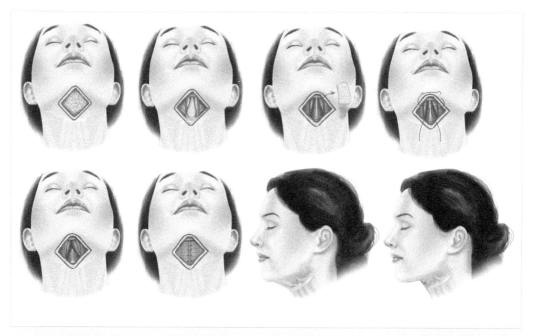

Fig. 17.4 Submental muscular medialization and suspension (SMMS) technique (left to right, top to bottom). Exposure of preplatysmal fat; excision of preplatysmal fat; exposure of subplatysmal fat with exposure of digastric muscles and mylohyoid fascia; suture medialization of the digastric muscles with suspension to the mylohyoid fascia; suture medialization of the platysma; pre-SMMS; post-SMMS.

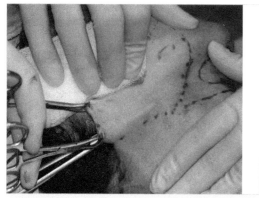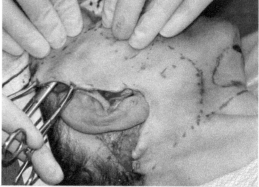

Fig. 17.5 Undermining of the facial skin from laterally to medially in a subdermal plane. The assistant is shown providing countertraction.

The skin is then undermined using facelift scissors beginning at the tragus, leaving as much subdermal tissue as possible attached to the deep tissue (▶ Fig. 17.5). A thin tragal flap minimizes tragal contracture during the postoperative healing phase. The remainder of the facial skin is then fully undermined in a supraSMAS (subdermal) layer to a point averaging 5 cm from the incision, following the preoperative marking plan (▶ Fig. 17.6). Care is taken to avoid damaging the subdermal vascular plexus. Countertraction is provided by the assistant. Hemostasis is achieved with bipolar cautery under direct visualization. The extent of skin undermining is generally limited to

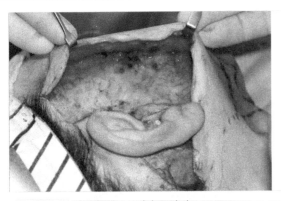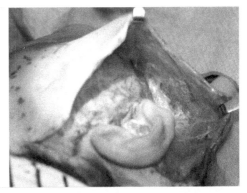

Fig. 17.6 Elevated flap in a subdermal plane

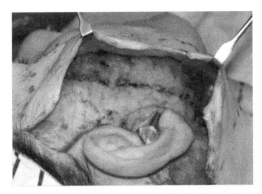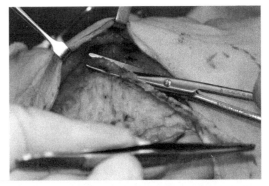

Fig. 17.7 SMASectomy showing removal of strip of superficial musculoaponeurotic system (SMAS) down to parotid fascia, extending from the angle of mandible to lateral canthus.

around 4 to 5 cm. This preserves the vascular supply in most patients.

With the skin flap adequately elevated, SMA Sectomy is performed (▶ Fig. 17.7). A 1-cm-wide strip of SMAS is excised in from the preauricular area down to infraauricular fascia. The SMAS can then be grasped and pulled ensuring adequate mobility and repositioning of the tissues. Undermining of the SMAS about 2 cm will allow further mobilization and repositioning of the SMAS for optimal results (▶ Fig. 17.8). Anchoring sutures of 2–0 Mersilene are used to anchor the SMAS in two positions. The first suture is placed in the strong preauricular fascia directly at the tragal–lobule juncture (▶ Fig. 17.9). The second is placed through the posterior periosteum of the zygomatic arch (▶ Fig. 17.10). Then sutures of either 2–0 polydioxanone (PDS) or 2–0 Vicryl are placed in the region superior to the arch suture and between the two Mersilene sutures. The placement of these sutures may be continued inferiorly into the mastoid region if cervical SMAS movement is possible. The SMAS suspension will elevate the jowl, neck, and nasolabial fold. The extent of nasolabial fold and mid-cheek improvement is dependent upon the extent of SMAS undermining.

The skin is draped in a posterior–superior vector and secured at the highest postauricular point with an interrupted 2–0 nylon or surgical staple (▶ Fig. 17.11). This is followed by a second securing suture or staple at the junction of the horizontal temporal incision and the superior extent of the preauricular incision. The redundant skin is then resected in a manner creating minimal skin tension (▶ Fig. 17.12). If any dimpling or bunching of skin is noted, further undermining can be performed. The neotragal skin is left redundant to avoid forward displacement of the tragus by skin contracture. The earlobe is placed in a position that is about ½ to ¾ cm superior to the position where it naturally lies in the unrepaired state (▶ Fig. 17.13). This overcorrection helps prevent

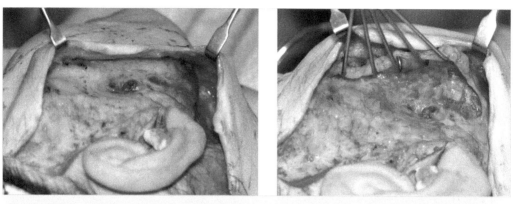

Fig. 17.8 Left, immediately after SMASectomy. Right, 1 to 2 cm of sub-SMAS (superficial musculoaponeurotic system) dissection.

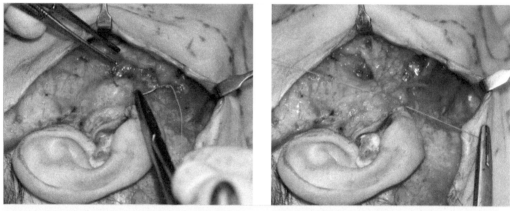

Fig. 17.9 Anchor suture with 2–0 Mersilene in the preauricular fascia adjacent to the lobule.

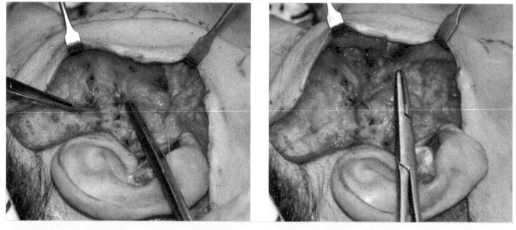

Fig. 17.10 Second anchoring suture with 2–0 Mersilene through periosteum of zygomatic arch.

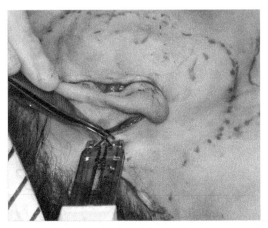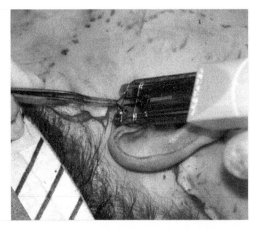

Fig. 17.11 Flap advanced in a posterior–superior vector with securing staples at the highest postauricular point (left) and at the junction of the horizontal temporal incision and the superior extent of the preauricular incision (right).

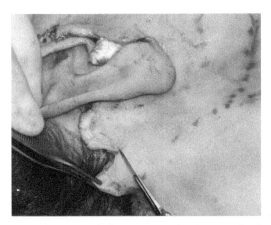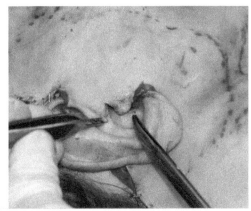

Fig. 17.12 Removal of excess occipital and preauricular skin (left). Neotragal skin is left redundant (right) to avoid forward displacement of the tragus by skin contracture.

the lobe from stretching too far inferiorly during the natural healing process, thus preventing the pixie earlobe deformity. The skin along the post-auricular occipital hair is reapproximated with the surgical staples. The skin edges in the non-hair-bearing postauricular areas are approximated with 5–0 plain gut suture in a running interlocking fashion, using 5–0 Monocryl for additional deep support as necessary. The postauricular closure, above the posterior portion of the earlobe and below the level of the hairline, is performed in a manner that leaves 1 cm gaps between sutures, thus aiding any fluid drainage. A size 7 round JP drain is placed posterior to the incision on the right within the hair-bearing scalp and tunneled

under the neck to the left. The preauricular and tragal skin is closed using 5–0 plain gut in a running interlocking fashion. The hair-bearing temporal scalp incision is closed with staples. The submental incision may be closed with 5–0 plain gut suture in a running interlocking fashion.

Any collected blood is expressed from under the flaps via the postauricular closure gaps. A dressing is then applied with 4 × 4 gauze pads and a Kerlix gauze wrap that applies only very gentle pressure over the preauricular area, lower face, and neck. Lastly, a light elastic wrap is placed over the dressing using Coban self-adherent wrap. The elastic wrap is removed 4 hours after placement.

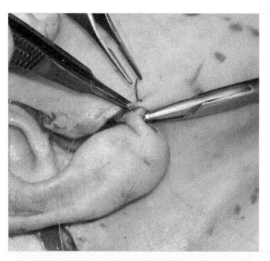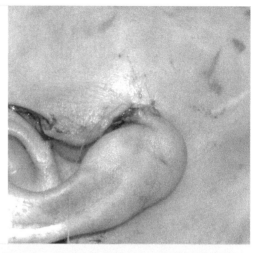

Fig. 17.13 Ear lobe is placed about ½ cm superior to the position where it naturally lies in the unrepaired state. This overcorrection prevents the lobe from being pulled too far inferiorly during the natural healing process.

The patient is evaluated prior to discharge and again the following day. The remaining dressing is removed and the incisions are cleaned with hydrogen peroxide and dressed with Vaseline®. The JP drain is removed if output is less than 30 mL. The patient is instructed to keep the head of the bed elevated 30 degrees, avoid strenuous activities, not bend over, and not turn his or her head (▶ Fig. 17.14).

17.3.2 Optimizing Results

Incision placement is one of the most important points to consider for optimal results. For the temporal incision line, it's important to preserve the temporal hair tuft, keeping the horizontal portion at the superior level of the ear. We extend the vertical portion into the hair-bearing scalp to hide the remainder of the incision. Sometimes a small amount of redundant hair-bearing scalp needs to be excised, but this is often negligible and has little effect on the anterior hairline. In female patients, a posttragal incision is nearly always used unless it interferes with a hearing aid. In male patients, a pretragal incision is often used to prevent draping bearded skin over the tragus. Postauricularly, the incision is hidden within the postauricular sulcus and carried along the posterior hairline.

Great attention is paid to both elevation and placement of the tragus and earlobe. Tragal skin is elevated in a very superficial, almost dermal plane, thereby leaving as much deep tissue as possible to prevent postoperative contracture. When closing the skin, the neotragal skin is left redundant to avoid forward displacement of the tragus by skin contracture. The earlobe is placed in a position that is about ½ to ¾ cm superior to the position where it naturally lies in the unrepaired state. This overcorrection usually prevents the lobe from being pulled too far inferiorly during the natural healing process.

During mobilization and plication of the SMAS, there are two important anchoring sutures that are placed. The first is placed through the fascia immediately anterior to the junction of the tragus and lobule. The second suture is placed through periosteum of the zygomatic arch about 1 cm anterior to the incision line. The senior author currently prefers permanent Mersilene for these anchoring sutures, and PDS is used for plication of the remaining SMAS.

Two important securing sutures are placed when re-draping the elevated skin flap, one at the most superior postauricular point and one at the junction of the horizontal temporal and preauricular incisions. These sutures anchor the skin for trimming. A skin staple is often placed as a temporary anchor that can be removed during skin closure.

17.4 Complications

17.4.1 Minimizing Risk and Complications

Complications occur in any surgical procedure and the facelift is no exception. Hematoma formation is possible but can be minimized with meticulous surgical hemostasis, proper patient selection, and

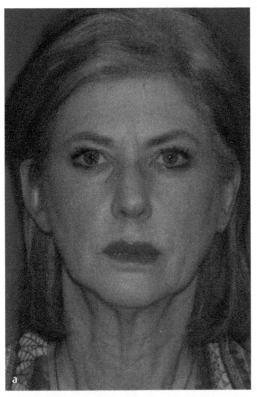 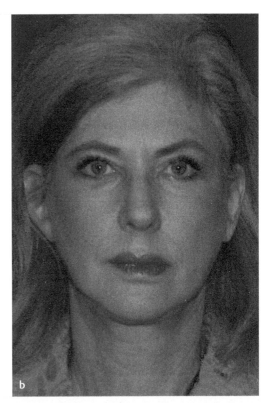

Fig. 17.14 Before **(a)** and after **(b)** superficial musculoaponeurotic system (SMAS) facelift.

the cessation of all medications, herbs, vitamins, and red wine that may cause bleeding 2 weeks prior to surgery. A Jackson Pratt drain will help to reduce the risk of early postoperative hematoma formation. On occasion, two drains will be used in patients who either have a greater amount of bleeding intraoperatively or are high risk (male patients, use of anticoagulants, etc.). Drains are kept on wall suction during the procedure and in the recovery area until discharge; bulb suction is used for home care. Postoperatively, it is important to counsel patients again on the importance of avoiding head movement, bending over, or any strenuous activity.

Flap necrosis can occur at the distal ends of flaps where blood supply is most tenuous. Most commonly, necrosis occurs in the mastoid region followed by the tragal skin because the flap is the thinnest at these sites, and these areas are farthest from the blood supply.[15] This would most commonly be an issue in tobacco users. We do not consciously accept smokers that use over three to five cigarettes per day as patients. Caution should be exercised in patients with tobacco use, diabetes,

collagen vascular disease, or Raynaud disease. However, the senior author does not consider these situations or conditions necessarily absolute contraindications to facelifting. Tobacco users should be counseled to reduce or discontinue use at least 2 weeks prior to surgery. We do not accept candidates who smoke over one-half pack per day. It is helpful to evaluate serum antinuclear antibody in those patients who either have a collagen vascular disease or who have relatives with the diseases. If levels are high, we generally put off surgery until they decline below 1:60. Undermining is limited in light smokers, diabetics, or those with vascular disease.

Deep infection is rare, as is cellulitis. Antibiotic prophylaxis is used routinely and should cover *Staphylococcus* and *Streptococcus*.

17.4.2 Early Identification of Complications

Prior to discharge, patients are evaluated in the recovery area when fully awake. Early hematoma formation can sometimes be difficult to detect with the dressings in place, but the face may show asymmetric swelling associated with dark bruising of the skin or buccal mucosa. Motor function is also assessed at this time. There may be some temporary weakness from the local anesthesia. Given the limited sub-SMAS dissection of the SMAS facelift, nerve injury is exceedingly rare. And the senior author has not seen any permanent paralysis in over 30 years of practice. Temporary weakness can occur. The most commonly injured branch of the facial nerve during facelift surgery is the frontal branch, which becomes superficial at the zygomatic arch and travels just beneath the subcutaneous tissues underlying the SMAS layer. The nerve travels 1.5 to 2 cm in front of the auricle and halfway between the lateral orbital rim and the temporal tuft of hair.[16] The majority of facial nerve weakness immediately after surgery is due to the local anesthetic, stretch, or compression. These nerve injuries usually resolve with time.[15]

After discharge, it is important to maintain communication with the patient. Patients are seen daily until the drain is ready to be removed, and the patient is called nightly for the first week (including day of surgery). Patients may not be aware of what is abnormal, and identifying and treating the complication early can have a significant impact on the final outcome. Additionally, regular communication helps ally patient fear. It also helps facilitate identification of any issues that might occur.

17.4.3 Management of Complications

Hematoma is the most common complication associated with a facelift. In the early postoperative period, small hematomas can often be expressed through the postauricular gap. Large hematomas, although rare, may need evacuation and intraoperative hemostasis. Delayed hematomas can occur up to 2 weeks postoperatively, and can be managed with needle aspiration. It is also important to review the patient's medications to ensure they are not taking anything that may interfere with clotting.

Flap necrosis can often be suspected early by duskiness or ecchymosis of the distal flap. If this is detected, then topical Nitrobid ointment four to six applications daily may help. We often instruct patients to make sure the skin is clean prior to each application. It's important to educate the patient that these areas will have delayed wound healing compared to the rest of the flap. Any eschar formation can be managed with application of hydrogen peroxide at home and possible conservative in-office debridement. Some surgeons prefer to delay debridement until the eschar starts to separate.

Nerve injury may be sensory or motor. Sensory reduction is common and not considered a complication; rather a normal consequence of surgery that requires only patient reassurance. Facial motor nerve injury is extremely uncommon but will be evident in the immediate postop period. It's important to reassure the patient that this is likely due to local anesthetic or stretch injury and should resolve in a matter of hours to days. Buccal branch weakness can be seen with extensive SMAS deep undermining. This usually resolves over time but can take several months. If there is significant frontal branch weakness limiting eye closure, maintaining hydration with eye drops and/or lubricant, as well as taping the eye shut during sleep, is important to protect the cornea. Frontal nerve injury from cautery or stretching can take months to a full year for recovery. Postoperative brow balance can be improved with botulinum toxin neuromodulation of the opposing frontal muscle.

Infections are very rare. If an early cellulitis develops, have a high index of suspicion for methicillin-resistant *Staphylococcus aureus*, and place the patient on an antibiotic with appropriate coverage. Abscess formation should be treated as soon as possible with a small incision and drainage in order to prevent spread of the infection along dissection planes. These infections can usually be treated without permanent sequela.

Minimizing complications starts with presurgical patient screening and presurgical instructions. Careful, meticulous surgical technique will help minimize intraoperative and early postsurgery complications. Early diagnosis and treatment of complications can minimize the potential for long-term complications.

References

[1] Hollander E. Plastiche (kosmetische) Operation: Kristische Darstellung ihres gegenwartigen Standes. In: Klemperer F, eds. Neue Deutsche Klinik. Berlin: Urban and Schwartzenberg; 1932

[2] Hamra ST. The deep-plane rhytidectomy. Plast Reconstr Surg. 1990; 86(1):53–61, discussion 62–63

[3] Ramirez OM, Mallard GF, Musolas A. The extended subperiosteal facelift: a definitive soft tissue remodeling for facial rejuvenation. 1991; 88(2):227–36

[4] Hamra ST. Composite rhytidectomy. Plast Reconstr Surg. 1992; 90(1):1–13

[5] Barton FE, Jr. The "high SMAS" facelift technique. Aesthet Surg J. 2002; 22(5):481–486

[6] Stuzin JM, Baker TJ, Gordon HL, Baker TM. Extended SMAS dissection as an approach to midface rejuvenation. Clin Plast Surg. 1995; 22(2):295–311

[7] Baker DC. Lateral SMASectomy. Plast Reconstr Surg. 1997; 100(2):509–513

[8] Saylan Z. The S-lift: less is more. Aesthetic Surg J. 1999; 19: 406–409

[9] Tonnard PL, Verpaele A, Gaia S. Optimising results from minimal access cranial suspension lifting (MACS-lift). Aesthetic Plast Surg. 2005; 29(4):213–220, discussion 221

[10] Langsdon P, Shires C, Gerth D. Lower face-lift with extensive neck recontouring. Facial Plast Surg. 2012; 28(1):89–101

[11] Langsdon PR. Management of the lower third of the face and neck. Facial Plast Surg. 2012; 28(1):1–2

[12] Langsdon PR, Velargo PA, Rodwell DW, III, Denys D. Submental muscular medialization and suspension. Aesthet Surg J. 2013; 33(7):953–966

[13] Langsdon PR, Moak S. Use of "submental muscular medialization and suspension" to improve the cervicomental angle. Facial Plast Surg. 2016; 32(6):625–630

[14] Langsdon PR, Renukuntl S, Obeid AA, Smith AM, Karter NS. Analysis of Cervical Angle in the Submental Muscular Medialization and Suspension Procedure. JAMA Facial Plast Surg. 2019; 21(1):56–60

[15] Gillman GS. Facelift (rhytidectomy). In: Myers EN, ed. Operative Otolaryngology: Head and Neck Surgery. Philadelphia: Saunders; 2003: 845–855

[16] Perkins S, Dayan S. Rhytidectomy. In: Papel ID, ed. Facial plastic and reconstructive surgery. New York: Thieme; 2002: 153–170

18 Hair Transplantation

Alfonso Barrera and Christian Arroyo

Summary

In this chapter we present how to safely perform hair transplantation and how to prevent complications, as well as how to treat the most frequent complications. There are two main techniques for donor hair harvesting: (1) Follicular unit transplantation (FUT) which refers to horizontal donor ellipse harvesting, subsequently carefully separating the individual follicular units and then transplanting them. (2) Follicular unit extraction (FUE) in which each individual follicular unit is harvested one by one using a 0.8 to 1.0 mm punch by manual, motorized, or robotic means. Then the actual transplantation is done in the same fashion with either method, one by one. Our personal preference is FUT, that is, the horizontal donor ellipse (Strip). We have described step by step how we do this safely. Unfavorable results are generally due to poor planning and execution of the procedure. The most frequent are: too low or too straight design for the front hairline, grafts that are too large giving a plug-like appearance, scarring alopecia due to tight closure of the donor ellipse or overharvesting with FUE, and poor hair growth. All of them can be avoided by proper planning and technique. We have given our recommendations of how to consistently obtain natural looking results, avoid complications, and how to treat them.

Keywords: follicular unit transplantation (FUT), follicular unit extraction (FUE), hair transplantation, hair follicular units, scarring alopecia, hair grafting, complications in hair transplantation

18.1 Introduction

Hair is an important component of facial aesthetics in both males and females. The hairline helps adorn and frame the face as well as assist in establishing facial proportions. Having good hair density provides youthful appearance, and the lack of it makes us look older. We will describe here our preferred technique in hair transplantation and how to prevent and treat most complications.

We must give credit to Norman Orentreich[1] as we learned so much from him. In the late 1950s he introduced and popularized the punch grafts (hair plugs) and described what we know as the donor "dominance concept" which is key for hair transplantation: The genetics of hair is at the roots of each individual hair follicle, the hair roots harvested from the donor area (occipital and temporal areas) and transplanted to the areas of baldness will continue to grow hair for as long as it was going to do so in the donor area. This is key and very important as hair in the donor areas is the most durable hair we have.

Male pattern baldness and female pattern alopecia is an inherited trait and therefore generally caused by the genes of each individual person. This makes the hair roots sensitive to dehydrotestosterone (DHT), resulting in hair loss when this hormone is present. In males, it typically starts in adolescence and progresses as we age. In females, it varies, tends to be more gradual and starts usually in the third or fourth decades of life.

Most men who lose their hair, do so primarily on the top of the head and not on the temporal and occipital areas. In women, it tends to be more generalized with less loss in the lower occipital and temporal areas. To date we have no method for creating new hair; all current techniques for hair restoration involve redistributing the patient's existing hair. Therefore, candidates for hair transplantation are limited to those who have a favorable ratio of donor hair density relative to the size of the area to be transplanted. Several centers worldwide are working on tissue engineering in an attempt to clone hair follicles or culture and multiply hair follicles in the laboratory setting. When this is successful, we will be able to treat patients with limited donor hair and will need only harvest a sample of their hair follicles.

Male pattern baldness is a progressive condition. The rate of hair loss may slow down after an individual is about 40 to 50 years of age, but it never stops completely. Thus, the preoperative plan must ensure a natural-looking result both short and long term.

As with any other elective procedure, make sure the patient is low risk when scheduling. If any doubts about their health, get clearance from their primary care physician. Make sure he or she is not taking anticoagulants, and if they are, make sure it is safe to discontinue them. The treatment of any medical problems should be optimized prior to any elective hair procedure. For example: If they have hypertension, it should be under control; if diabetic, make sure it is well controlled, etc.

18.2 Current Hair Transplantation Technique

First we should mention that there are two main techniques for donor hair harvesting:

1. Donor strip: This is often referred to in the hair transplantation literature as follicular unit transplantation (FUT). A horizontal donor ellipse is taken from the occipital scalp and often part of the temporal areas. The resulting donor site is then closed primarily. Out of the harvested ellipse, careful dissection under magnification is done to separate the individual hair follicles to subsequently transplant them individually.

2. Follicular unit extraction (FUE) requires that a large area or the entire scalp is shaved and with a 0.8 to 1.0 mm in diameter punch, the follicular units are harvested one by one. This can be done manually, using motorized equipment, or with robotics. Subsequently, the follicular units are transplanted.

Here we will share with you our personal technique based on over 30 years of experience in which donor strip harvesting (FUT) was almost invariably used. We will also show how to minimize these complications and how to correct them.[2,3,4,5,6,7,8,9,10,11]

In addition, we will share with you our thoughts on FUE and how to prevent complications when doing the FUE technique.

When performing hair transplantation, we must think and plan long term. Even on young patients, we should plan on a mature hairline design, with some degree of frontotemporal recession. There is no magic measurement as to the distance from the eyebrows to the hairline, which varies depending on the craniofacial proportions. Sometimes 5 to 6 cm is fine, other times 8 to 10 cm. The main objective is to mimic a natural, mature hairline.

The hairline should also be slightly irregular without rows or lines, we want a no line hairline. In addition, only single hair grafts should be used at the hairline.

By doing the donor strip technique under 3.5-loupe magnification, incising parallel to the hair follicles and closing primarily without tension, we are able to have almost invariable, minimally detectable scarring. Once we harvest the donor strip, by using background lighting and magnification we can see each hair root well from top to bottom and thus we are able to keep at least 95% intact as we dissect them, this way increasing the viability and growth of the hair grafts. Some patients have limited donor hair, so we don't want any to go waste.

We prefer having the patient in the supine position, under IV sedation with midazolam (Versed, Dormicum), fentanyl (Sublimaze), and occipital and supraorbital nerve blocks with 0.5% bupivacaine (Marcaine) with epinephrine 1:200,000. Other surgeons use a combination of local anesthesia and mild oral sedation rather than IV sedation. If the patient is a small child, of course general anesthesia may be better. We generally do these cases in our AAAASF facility (**Video 18.1**).

Once the area is locally well anesthetized, we use tumescence infiltration along the donor ellipse. This provides hemostasis and we also feel it assists in the graft dissection.

Our tumescence solution consists of 120 mL of normal saline with 20 mL of 2% plain Xylocaine plus 1 mL of epinephrine 1:1,000 plus 40 mg of triamcinolone (Kenalog). The same solution is used to infiltrate both the donor and the recipient area. By adding Kenalog we have found significantly less postoperative pain, and significantly less postoperative edema.

The occipital/temporal area is generally where the hair is the thickest and the most permanent (▶ Fig. 18.1, ▶ Fig. 18.2, ▶ Fig. 18.3, ▶ Fig. 18.4, ▶ Fig. 18.5, ▶ Fig. 18.6, ▶ Fig. 18.7, ▶ Fig. 18.8).

It is best to place the grafts at about 5 mm from each other initially, beginning at the front hairline and proceeding posteriorly.

As fibrinogen turns into fibrin (15–20 min later), the grafts become more secure in place. Then we go back anteriorly between the previously inserted grafts, getting them about 2.5 mm apart. If you try to pack them densely too soon, they often "Pop Out" which is very frustrating and time consuming as you would have to reinsert them.

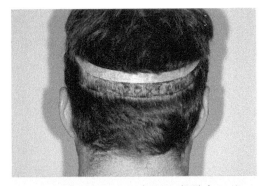

Fig. 18.1 Follicular unit transplantation (FUT) donor site. (Source: Chapter 6 Correction of Male Pattern Baldness. In: Barrera A, Uebel C, ed. Hair Transplantation: The Art of Follicular Unit Micrografting and Minigrafting. 2nd Edition. Thieme; 2013.)

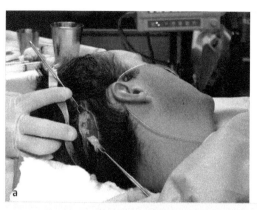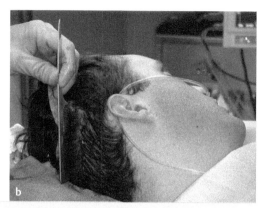

Fig. 18.2 (a) Harvesting right half of the donor ellipse incising parallel to hair follicles; **(b)** donor site closure with 3–0 Prolene simple running. (Source: Chapter 6 Correction of Male Pattern Baldness. In: Barrera A, Uebel C, ed. Hair Transplantation: The Art of Follicular Unit Micrografting and Minigrafting. 2nd Edition. Thieme; 2013.)

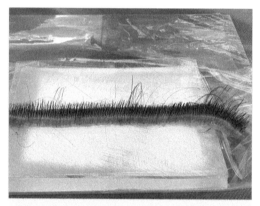

Fig. 18.3 Donor ellipse, notice accuracy of incision as it relates to the hair follicles.

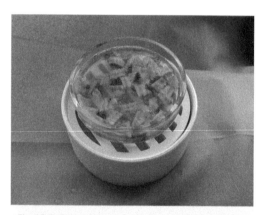

Fig. 18.5 One- to 2-mm slices of scalp submerged in chilled normal saline solution. (Source: Chapter 6 Correction of Male Pattern Baldness. In: Barrera A, Uebel C, ed. Hair Transplantation: The Art of Follicular Unit Micrografting and Minigrafting. 2nd Edition. Thieme; 2013.)

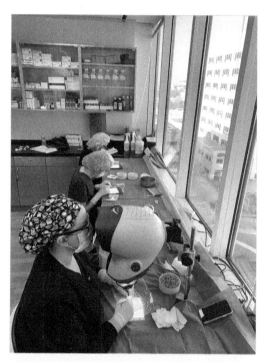

Fig. 18.4 Members of our surgical team dissecting the donor ellipse into follicular unit grafts.

Again, as fibrinogen turns into fibrin we go back time and time again to place more grafts in between, getting them closer and closer to each other until we are about 1 to 1.5 mm between grafts (▶ Fig. 18.9, ▶ Fig. 18.10, ▶ Fig. 18.11, ▶ Fig. 18.12).

The donor site sutures (3–0 Prolene) are removed in the 10th postoperative day.

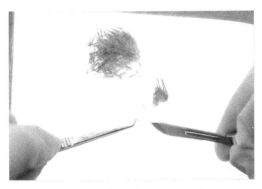

Fig. 18.6 Dissection of the slices into follicular unit grafts. (Source: Part I Fundamentals. In: Barrera A, Uebel C, ed. Hair Transplantation: The Art of Follicular Unit Micrografting and Minigrafting. 2nd Edition. Thieme; 2013.)

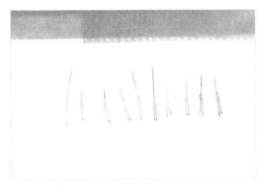

Fig. 18.7 Close-up of 1–2 and 3 hair follicular unit grafts. (Source: Part I Fundamentals. In: Barrera A, Uebel C, ed. Hair Transplantation: The Art of Follicular Unit Micrografting and Minigrafting. 2nd Edition. Thieme; 2013.)

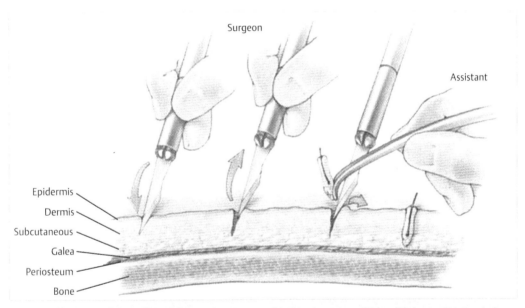

Fig. 18.8 Illustration of the Stick-and-Place technique, a small incision is made and immediately a graft is inserted. (Source: Part I Fundamentals. In: Barrera A, Uebel C, ed. Hair Transplantation: The Art of Follicular Unit Micrografting and Minigrafting. 2nd Edition. Thieme; 2013.)

The hair begins to grow at 3 to 4 months and looks good at 6 months. It takes 12 months for the ultimate result.

Here is an example of the results that we can predictably obtain with today's technology.

The hair transplantation procedure works every time. By handling the grafts gently and atraumatically, up to 90% of the grafts should grow good healthy hair. In addition, the number of hair grafts done will impact the result. In patients who want as much density as possible, assuming they have plenty of donor hair we can do the procedure several times. We prefer to wait a year between sessions, so we can see what we accomplished the first time, and let the scalp recover completely. A year later or any time thereafter we can go over the area again grafting in between the previous grafts, further increasing the hair density (▸ Fig. 18.13a–k).

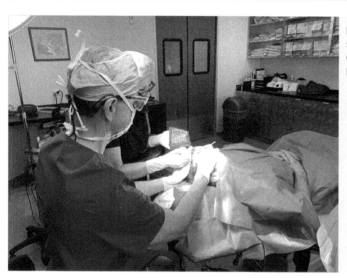

Fig. 18.9 All grafts inserted by the surgeon himself, this is how we always do this in our practice, in all our patients.

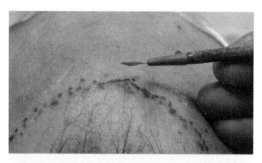

Fig. 18.10 22.5-degree sharpoint is our favorite blade for scalp hair transplantation.

18.3 Unfavorable Results in Hair Transplantation

Now, we will focus on "Unfavorable Results in Hair Transplantation," how to prevent them and how to correct them.[12,13,14,15,16,17,18,19]

Most of them have to do with poor planning and execution of the procedure.

18.3.1 Hairline That Is Too Low and/or Too Straight

A mature man's hairline is usually not less than 8.0 to 8.5 cm from the mid-glabellar area, is symmetric, and exhibits bilateral temporal recession. The most common problems associated with hairline design are blunted temporal angles or hairlines placed too low on the forehead. Correction usually involves surgical excision, redesign, and elevation

or reorientation of the hairline. In most cases, the hairline can be redesigned in a single surgical session and hair grafts can be concomitantly incorporated into the surgical plan as part of a comprehensive approach to correction.

Invariably, a pluggy hairline appearance also coexists and the linear excision also serves as an excellent method to directly eliminate the offending large plug appearance. A simple linear excision of the hairline itself is performed to accomplish this goal. Care should be taken to avoid too wide of an excision. The frontal scalp is typically more difficult to advance than assumed based on preoperative assessment, and a tight closure at the anterior hairline will lead to a wide scar. As stated above with regard to plug correction, a second and possible third session of plug reduction and grafting is often necessary to obtain the optimal result (▶ Fig. 18.14a–j).

18.3.2 Grafts Too Large (Too Many Hairs Per Graft) Giving a Clumpy (Pluggy) Appearance

The essential problem with the unnatural appearing hair graft is the size of the graft which renders it "pluggy" in appearance. Thus, the most direct approach to this problem is to reduce the size of the graft. The concept of grafting anterior to the pluggy hairline alone to achieve improvement does not work and fails to address the basic dense plug problem. The current technique is to employ a punch that is approximately 0.5 to 0.75 mm smaller than the estimated size of the unsightly plug. As an example, if

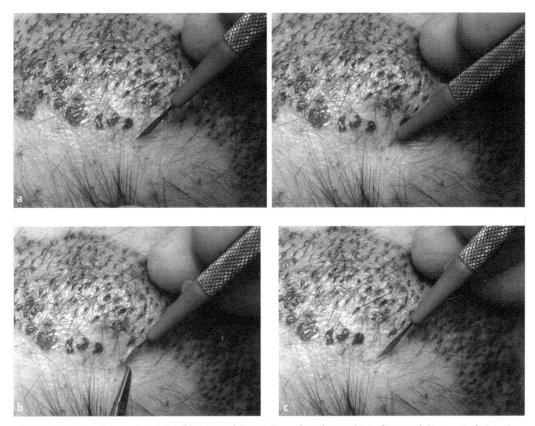

Fig. 18.11 (a) Creating a recipient site. (b) Assistant bringing the graft to the site. (c) Graft inserted. (Source: Technique. In: Barrera A, Uebel C, ed. Hair Transplantation: The Art of Follicular Unit Micrografting and Minigrafting. 2nd Edition. Thieme; 2013.)

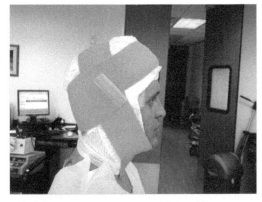

Fig. 18.12 Dressing consists of adapticimpregnated with antibiotic ointment, that is, Polysporin, Kirlex, and a 3-inch Ace bandage, worn for 2 days.

4-mm plugs are being reduced, a 3.5- to 3.25-mm punch would typically be chosen for plug reduction and subsequent recycling (PR&R). The reason for this

is to remove a substantial amount of the plug hairs and leave behind a few hairs that will look soft and natural.

The actual technique of plug removal is very straightforward. The hair in the plugs to be reduced are trimmed to approximately 3 mm in length and the punch removal is performed eccentrically to leave a crescent or sliver of the remaining original plug to leave behind approximately three to four hairs. The punch excision should be deep enough to include 1 to 2 mm of subpapillary fat. These removed plugs are then recycled into follicular unit grafts. The yield of salvaged follicular unit grafts is approximately 50 to 70%.

The hair recycled from the removed plugs, as well as additional hair concomitantly harvested from the occipital region, can be densely transplanted anterior, posterior, and most importantly adjacent to the plug reduction sites. In the majority of cases, the plug reduction sites are not sutured closed. The final appearance of the healed scar following plug

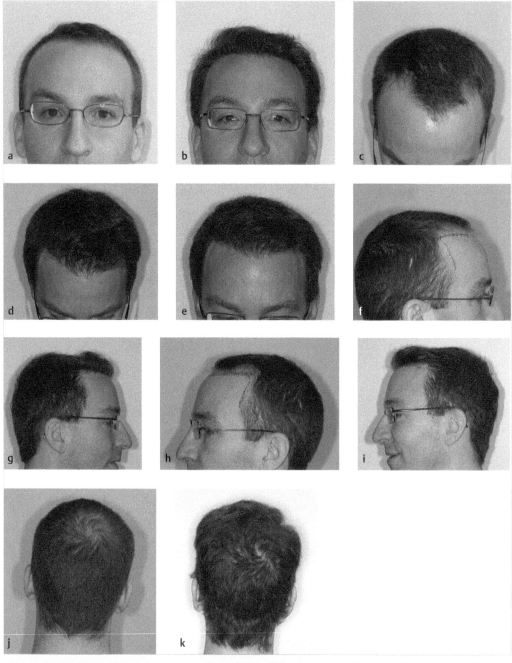

Fig. 18.13 (a–k) Thirty-nine-year-old man, before and a year after two sessions of hair transplantation. Total 5,300 grafts. (The images are provided courtesy of Alfonso Barrera.)

reduction is essentially indistinguishable whether the site was sutured or left to heal by secondary intention. Depending on the size of the punch removal, suture closure may be appropriate.

While each patient's distribution of plugs is unique, the final surgical plan is always to create a zone of natural appearing hair at the leading edges, anteriorly as well as posteriorly while tak-

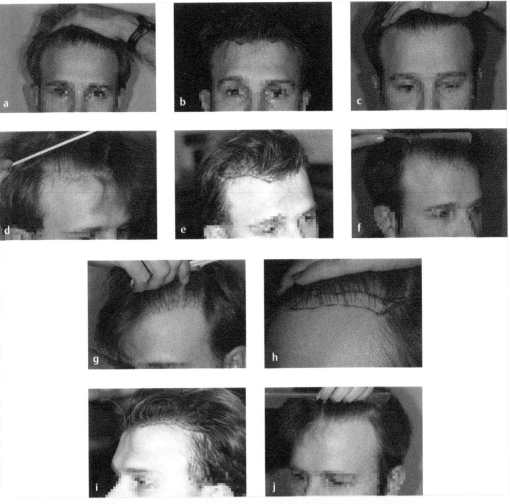

Fig. 18.14 (a–j) This is an example of a previous hair transplantation made with the anterior hairline, too low and the grafts too large, resulting in an unnatural appearance and a pluggy look. The photos show the sequence of excision and cephalic advancement of forehead skin to recreate a slight frontotemporal recession. In addition, adding single-haired follicular unit grafts. (Source: Chapter 11 Revision of Unfavorable Results. In: Barrera A, Uebel C, ed. Hair Transplantation: The Art of Follicular Unit Micrografting and Minigrafting. 2nd Edition. Thieme; 2013.)

ing advantage of the centrally located plugs of higher hair density. In some instances, the patient may prefer to soften all plugs previously grafted, or just have them removed completely.

Although a single session will provide significant improvement, two and sometimes three sessions of plug reduction may be needed to adequately convert the unnatural hair transplant into a result that does not draw curious attention. In general, a second session is performed 6 to 8 months following the first procedure. Occasionally a "faster track" approach can be employed and additional

plug reduction and grafting is performed within the first 2 months following the initial corrective procedure (▶ Fig. 18.15, ▶ Fig. 18.16).

18.3.3 Scarring Alopecia of the Donor Site

This is primarily due to excessively tight closures in the donor site areas (occipital and temporal areas).

Results in varying degrees of widened scars, which can be large especially if necrosis occurs (▶ Fig. 18.17).

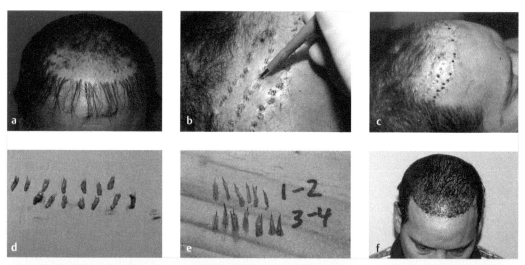

Fig. 18.15 (a–f) Example of the technique for plug reduction and recycling (PR&R) using a 2.5-mm punch, removing most of the hairs from the previous hair plugs, recycling the hair from the plugs, plus additional hair grafts to further camouflage the deformity. (Source: Chapter 28 Hair Restoration. In: Cohen M, Thaller S, ed. The Unfavorable Result in Plastic Surgery: Avoidance and Treatment. 4th Edition. Thieme; 2018.)

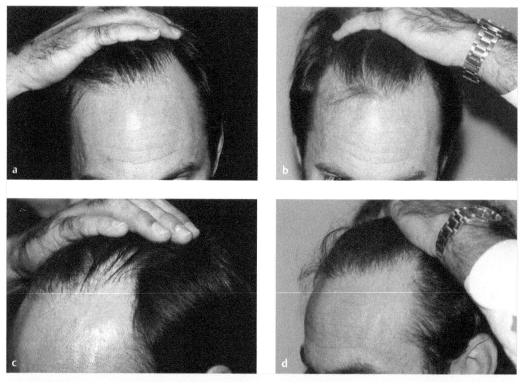

Fig. 18.16 (a–d) Actual example of plug reduction and recycling. (Source: Chapter 28 Hair Restoration. In: Cohen M, Thaller S, ed. The Unfavorable Result in Plastic Surgery: Avoidance and Treatment. 4th Edition. Thieme; 2018.)

The way to prevent this is by harvesting long and narrow donor strips as opposed to short and wide strips.

By long we mean 15 to 20, up to 30 cm in length depending on the number of grafts being done on that particular case.

With narrow meaning 1 cm in width, at this width we can usually close the donor site without any undermining. In selected cases with a lot of laxity you could of course go wider, but keeping this recommendation in mind will keep you in the safe zone.

In secondary or tertiary hair transplantation, when scarring is present and less elasticity (laxity) in the donor area, you may need to go even narrower than 1 cm in width. In addition, if you find yourself in the situation in which it is just too tight

to close the donor area, which will happen once in a while, the best solution is to do extensive undermining in the caudal direction. In this case, you would have to go below the retroauricular hairline to the mid neck, to be able to gain enough mobility to solve the problem (▶ Fig. 18.18).

FUE can be done manually, motorized (powered), or using robotics. In either way we must minimize scarring by not overharvesting from small areas, and using punches ideally not larger than 0.8 mm in diameter. Harvesting must be done over a larger "safe area" and avoid harvesting too close to each other.

Proponents of FUE claim and advertise "that with their technique there are no scarring, certainly no linear scars." Let me tell you, there is donor site scarring with both FUE and FUT techniques even when doing them well.

See examples with both techniques in ▶ Fig. 18.19 and ▶ Fig. 18.20.

18.3.4 Poor Hair Growth After Hair Transplantation

Naturally the type and qualities of hair varies from patient to patient, some patients have thicker fuller hair than others. The texture, color, hair shaft diameter, curl (genetically determined) will result in a thicker or thinner look.

Of course, the number of grafts done and the percentage of graft survival are important.

The most common cause of poor hair growth is inaccuracy in the follicular hair graft dissection. The grafts must of course be handled gently and atraumatically. It is also very important to keep them in a chilled saline solution. Do not let them desiccate. Transplant them ASAP all within 4 to 5 hours ideally.

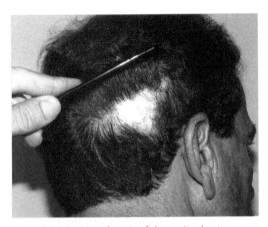

Fig. 18.17 Scarring alopecia of donor site due to excessive tension at the time of donor site closure. (Source: Chapter 28 Hair Restoration. In: Cohen M, Thaller S, ed. The Unfavorable Result in Plastic Surgery: Avoidance and Treatment. 4th Edition. Thieme; 2018.)

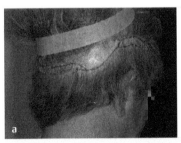 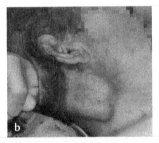 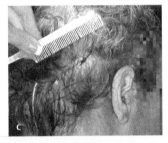

Fig. 18.18 (a–c) Example of correction of scarring alopecia from previous hair transplantation with excessive tension at the closure resulting in necrosis and the resultant alopecia. It can be reconstructed by hair grafting, or it can be excised by doing extensive undermining and closed. (Source: Chapter 28 Hair Restoration. In: Cohen M, Thaller S, ed. The Unfavorable Result in Plastic Surgery: Avoidance and Treatment. 4th Edition. Thieme; 2018.)

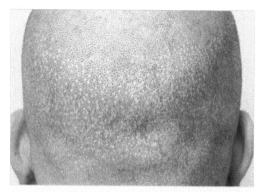

Fig. 18.19 Scarring from follicular unit extraction (FUE).

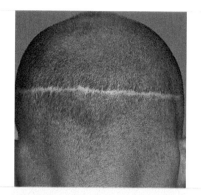

Fig. 18.20 Scarring from follicular unit transplantation (FUT).

Excessively dense graft packing (over 50/cm^2) in one session I feel decreases the percentage follicular unit graft ultimate hair growth. They need a little space in between (1–1.5 mm) to thrive. A year later you can go between them and add more density safely.

18.4 Conclusion

This chapter represents the authors' current technique of hair transplantation, their views and recommendations on how to prevent and correct unfavorable results.

When the surgeon is faced with correcting these types of problems, creativity and a variety of techniques can help as described above. The exact techniques used in an individual patient will be as varied as the presenting problem itself. Most patients with unsightly hair transplantation results can be helped as long as there is remaining donor hair.

With either FUT or FUE techniques, patients should *not* plan on wearing very short hair on the donor area. As mentioned above *both* techniques can result in visible scarring.

References

[1] Orentreich N. Autografts in alopecias and other selected dermatological conditions. Ann N Y AcadSci. 1959; 83:463–479

[2] Barrera A. Micrograft and minigraftmega session hair transplantation results after a single session. Plast Reconstr Surg. 1997; 100(6):1524–1530

[3] Barrera A. Refinements in hair transplantation: micro and minigraftmega session. Perspect Plast Surg. 1998; 11(1):53–70

[4] Barrera A. Hair transplantation: the art of micrografting and minigrafting. St Louis, MO: Quality Medical Publishing, Inc.; 2002

[5] Barrera A. Hair grafting tips and techniques. Perspect Plast Surg. 2001; 15(2):147–158

[6] Barrera A. Advances in hair restoration. AesthSurg J. 2003; 23(4):259–264

[7] Barrera, A. Clinical decision-making in hair transplantation. In: Nahii F, ed. The Art of Aesthetic Surgery: Principles and Technique, Vol. II. Quality Medical Publishing; 2005: 1691–1724

[8] Barrera A. Applied anatomy in hair transplantation. In: Nahii F, ed. The Art of Aesthetic Surgery: Principles and Technique. Quality Medical Publishing; 2005:1679–1689

[9] Barrera A. Clinical decision making in hair transplantation. In: Nahii F, ed. The Art of Aesthetic Surgery: Principles and Technique, Vol. I, 2nd ed. Quality Medical Publishing; 2011:604–633

[10] Vogel JE, Jimenez F, Cole J, et al. Hair restoration surgery: the state of the art. AesthetSurg J. 2013; 33(1):128–151

[11] Barrera A, Uebel C. Hair transplantation: the art of follicular unit micrografting and minigrafting. 2nd ed. St Louis, MO: Quality Medical Publishing Inc.; 2014

[12] Vogel JE. Correction of cosmetic problems secondary to hair transplantation. In: Unger W, Shapiro R, Unger R, Unger M, eds. Hair Transplantation. 5th ed. London: Informa Healthcare; 2010:291–296

[13] Vogel JE. Hair restoration complications: an approach to the unnatural-appearing hair transplant. Facial PlastSurg. 2008; 24(4):453–461

[14] Vogel JE. Correcting problems in hair restoration surgery: an update. Facial Plast Surg C lin North Am. 2004; 12(2): 263–278

[15] Vogel JE. Correction of the cornrow hair transplant and other common problems in surgical hair restoration. Plast Reconstr Surg. 2000; 105(4):1528–1536, discussion 1537–1541

[16] Brandy DA. Corrective hair restoration techniques for the aesthetic problems of temporoparietalflaps. DermatolSurg. 2003; 29(3):230–234, discussion 234

[17] Bernstein RM. The art of repair in surgical hair restoration—part II: the tactics of repair. DermatolSurg. 2002; 28:10

[18] Epstein JS. Revision surgical hair restoration: repair of undesirable results. PlastReconstrSurg. 1999; 104(1):222–232, discussion 233–236

[19] Lucas MWG. Partial retransplantation: a new approach in hair transplantation. J Dermatol Surg Oncol. 1994; 20(8): 511–514

19 Blepharoplasty

Fred G. Fedok and Sunny S. Park

Summary

Upper and lower blepharoplasty are among the most popular and safe surgical procedures. Blepharoplasty is performed for both cosmetic and functional indications in a wide variety of ages. Although the incidence of complications is low, complications can and do occur. The avoidance of complications involves an optimal assessment of the patients underlying anatomy and the selection of appropriate blepharoplasty and ancillary procedures.

Keywords: blepharoplasty, complications, lid tightening, ectropion, chemosis

19.1 Introduction

Blepharoplasty is one of the most common cosmetic procedures performed in the United States.[1] Although it may be considered one of the least invasive cosmetic surgeries, it is not without complications. These complications can range from mild issues that resolve spontaneously to devastating and permanent damage to associated structures. In this chapter, blepharoplasty-related complications and their recognition and management will be presented. In addition, preventative measures will be discussed in order to minimize the incidence of these complications.

19.2 Patient Evaluation

A thorough preoperative patient evaluation is an important first step to limit the risk of postoperative complications. For example, systemic diseases such as thyroid disease should be investigated as it can affect eyelid position and eyelid edema.[2] In addition, ocular, facial, and skin abnormalities such as dry eyes, narrow chamber angles, facial nerve dysfunction, blepharitis, eczema, rosacea, blepharospasm, and visual acuity/visual field are among the issues that should be noted and documented.

Identifying abnormal and undesirable periorbital anatomical characteristics in the patient is necessary in order to choose the appropriate surgical technique. When preparing for an upper blepharoplasty, various anatomical attributes should be assessed. For example, the amount of skin, symmetry of eyelid creases, the amount and location of protruding fat, presence of orbital hollowing, blepharoptosis, lid position, and position of the lacrimal gland and eyebrow all need to be noted. These findings should be discussed with the patient preoperatively and adjunct procedures offered as necessary. If these undesirable periorbital anatomical characteristics are undiagnosed, the surgical results may be suboptimal.

In the examination of the lower eyelid, the amount and location of fat pseudoherniation, excess skin, the presence of tear trough deformity, the presence of a negative vector midface or midface deficiency, and malar bags/festoons should be noted. These findings may determine the type of surgery performed. Patients with negative vector and midface deficiency should be educated on the limitations of surgery and outcome due to their anatomical features. The lower eyelid support should be assessed. If laxity is noted, a horizontal shortening or other tightening procedure may be necessary at the time of the blepharoplasty to prevent postoperative lid malposition.

19.3 Common Postoperative Problems: Their Avoidance and Correction

19.3.1 Upper Eyelid Blepharoplasty Complications

Brow Ptosis

The preoperative recognition of a ptotic brow is essential for a satisfactory upper blepharoplasty result. The patient may require a brow lift instead of, or in addition to, an upper blepharoplasty procedure. It is observed that when the upper eyelid skin is removed, the distance between the eyebrow and the eyelid margin is shortened. Consequently, an uncorrected brow ptosis may be more noticeable after surgery, resulting in a seemingly less effective blepharoplasty.[3] Therefore, when brow ptosis is noted, patients should be advised on procedures available to reposition the eyebrow prior to or at the same time as an upper blepharoplasty (▶ Fig. 19.1).

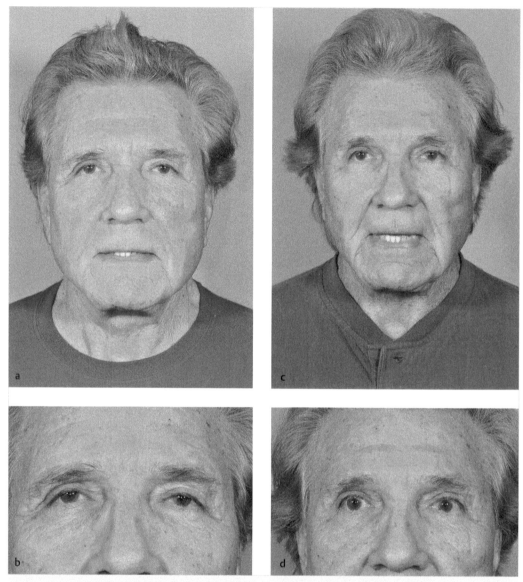

Fig. 19.1 Patient who presented for upper eyelid concerns following two previous upper blepharoplasty procedures and was determined to have significant brow ptosis. **(a, b)** Preoperative images of patient. **(c, d)** Postoperative images of patient after bilateral mid-forehead lift only.

Blepharoptosis

If upper eyelid ptosis is noted preoperatively, it should be evaluated and documented with specific measurements. This includes assessing the height of palpebral fissure, the distance between the upper eyelid margin to the corneal light reflex (MRD1) and levator muscle function. These findings should be discussed with the patient and if clinically significant, a ptosis repair procedure should be considered to be performed at the same time as upper blepharoplasty. The documented findings may also be helpful to secure insurance coverage of the procedure (▶ Fig. 19.2, ▶ Fig. 19.3). A transient postoperative blepharoptosis can also be seen soon after blepharoplasty surgery and is thought to be caused by edema, diminished levator or Müeller muscle function, or hematoma formation.[4,5,6] This transient phenomenon usually

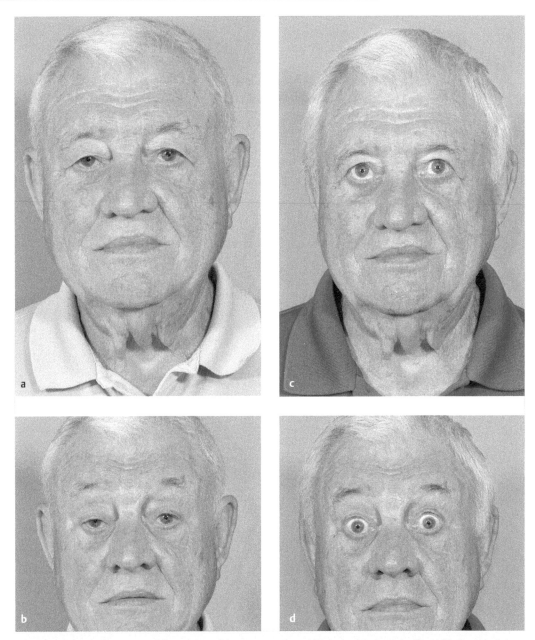

Fig. 19.2 Patient who presented for upper eyelid concerns and was determined to have significant blepharoptosis in addition to dermatochalasis. **(a, b)** Preoperative images of patient. **(c, d)** Postoperative images of patient after bilateral upper blepharoplasty and ptosis repair. Note improved upper eyelid opening after surgery in **d** compared to **b**.

resolves spontaneously. On the other hand, if postoperative ptosis persists for more than 3 to 6 months, an inadvertent disinsertion of the levator aponeurosis may have occurred during resection of the orbicularis muscle or preaponeurotic fat.[3] In order to correct this problem, a secondary levator advancement procedure may be needed. To avoid this particular complication, it is important to recognize that the levator muscle is immediately posterior to the central fat pad and a prudent dissection should be performed during blepharoplasty surgery.

Fred G. Fedok, MD FACS - Ptosis evaluation

Patient name _____

Measurements

Lid height - Bottom UL - Top LL - 8–10 mm

od _____   os _____

Levator function - > 11 mm (stabilize brow)

od _____   os _____

EL crease - Margin to crease, looking down - 7–8 males, 9–10 females

od _____   os _____

MRDI - Central UL to pup light reflex (mL - 4.00 – 4.5 mm)

od _____   os _____

2.5% neosysnephrine testing—1 drop – 5 min - > 2–3 mm —> Müller or plan overcorrection

od _____   os _____

Examiner _____   Date _____

Fig. 19.3 Simple form used to document findings of ptosis evaluation.

Persistent Dermatochalasis

Inadequate removal of excess upper eyelid skin will result in persistent dermatochalasis. Although this may be considered a suboptimal result, it behooves the surgeon to maintain a conservative approach in removing excess skin in upper blepharoplasty as lagophthalmos from overly aggressive skin excision may be difficult to correct. It is, therefore, best to educate patients on the importance of conservative skin excision and that in this situation less is better. Patients should also be instructed that later additional skin removal as an in-office procedure, if needed, is always a possibility without a compromise of the final cosmetic result.

To assess how much skin can be safely removed during upper blepharoplasty, the "pinch" technique may be considered as a safe and effective method to be used during preoperative marking. First, the patient is placed in an upright position. Planning markings are made with a surgical marking pen. The inferior aspect of the proposed eyelid incisions is marked first. At the central portion of the eyelid, this marking and subsequent incision is usually placed at or just inferior to the supratarsal crease, or 8 to 10 mm from the ciliary margin. Medially, this incision is carried to the level of the puncta, but no further medially to avoid webbing of the incision. Laterally, in females, the incision is commonly carried to approximately 1 cm over the orbital rim and usually placed in a lateral eyelid crease. In males, the lateral extent of the incision is planned to terminate with only a minimal crossing onto the lateral orbital rim.

In marking the skin, one must verify that eye closure will be complete with the amount of skin excised, and hence, there should be a certain conservatism during the planned marking of the skin (▶ Fig. 19.4). The excess eyelid skin is grasped with smooth forceps. The tines of the forceps are adjusted to approximate the amount of skin to be removed while maintaining the lower tine of the forceps on the planned inferior incision and gently pinching the skin. This is repeated at several positions along the eyelid to determine some of the points for the placement of the upper eyelid incision.[7] While holding the excess skin between the forceps' tines, the eyelid should be observed to still be able to be closed. The incisions should be planned to be limited to the thinner upper eyelid skin and to not extend into the thicker infrabrow skin. Often the thinner eyelid skin that can be removed has a different color and texture than the surrounding skin. The position of the brow should also be noted and should not be disturbed by this process. The amount of skin between these superior and inferior incisions varies between patients. Even in the same patient it can vary between the left and right eyes. It is important to avoid excess skin excision as this can cause lagophthalmos and problems with dryness. Note that when the eyes are closed, there should be complete closure of the eyelids. The lateral aspect of the incision should be designed along a diagonal (parallel to the crow's feet) so that lateral hooding is reduced during skin excision.

Scarring

Significant postoperative scarring of the upper eyelid skin is unusual after blepharoplasty as the overlying skin is very thin and heals very fast compared to other parts of the body. Darker pigmented skin types, however, are more prone to pigmentary changes and hypertrophy after surgical procedures. Therefore, the use of current CO_2 laser technology for making skin incisions on darker pigmented skin such as Asian and Black patients should be avoided.[8] In addition, extending the incision lateral to the orbital rim should be minimized in these patients to avoid the creation of a noticeable scar.

Once an incision is made, a meticulous closure is crucial. Similarly, removing the sutures in a timely fashion, usually in about 3 to 7 days, and using a nonreactive suture, such as polypropylene, are important in minimizing chances of scarring and granuloma formation.

Lagophthalmos

Lagophthalmos can occur after upper eyelid blepharoplasty because of several reasons. It occurs most commonly after the removal of too much upper eyelid skin. As a general guideline, the amount of remaining intact skin after blepharoplasty excision should be anticipated during surgical marking as noted previously. It is recommended that at least 20 mm of skin should be retained between the inferior aspect of the eyebrow and the lid margin to prevent lagophthalmos. If it is recognized that too much skin has been removed at the time of surgery, the excised skin can be immediately sutured back in place as a skin graft. Alternatively, if excessive excision is of lesser concern during the surgery, the removed skin may be stored in saline gauze and refrigerated. If considering this there are some associated risks that should be carefully considered. (Considering the risks the first editor does not use this technique.) This can be used 1 to 2 weeks after surgery if needed.[9]

Lagophthalmos can also be seen without excessive removal of skin. Postoperative middle lamellar cicatrix formation may occur when the orbital septum is inadvertently included during levator aponeurosis advancement, eyelid crease formation, or wound closure.[9] The resolution of this type of lagophthalmos may require the surgical lysing of adhesions between the orbicularis muscle, the septum, and levator aponeurosis.

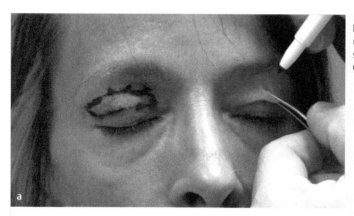

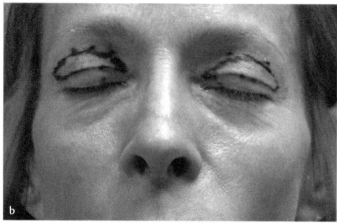

Fig. 19.4 (a, b) Surgical marking for upper blepharoplasty. See text for description. (Adapted from Fedok and Carniol 2013.[7])

Minor degrees of lagophthalmos will usually resolve over a few weeks as edema subsides and orbicularis function recovers. In the meantime, the ocular surface should be protected by advising eye lubricants and ointments while closely monitoring patients. Taping the eyelids at night may also help prevent excessive drying related to the lagophthalmos. If this is ineffective, a consultation with a cornea specialist may be warranted. If lagophthalmos does not improve with time, additional surgery, including skin grafts or other procedures, may be required.

Dry Eye

Transient vision changes frequently occur after blepharoplasty and arecommonly caused by dry eyes resulting from ocular surface exposure. With time and the help of therapeutics, these dry eye symptoms usually improve in 4 to 6 weeks. Patients already with dry eyes from pre-existing conditions such as diminished blink reflex, upper or lower eyelid malposition, and lagophthalmos may experience the most discomfort and blurred vision, postoperatively.[9] Therefore, patients should be educated on these conditions preoperatively to establish their postoperative expectations. Although most dry eye cases are short lived and will resolve on their own, having an ophthalmologic assessment may hasten the resolution of these postoperative complications with the use of "bandage" contact lenses and punctal plugs.

Asymmetric Creases/Malposition of Incision

Identifying natural creases on the upper lid and properly marking the incisions are important in preventing postoperative eyelid crease asymmetries. A low positioned crease can be elevated by making an incision in the desired area and undermining the unwanted eyelid crease. The skin is closed by including the levator aponeurosis just above the superior edge of the tarsal plate.[9] Lowering a crease that is too high is more difficult and may involve an

Alloderm graft, an advancement of preaponeurotic fat, or placing free fat pearls to prevent readhesion at the higher level.[3,9] If asymmetry is present after surgery, hyaluronic acid filler may be a safe, nonsurgical alternative to repair.[10]

Postoperative asymmetric crease is the most common complication after performing Asian blepharoplasty. Therefore, it is important to discuss with the patient, in depth, the desired position and shape of the crease. Careful placement of the incision in the upper eyelid is especially crucial in this population. Even a mild 1 to 2 mm ptosis should be corrected before attempting to create a double eyelid crease.[11]

19.3.2 Lower Eyelid Blepharoplasty Complications

Eyelid Retraction/Ectropion

Retraction and ectropion of the lower eyelid are among the most significant, common, and difficult to treat complications that occur after blepharoplasty. Hence, the best solution is avoidance. Avoidance is first accomplished by adequately evaluating the patient's risk of developing these complications. The tone and support of the lower eyelid should be assessed with the distraction test and snap test. Other important factors include the globe position and the structure of the midface. If the patient has unfavorable anatomy, the type of blepharoplasty performed and whether a canthopexy, canthoplasty, or other lid-tightening procedure should be performed in conjunction with the blepharoplasty procedure.

Ectropion can be caused by removing an excess amount of lower eyelid skin or it can be the result of an untreated preexisting lower eyelid laxity. For patients with significant excess skin, transcutaneous lower eyelid blepharoplasty should be considered with a conservative excision of only a few millimeters of skin. The amount of skin to be removed should be ascertained while the patient is looking in an up-gaze position with an opened mouth. A pinch skin excision with transconjunctival blepharoplasty is another option to lower the risk of lid retraction and ectropion[12] (▶ Fig. 19.5).

Retraction and ectropion are difficult complications to manage and treat as they affect both the function and cosmesis of the lower eyelid. Retraction is frequently caused by scarring in the middle lamella which then shortens and pulls the lid inferiorly. Conservative management consists of massaging and/or administering steroid injections in the area of the retraction. If these do not ameliorate the retraction, additional surgery may be necessary. This additional surgery involves releasing the cicatrix in the middle lamella and placing an autologous tissue or an acellular dermis as a spacer. In severe cases, a skin graft may be needed. Again, as an alternative to surgical intervention, hyaluronic acid fillers may improve the retraction.[13]

Lagophthalmos

Lagophthalmos may result after lower blepharoplasty from retraction and/or ectropion. As previously discussed above, supportive care with eye drops and lubricants are crucial in order to prevent keratitis. Additional surgery may be necessary if a conservative approach does not alleviate the problem.

Chemosis

Chemosis can occur as a result of dissection in the periorbital tissue and globe exposure from an inadequate blink and lagophthalmos. Although more common in patients with rosacea and hypervascularity, it can cause significant ocular discomfort to all types of patients.[9] Similar to the treatment of dry eyes, nonpreservative artificial tears and lubricating ointments are recommended. Symptoms usually improve within a few days to weeks, but if not, topical and oral steroids may be added. In refractory postoperative chemosis, a variety of surgical techniques can be used to alleviate symptoms. These include limbal peritomy conjunctivoplasty, temporary tarsorrhaphy, drainage conjunctivotomy, perilimbal needle manipulation, and snip conjunctivoplasty. Early surgical intervention should be considered to break the chain of events that could lead to chronic, harder-to-manage chemosis.[14]

19.3.3 Uncommon/Catastrophic Blepharoplasty Complications

Globe Injury

Although rare, globe injury may occur during blepharoplasty. The risk of injury is increased in patients with proptosis and patients with filtering blebs from glaucoma surgery. Globe injury is not limited to any one specific tool as it can occur with a laser, scalpel, and needle used for local anesthesia.[8] To reduce the incidence of such injuries, a corneal shield is sometimes employed. When a globe injury is suspected, an urgent consultation with an ophthalmologist is warranted. Otherwise, minor abrasions can be treated with lubricants, antibiotic drops, and ointments.

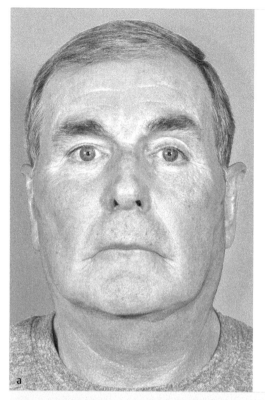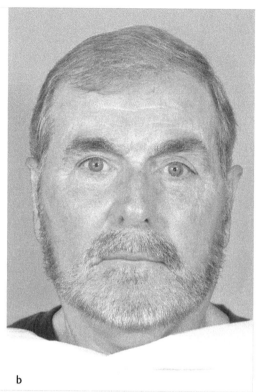

Fig. 19.5 **(a)** Clinical image of patient with history of past left-side Bell palsy who developed persistent lateral retraction and exposure symptoms of left lower eyelid after bilateral lower blepharoplasty. **(b)** Patient 4 months after surgical correction of problem with left lateral tarsal suspension procedure.

Retro-orbital Hematoma

A retro-orbital hematoma can lead to vision loss. The incidence of orbital hemorrhage after a cosmetic blepharoplasty is 1:2,000 (0.05%). The incidence of orbital hemorrhage resulting in permanent vision loss is 1:10,000 (0.01%).[15] This most commonly presents within the first 24 hours of surgery but can still occur several days after surgery. It is believed that hematoma most commonly occurs due to manipulation of orbital fat after entering the septum. As a result, bleeding can extend posteriorly leading to ischemic optic neuropathy.[16,17]

Acute retro-orbital hematoma is an emergency as permanent vision loss can occur without prompt treatment. Patients will have severe pain, an edematous dark purple periorbital hematoma, and brisk incisional bleeding. With elevated intraocular pressure, topical ocular hypotensive agents should be instilled along with an urgent ophthalmologic consultation. Intravenous osmotic agents may be given as well. If hematoma is suspected,

patients should be taken to the OR immediately for evacuation of the hematoma. If there is proptosis, changes in vision and/or abnormal pupillary reactivity, a cantholysis and inferior cantholysis should be performed at the bedside to release the developing orbital compartment syndrome. This relieves the pressure on the optic nerve and ocular blood flow which may prevent permanent anoxic damage. If appropriate intervention is performed within 1 to 2 hours, permanent optic nerve and retinal ischemic damage can be prevented.[18]

Prevention of hematoma is accomplished with meticulous intraoperative hemostasis. If there is any excision of the orbital fat, cautery should be used to ensure there is no bleeding at the edge of the fat which may retract posterior to the septum. Blood pressure needs to be controlled intra-and postoperatively. Patients are commonly advised to stop all blood thinners, whether prescribed or over the counter, 1 to 2 weeks before surgery. Alcohol intake and strenuous activity should be limited. Postoperatively, head elevation and the use of ice packs in the first 3 to 4 days of surgery are helpful in minimizing the risk of hematoma.

19.4 Conclusion

Although blepharoplasty is a popular and safe procedure, complications can and do occur. Patient evaluation and identification of risk factors are important in the avoidance of complications. The appropriate incorporation of ancillary procedures such as lid-tightening procedures is necessary when patient's present with unfavorable physical findings such as lid laxity.

Many of the common significant unfavorable outcomes of blepharoplasty have been reviewed along with their etiologies and remedies. Lesser postoperative problems such as fixed and dynamic rhytids, bruising, edema, and subconjunctival hemorrhage have not been covered because of their low morbidity and self-limited nature. **Video 19.1** demonstrates upper eyelid blepharoplasty technique.

References

[1] AAFPRS Membership Survey 2019. Link: https://www.aafprs.org/Media/Press_Releases/New%20Stats%20AAFPRS%20Annual%20Survey.aspx. Accessed July, 2020.

[2] Knopf H. Refractive distractions from drugs and disease. Ophthal Clin North Am. 1993; 6:599–605

[3] Whipple KM, Korn BS, Kikkawa DO. Recognizing and managing complications in blepharoplasty. Facial Plast Surg Clin North Am. 2013; 21(4):625–637

[4] Adams BJS, Feurstein SS. Complications of blepharoplasty. Ear Nose Throat J. 1986; 65(1):6–18

[5] Baylis HI, Sutcliffe T, Fett DR. Levator injury during blepharoplasty. Arch Ophthalmol. 1984; 102(4):570–571

[6] Rainin EA, Carlson BM. Postoperative diplopia and ptosis:a clinical hypothesis based on the myotoxicity of local anesthetics. Arch Ophthalmol. 1985; 103(9):1337–1339

[7] Fedok FG, Carniol PJ. Upper blepharoplasty. In: Fedok FG, Carniol PJ, eds. Minimally Invasive and Office-Based Procedures in Facial Plastic Surgery.New York: Thieme;2013, Chapter 22

[8] Oestreicher J, Mehta S. Complications of blepharoplasty: prevention and management. Plastic Surgery International;. 2012. DOI: 10.1155/2012/252368

[9] Klapper SR, Patrinely JR. Management of cosmetic eyelid surgery complications. Semin Plast Surg. 2007; 21(1): 80–93

[10] Mancini R, Khadavi NM, Goldberg RA. Nonsurgical management of upper eyelid margin asymmetry using hyaluronic acid gel filler. Ophthal PlastReconstrSurg. 2011; 27(1):1–3

[11] Chen WPD. Techniques, principles and benchmarks in Asian blepharoplasty. Plast Reconstr Surg Glob Open. 2019; 7(5): e2271

[12] Fedok FG, Perkins SW. Transconjunctival blepharoplasty. Facial Plast Surg. 1996; 12(2):185–195

[13] Zamani M, Thyagarajan S, Olver JM. Functional use of hyaluronic acid gel in lower eyelid retraction. Arch Ophthalmol. 2008; 126(8):1157–1159

[14] Jones YJ, Georgescu D, McCann JD, Anderson RL. Snip conjunctivoplasty for postoperative conjunctival chemosis. Arch Facial PlastSurg. 2010; 12(2):103–105

[15] Hass AN, Penne RB, Stefanyszyn MA, Flanagan JC. Incidence of postblepharoplasty orbital hemorrhage and associated visual loss. Ophthal PlastReconstrSurg. 2004; 20(6):426–432

[16] Anderson RL, Edwards JJ. Bilateral visual loss after blepharoplasty. Ann PlastSurg. 1980; 5(4):288–292

[17] Goldberg RA, Marmor MF, Shorr N, Christenbury JD. Blindness following blepharoplasty: two case reports, and a discussion of management. Ophthalmic Surg. 1990; 21(2):85–89

[18] Hayreh SS, Weingeist TA. Experimental occlusion of the central artery of the retina. I. Ophthalmoscopic and fluorescein fundus angiographic studies. Br J Ophthalmol. 1980; 64 (12):896–912

Index

Note: Page numbers set **bold** or *italic* indicate headings or figures, respectively.